ELASTIC
FIBER
MATRICES

Biomimetic Approaches to
Regeneration and Repair

ELASTIC
FIBER
MATRICES
Biomimetic Approaches to Regeneration and Repair

ANAND RAMAMURTHI
CHANDRASEKHAR KOTHAPALLI

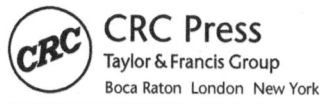

CRC Press
Taylor & Francis Group
Boca Raton London New York

CRC Press is an imprint of the
Taylor & Francis Group, an **informa** business

CRC Press
Taylor & Francis Group
6000 Broken Sound Parkway NW, Suite 300
Boca Raton, FL 33487-2742

ISBN-13: 978-1-1383-2268-4 (pbk)

Visit the Taylor & Francis Web site at
http://www.taylorandfrancis.com

and the CRC Press Web site at
http://www.crcpress.com

Contents

Preface

S OFT CONNECTIVE TISSUES (e.g., skin, blood vessels, lung, and urogenital tissues) contain architecturally distinct extracellular matrix (ECM) structures determined by tissue type, location, and function. The elastic matrix is composed of hydrophobic, cross-linked elastin protein, microfibrils, and numerous other proteins and glycoproteins. It is a critical structural component of the ECM, which serves to maintain the native structural configurations of elastic tissues, imparts tissue distensibility, and facilitates their ability to recoil after removal of stretching forces. In addition, the elastic matrix regulates cell signaling pathways involved in morphogenesis, injury response, and inflammation via biomechanical transduction and is thus a vital regulator of tissue homeostasis.

The dysregulated activity or chronic overexpression of proteases—enzymes that critically regulate cellular and physiologic processes and essential to tissue remodeling in healthy tissues—underlies the etiology and progression of major tissue degenerative diseases, including those that involve elastic matrix disruption and loss. While in situ regenerative repair of disrupted tissues promises to provide an alternative to clinical tissue transplantation, restoring the complex ECM architecture in a proteolytic tissue milieu presents several challenges. One significant problem concerns the generation of elastin and elastic matrix structures due to inherent deficiencies in post-neonatal cells, more so by diseased cells, in synthesizing and assembling elastin precursors into elastic fibers and higher order matrix structures (e.g., sheets and meshes). This deficiency also has negative implications to our ability to tissue engineer elastic tissue constructs on demand using patient-derived adult cell types, to replace those compromised by disease. The development of technologies for biomimetic de novo elastic matrix assembly, or alternately in situ regenerative repair of elastic matrix has thus been an area of research emphasis over the past several years. *Elastic Matrix: Biomimetic Approaches to Regeneration and Repair* presents the current status of numerous aspects of this broad discipline. With individual chapters contributed by leading researchers worldwide in the field, our book not only represents an exclusive and comprehensive resource on the subject but also (1) details state-of-the-art approaches to elastic matrix regeneration and repair, (2) presents a critical analysis of the merits and limitations of available technologies, and (3) offers perspectives on future technological needs and advances, and clinical translation and commercialization of these technologies.

The contributors have been carefully selected to provide the benefit of their respective expertise in the included topics such as (1) architectural diversity of elastic matrices in different elastic tissue types and pathological aberrations of the complex process of elastic matrix assembly, (2) matrix replacement strategies based on the use of synthetic or biologic elastomers, (3) pharmacologic approaches to preserving and regenerating elastic matrix structures, (4) cellular and biomolecular strategies to enhance elastin deposition and elastic fiber assembly, (5) gene therapies targeting genetic aberrations underlying congenital elastic matrix defects and acquired proteolytic diseases, (6) biomaterial-based strategies using scaffolds and nano-carriers for spatiotemporal control over the presentation of cells and biomolecules at the site of matrix repair, and release of these biomolecules, to direct biomimetic assembly and structural organization of clinically relevant native elastic matrix-like superstructures.

As editors, we believe that the chapters reflect the current status of this important field, in a timely fashion. We expect this book to be highly resourceful for established investigators, clinicians, students, entrepreneurs and nonspecialists alike, by providing a thorough understanding of the various facets of this field. Finally, we anticipate that readers from various disciplines, including but not limited to physiology, cell and molecular biology, pharmacology, biochemistry, and bioengineering, will benefit from the scope and variety of topics covered in this book.

Anand Ramamurthi
Cleveland Clinic Lerner Research Institute

Chandrasekhar Kothapalli
Cleveland State University

Acknowledgments

WE EXPRESS OUR THANKS to all our colleagues from the United States and abroad for their timely and high-quality contributions to this volume. We also thank the staff of CRC Press, including Dr. Gagandeep Singh (editorial manager, engineering/environmental services), Hayley Ruggieri (project coordinator, editorial project management), Marsha Pronin (project coordinator, editorial project development), Rachael Panthier (production editor), Kyra Lindholm (editorial assistant), and B. Sundaramoorthy (associate project manager, Lumina Datamatics, Pvt. Ltd.), for all their help and guidance in bringing this book to print.

We thank all of our author colleagues for agreeing to be part of this undertaking and for their timely contributions of high quality and introspective articles, and our respective academic institutions for their support to this academic endeavor. Finally, sincere thanks are due to our families – our parents, spouses, and children – for their unwavering support and encouragement as we pursue our academic and research endeavors.

Editors

Anand Ramamurthi is an associate professor of molecular medicine and biomedical engineering at the Cleveland Clinic with adjunct appointments at the University of Akron (Integrated Biosciences Program), and Case Western Reserve University (BME). He earned his PhD in chemical engineering, from Oklahoma State University, Stillwater, Oklahoma, in 1999 and subsequently completed a postdoctoral fellowship at the Cleveland Clinic funded by an award from the American Heart Association (AHA).

Prior to 2010, Dr. Ramamurthi was a tenured faculty in the Departments of Bioengineering at Clemson University and Regenerative Medicine and Cell Biology at the Medical University of South Carolina, Charleston, South Carolina, respectively. In the past 13 years, he has directed a research program that focuses on developing technologies for enabling biomimetic regeneration and repair of ECM structures, specifically the poorly regenerated elastic matrix component, both in vitro and in situ at sites of chronic matrix disruption (e.g., aortic aneurysms and pelvic organ prolapse). His research has resulted in several book chapters, 50 peer-reviewed publications in top journals in the biomaterials, tissue engineering, and regenerative medicine fields, nearly 200 conference abstracts and proceedings and several awarded and filed patents. His research has been funded by the National Institutes of Health, National Science Foundation, American Heart Association, and Industry.

Dr. Ramamurthi is a member of several international professional societies in the cardiovascular sciences, biomaterials, and tissue engineering fields; he is a professional member of the AHA Council on arteriosclerosis, thrombosis, and vascular biology, and is an elected fellow of the AHA Council on basic cardiovascular sciences. He serves on several national committees such as that of the North American Vascular Biology Organization, on the editorial board of several scientific journals in the fields of tissue engineering, regenerative medicine, and vascular biomedicine, and actively reviews for the NIH, NSF, AHA, and several international scientific funding agencies, and nearly 25 journals including *Tissue Engineering, Biomaterials,* and *Acta Biomaterialia.* He serves on the external advisory committee of the NIH-supported Center for Biomedical Research Excellence (COBRE) in biomaterials for tissue regeneration in South Carolina, and on the Inventions Peer Review Committee of Cleveland Clinic Innovations, the commercialization wing of the Cleveland Clinic. Dr. Ramamurthi has been an invited speaker at several national conferences, and in 2007, he was the featured investigator at the Biomedical Entrepreneurship Meeting of the Upstate South Carolina Biomedical Cluster.

Chandrasekhar Kothapalli is an assistant professor in the Department of Chemical and Biomedical Engineering at Cleveland State University since 2011. He also holds adjunct appointments in the Department of Biomedical Engineering at the Lerner Research Institute in the Cleveland Clinic, and in the Division of General Medical Sciences at the Case Western Reserve University School of Medicine. He earned his PhD in bioengineering from the Clemson University—Medical University of South Carolina joint program in 2008, and performed postdoctoral work in the Biological Engineering Department at the Massachusetts Institute of Technology and in the Biomedical Engineering Department at the City University of New York. His research interests are in tissue engineering, matrix biology, microfluidics, simulations and modeling, axonal biology, stem cells, and cancer cell biology.

Dr. Kothapalli's research has resulted in 1 approved and 2 filed patents, 32 peer-reviewed journal publications and conference proceedings, 4 book chapters, and more than 60 conference abstracts and presentations. He is an active member of numerous professional societies in the biomedical and materials science fields and serves as a reviewer for numerous federal and private funding agencies, conferences, and journals in the field. Among his honors, he was a recipient of the Faculty Merit Award from CSU in 2013 and 2014, member of Sigma XI, and was the presidential scholar at the Medical University of South Carolina. His current research is supported by the US National Institutes of Health, National Science Foundation, and Institutional funds.

Contributors

Brian M. Balog
Department of Biology
University of Akron
Akron, Ohio

Aniqa Chowdhury
Department of Bioengineering
Clemson University
Clemson, South Carolina

Margot S. Damaser
Department of Biomedical
  Engineering
Lerner Research Institute
Cleveland Clinic
and
Advanced Platform Technology
  Rehabilitation R&D Center
  of Excellence
Louis Stokes Cleveland Veterans
  Affairs Medical Center
Cleveland, Ohio

Svenja Hinderer
Department of Cell and Tissue
  Engineering
Fraunhofer Institute for Interfacial
  Engineering and Biotechnology
Stuttgart, Germany

Aleksander Hinek
Cardiovascular Research Program
The Hospital for Sick Children
Toronto, Ontario, Canada

Dirk Hubmacher
Department of Biomedical
  Engineering
Lerner Research Institute
Cleveland Clinic
Cleveland, Ohio

Jyotsna Joshi
Department of Chemical
  and Biomedical Engineering
Cleveland State University
Cleveland, Ohio

Inkyung Kang
Matrix Biology Program
Benaroya Research Institute
Seattle, Washington

Saketh R. Karamched
Department of Bioengineering
Clemson University
Clemson, South Carolina

Chandrasekhar Kothapalli
Department of Chemical and
   Biomedical Engineering
Cleveland State University
Cleveland, Ohio

Beth A. Kozel
Department of Genetics and
   Genomic Medicine
Washington University School
   of Medicine
St. Louis, Missouri

Mervyn J. Merrilees
Department of Anatomy with
   Radiology
Faculty of Medical and Health
   Sciences
The University of Auckland
Auckland, New Zealand

Suzanne M. Mithieux
School of Molecular Bioscience
and
Charles Perkin Center
The University of Sydney
New South Wales, Australia

Nasim Nosoudi
Department of Bioengineering
Clemson University
Clemson, South Carolina

Jazmin Ozsvar
School of Molecular Bioscience
and
Charles Perkin Center
The University of Sydney
New South Wales, Australia

Vaideesh Parasaram
Department of Bioengineering
Clemson University
Clemson, South Carolina

Anand Ramamurthi
Department of Biomedical
   Engineering
Lerner Research Institute
Cleveland Clinic
and
Department of Molecular
   Medicine
Cleveland Clinic Lerner College
   of Medicine
Case Western Reserve University
Cleveland, Ohio

Katja Schenke-Layland
Department of Women's Health
Research Institute for Women's
   Health
Eberhard Karls University
Tübingen, Germany

Christian E. H. Schmelzer
Institute of Pharmacy
Martin Luther University
    Halle-Wittenberg
Halle, Germany

Nian Shen
Department of Cell and Tissue
    Engineering
Fraunhofer Institute for Interfacial
    Engineering and Biotechnology
Stuttgart, Germany

Balakrishnan Sivaraman
Department of Biomedical
    Engineering
Lerner Research Institute
Cleveland Clinic
Cleveland, Ohio

Ganesh Swaminathan
Department of Biology
University of Akron
Akron, Ohio

Naren Vyavahare
Department of Bioengineering
Clemson University
Clemson, South Carolina

Richard Wang
School of Molecular Bioscience
and
Charles Perkin Center
The University of Sydney
New South Wales, Australia

Anthony S. Weiss
School of Molecular Bioscience
and
Charles Perkin Center
and
Bosch Institute
The University of Sydney
New South Wales, Australia

Thomas N. Wight
Matrix Biology Program
Benaroya Research Institute
Seattle, Washington

CHAPTER 1

Assembly and Properties of Elastic Fibers

Christian E. H. Schmelzer

CONTENTS

1.1 INTRODUCTION

The evolutionary process of vertebrates required the development of flexible and extensible tissues. This fact appears to be reflected by extensive structural changes of the blood vessel walls, which were required for the conversion from an open to a closed circulatory system. The properties of elasticity and extensibility were implemented by the emergence of elastic fibers and are inevitable to the function of blood vessels that dilate and constrict to manage flow. Elastic fibers are integral components of the extracellular matrix (ECM) of virtually all force-bearing tissues such as arteries, lung, tendon, cartilage, or skin. The fibers are durable macromolecular assemblies of the ECM of jawed vertebrates including cartilaginous fishes and are composed of two morphologically distinguishable components: an outer microfibrillar mantle and an inner core of elastin that constitutes ~90% of the mature fibers.

Microfibrils are 10- to 12-nm-wide filaments that provide the tissues with characteristic biomechanical properties, partly, but not exclusively, with participation of elastin, which can be deposited on a microfibrillar scaffold. Microfibrils consist of fibrillins, large (~350 kDa) modular glycoproteins that have a remarkable high cysteine content of ~13%. Evolutionarily, microfibrils are one of the most ancient assemblies in the ECM. They emerged more than 600 million years ago and remained essentially unchanged over that period (Robertson et al. 2011). Fibrillins are widely distributed from cnidarians to mammals (Reber-Müller et al. 1995, Piha-Gossack et al. 2012), which underlines their biomechanical importance. In humans, there are three fibrillins, each of which comprises 43 Ca-binding epidermal growth factor (EGF)-like domains, five EGF-like domains, seven eight-cysteine-containing domains, and two so-called hybrid domains. The proteins have unique properties that provide long-range elasticity to dynamic connective tissues (Baldwin et al. 2013), but they also interact with cell-surface receptors such as integrins and regulate growth factor signaling (Sakamoto et al. 1996, Ramirez and Rifkin 2009). Despite the fibrillins, which are the major components of microfibrils, a number of other proteins are known to be associated with them. These include microfibril-associated glycoproteins (Gibson et al. 1989, 1996, Mecham and Gibson 2015), EMILINs (Bressan et al. 1993), and latent transforming growth factor-β binding proteins (LTBPs) (Sinha et al. 1998, 2002, Isogai et al. 2003).

In contrast to the fibrillin family, which has ancient roots in metazoan evolution, the second major protein, elastin, is absent in lower chordates and in all invertebrates (Sage and Gray 1979). It appeared relatively late in evolution and is a synapomorphy of gnathostomes. Cyclostomes, such as hagfish and lamprey, which are thought to have split off before the evolution of bones, lack elastin. However, studies on lamprey identified a protein termed lamprin, which shares some features with elastin but is distinct from it in various aspects including the types of cross-links (Robson et al. 1993, Fernandes and Eyre 1999). Elastin imparts elasticity and resilience to many tissues that undergo reversible deformation and these properties are critical for their long-term function. Elastin is an insoluble polymer of the soluble monomeric precursor tropoelastin. Tropoelastin has a highly repetitive sequence with 78% of the human type (isoform 2) composed of only four amino acids: glycine (~30%), alanine (~22.5%), valine (~13%), and proline (~12.5%). With few exceptions among vertebrates, tryptophan, histidine, and methionine residues are absent from tropoelastins (Keeley 2013).

In humans, tropoelastin is encoded by a single gene (ELN) on chromosome 7q11.23 (Fazio et al. 1991) and secreted as an ~62 kDa unglycosylated protein by elastogenic cell types including fibroblasts (Mecham et al. 1985), smooth muscle cells (Narayanan et al. 1976), chondrocytes (Brown-Augsburger et al. 1996), keratinocytes (Kajiya et al. 1997), and endothelial cells (Mecham et al. 1983, Damiano et al. 1984). Unlike other vertebrates, the human gene lacks exons 34 and 35 (nonhuman primates only lack exon 35), which have been lost during primate evolution (Szabo et al. 1999). Tropoelastin consists of alternating hydrophobic and more hydrophilic domains, which are encoded by separate exons, so that the domain structure of tropoelastin maps the exon organization of the gene. The hydrophilic domains contain Lys-Ala (KA) and Lys-Pro (KP) motifs that are involved in cross-linking during the formation of mature elastin. In the KA domains, lysine residues occur as pairs or triplets separated by two or three alanine residues, whereas in KP domains the lysine residues are separated mainly by proline residues (see Figure 1.1). The ELN primary transcript undergoes extensive alternative splicing and thus elastin's precursor tropoelastin occurs in several isoforms with molecular weights ranging between 60 and 75 kDa (Bashir et al. 1989). The splicing occurs in a cassette-like manner without affecting the reading frame. Thus, an exon is either included or deleted, but occasionally a splicing event may also divide an exon (Kozel et al. 2011). At least six exons of human tropoelastin have been reported to be alternatively spliced: 22, 23, 24, 27, 32, and 33. As can be seen from Figure 1.1, alternative splicing affects both hydrophobic and hydrophilic domains. In the case of exon 22, which is virtually always spliced out in human (Keeley 2013), the two cross-linking domains 21 and 23 are connected. However, deletion of exon 27 increases the hydrophobic distance between the adjacent cross-linking domains. Although some studies indicate that splicing could be tissue specific or correlate with developmental changes of cells (Parks and Deak 1990, Heim et al. 1991), the exact function of these sequence variations remains to be determined.

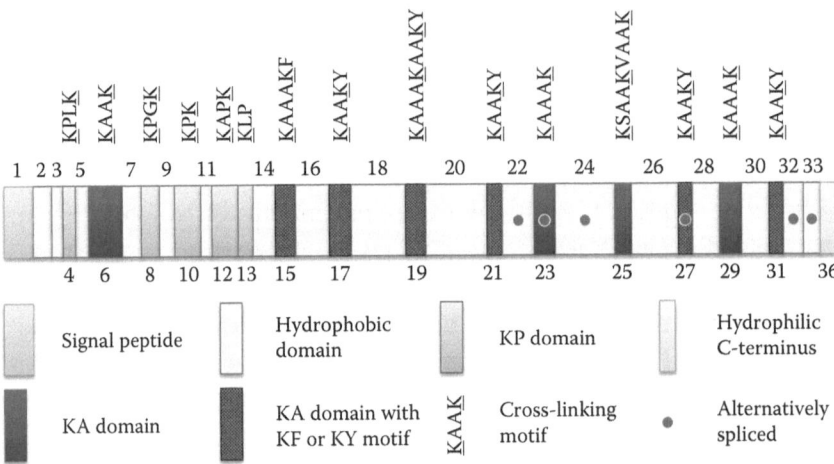

FIGURE 1.1 The domain structure of human tropoelastin. The domain numbering shown across the top (hydrophobic domains) and the bottom (hydrophilic domains) is based on exon assignment. Gray squares display hydrophobic domains and light and dark blue squares represent the 15 hydrophilic cross-linking domains. Filled circles indicate exons that are alternatively spliced. The sequence motifs of the cross-linking sites within the domains (lysine residues that are mainly separated by alanine or proline residues) are shown above the domain scheme. Human tropoelastin lacks exons 34 and 35 that were evolutionarily lost, but are present in nonprimate vertebrates.

Mature elastic fibers are organized in various structural configurations in different elastic tissues, for example, concentric fenestrated lamellae in the medial layer of the aorta, three-dimensional honeycomb-like structures in elastic cartilage, or networks of reticular fibers in the dermis. The structural configurations and elastin contents of several human tissues are listed in Table 1.1. It is apparent that differences in morphology are closely connected to the magnitude and direction of reversible deformation the connective tissues undergo. The amount of elastin highly varies between different connective tissues, but also between same tissues of different species (Scarselli 1961, Greenlee et al. 1966, Peters and Smillie 1971, Starcher 1977, Uitto 1979, Chrzanowski et al. 1980, Spina et al. 1983, Mikawa et al. 1986). In spite of its low content, for instance in intervertebral disk or skin (Mikawa et al. 1986, Cloyd and Elliott 2007), elastin is essential in maintaining the elasticity and tensile strength of these tissues.

TABLE 1.1   Structural Configuration of Elastic Fibers in Various Tissues and Elastin Content as Percentage of the Dry Weight

Human Tissue	Elastin (%)	Structural Configuration	References
Aorta	<57	Concentric lamellae	Scarselli (1961), Spina et al. (1983)
Elastic cartilage[a]	19	Honeycomb-like structures	Peters and Smillie (1971)
Elastic ligaments	<75	Rope-like fibers	Uitto (1979)
Intervertebrate disk (anulus fibrosus)	2	Densely clustered and randomly oriented	Mikawa et al. (1986)
Intervertebrate disk (nucleus pulposus)	2	Radial fiber network	Mikawa et al. (1986)
Lung	<30	Lamellar sheets surrounding the alveoli	Chrzanowski et al. (1980)
Skin (dermis)	<5	Rope-like fibers	Starcher (1977)
Tendon	4	Bundles of long fibers	Greenlee et al. (1966), Uitto (1979)

[a] Content determined for bovine elastin.

1.2 ELASTOGENESIS

The process that leads to a fully functional elastic fiber formation, also known as elastogenesis, is a highly complex multistep process involving a large number of proteins and other molecules, whose structural and functional interactions are yet not entirely understood. Elastic fiber formation starts at mid-gestation, reaches its maximum near birth, and completes during postnatal development (Keeley 1979, Mecham 2008). Starcher and Percival (1985) reported for rats that elastogenesis in the uterus starts again with every new pregnancy and elastin is rapidly removed after parturition. Apart from this noteworthy exception, it is generally accepted that virtually no new functional elastic fibers are formed in the adult tissues (Rucker and Dubick 1984). The two distinct structural components that together make up the elastic fiber, the microfibrils and the amorphous elastin core, are formed rather independently and thus their formation is discussed separately below. The major steps that are currently thought to be essential for the elastogenesis are illustrated in Figure 1.2.

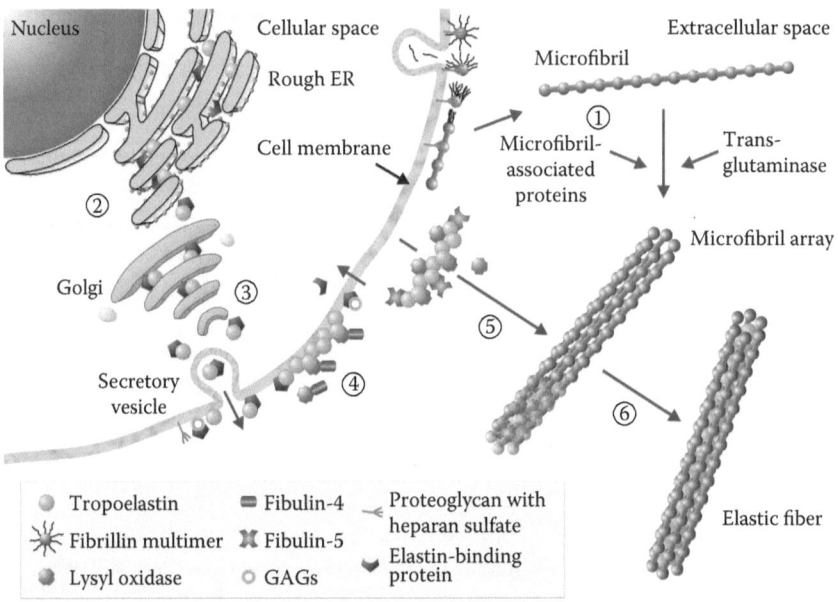

FIGURE 1.2   Schematic representation of the elastic fiber assembly: (1) Fibrillin and microfibril-associated proteins are secreted into the extracellular space, multimerize into bead-like structures and form the microfibrillar array. (2) Tropoelastin is synthesized on the rough ER where it binds to the chaperone protein EBP. (3) The EBP-tropoelastin complex is transported through the Golgi apparatus and secreted to the cell membrane. (4) Tropoelastin is released from the chaperone and forms globules at the cell surface, while EBP dissociates as a result of interaction with glycosaminoglycans. Fibulin-4 is important for the chain alignment of tropoelastin mediating the interplay with lysyl oxidase or lysyl oxidase-like enzymes. The oxidation of lysine residues initiates a series of condensation reactions forming covalent intra- and intermolecular cross-links. (5) After the cluster of tropoelastin molecules reaches a critical size, it is moved from the plasma membrane through the ECM. Fibulin-5 is thought to direct the premature elastin to fibrillin microfibrils. (6) The elastin aggregates fuse into larger assemblies and are further cross-linked to eventually form the elastic fiber.

1.2.1 Microfibril Formation

Elastogenesis is initiated by the assembly of microfibrils that probably serve as a scaffold for the subsequent elastin deposition. The ubiquitous components of the 10- to 12-nm-diameter microfibrils are the fibrillins (Ramirez 2000), which are secreted from cells of mesenchymal origin such as fibroblasts or smooth muscle cells. Fibrillin-1 is the major component of microfibrils in all tissues and expressed throughout life, whereas fibrillin-2 and fibrillin-3 are restricted to developing fetal tissues (Zhang et al. 1994, Charbonneau et al. 2010, Sabatier et al. 2011). Fibrillin-3 seems to perform unique functions in certain tissues such as the brain (Corson et al. 2004). During or after secretion of the precursors, profibrillins undergo N- and C-terminal cleavage by furin/PACE-like proprotein convertases at the consensus motif RXK/RR resulting in the ~320 kDa mature forms (Milewicz et al. 1995, Raghunath et al. 1999). This processing is required for the subsequent linear multimerization into bead-like structures through the C-terminal domain and their assembly at the cell surface (Marson et al. 2005, Hubmacher et al. 2008). Jensen et al. (2014) have recently shown that the presence of the N-terminal propeptide is essential for the secretion of fibrillin-1 as it prevents premature intracellular assembly, but the subsequent cleavage of the propeptide is crucial for the proper microfibril assembly. There is evidence that the multimerization promotes the affinity of the fibrillin beads to fibronectin, the N-terminus of fibrillin-1, and especially to heparin/heparan sulfate (Sabatier et al. 2014). The beads probably interact first with heparan sulfate-containing proteoglycans at the cell surface via C-terminal binding sites and then undergo focal adhesion formation. This process is followed by interactions between the N- and C-termini of fibrillin molecules that mediate the assembly of the multimeric beads in a parallel head-to-tail fashion and their lateral interaction (Reinhardt et al. 1996, Lin et al. 2002). The growing microfibrils are subsequently transported to a fibronectin network, which is thought to play an important role in stabilizing the newly formed microfibrils and/or promoting their interaction with other microfibril proteins (Sabatier et al. 2014). The fibrillin network can undergo cross-linking, which further stabilizes the three-dimensional bundle structure. The cross-links reported to date are intermolecular disulfide bonds (Reinhardt et al. 2000) and ε(γ-glutamyl)lysine cross-links that are catalyzed by members of the *transglutaminase* family (Qian and Glanville 1997). Fibrillin-1 can also interact with cells through integrins such as $\alpha_5\beta_1$ and $\alpha_v\beta_3$, but it remains to be determined whether these interactions are required for microfibril assembly or tissue-specific functions (Bax et al. 2007).

1.2.2 Formation of the Elastic Fiber Core

1.2.2.1 Synthesis of Tropoelastin and Secretion

As mentioned above, the pre-mRNA of tropoelastin undergoes alternative splicing, giving rise to several different isoforms. After the mRNA is exported from the nucleus, translation occurs on the surface of the rough endoplasmic reticulum (ER) and the N-terminal signal peptide is cleaved off. Before tropoelastin is transported through the Golgi apparatus to the cell surface, it is hydroxylated at prolyl residues by the prolyl 4-hydroxylase. Unlike collagens, for which the role of hydroxyproline—the stabilization of the triple-helical structure—is well understood, virtually nothing is known about the exact function of this modification in elastin. However, it had been shown in several studies that a high hydroxylation degree is detrimental for the self-assembly of tropoelastin (Bochicchio et al. 2013) and thus can impede elastic fiber formation (Urry et al. 1979).

Intracellularly, tropoelastin binds to the elastin-binding protein (EBP), a 67 kDa β-galactosidase splice variant that is part of the elastin receptor complex (ERC). The ERC consists of two further subunits, the membrane-associated proteins cathepsin A/protective protein (PPCA) and neuraminidase-1 (Neu-1). The EBP protects the newly synthesized tropoelastin from degradation and coacervation inside the cell and furthermore delivers it to the cell surface (Privitera et al. 1998, Duca et al. 2007, Blanchevoye et al. 2013). When the complex of EBP and tropoelastin is secreted, it associates with the other subunits of the ERC and probably also interacts with glycosaminoglycans. This interaction causes conformational changes in the EBP that leads to the release of tropoelastin from its chaperone (Privitera et al. 1998, Blanchevoye et al. 2013). The EBP is recycled back into the intracellular endosomal compartments and associates with newly synthesized tropoelastin. Its reuse is thought to be important for elastogenesis (Hinek et al. 1995).

1.2.2.2 Microassembly

Tropoelastin subsequently undergoes self-association in an endothermic, entropically driven process of liquid–liquid phase separation termed coacervation. In this process, also called microassembly, hydrophobic domains of the precursor tropoelastin, especially the domains encoded by exons 17–27, interact with each other (Dyksterhuis et al. 2007) leading to the formation of distinct globular aggregates on the cell surface (Clarke et al. 2006, Kozel et al. 2006). The behavior of droplet formation can also be observed in vitro from full-length tropoelastin or smaller polypeptides as their solutions become turbid on reaching a critical transition temperature (Vrhovski et al. 1997, Bellingham et al. 2001). The rate at which these droplets are formed as well as their sizes and properties depend on tropoelastin concentration, ionic strength, pH, and temperature (Yeo et al. 2011). It has long been assumed that coacervation is essential for elastogenesis. However, several studies, among them one carried out by Kozel et al. (2003) using deletion constructs of tropoelastin, suggest that this process might not be the initial step of elastin formation. Instead, interactions of the C-terminal region of tropoelastin, especially the domain 30, with microfibrillar proteins seem to be required for the assembly of the elastic fiber (Kozel et al. 2003, Sato et al. 2007). Another important sequence comprising the polybasic motif KXXXRKRK is located in the C-terminal domain that is encoded by the highly conserved exon 36. It has been shown that tropoelastin lacking this sequence is less efficiently incorporated into mature elastin and shows abnormal cross-linking (Hsiao et al. 1999, Kozel et al. 2003). Proteoglycans may interact with this domain facilitating the correct alignment of the tropoelastin monomers (Broekelmann et al. 2005). The alignment of tropoelastin and the subsequent cross-linking is further promoted by fibulin-4, which mediates the association between tropoelastin and the extracellular Cu^{2+}-dependent amine oxidase, lysyl oxidase (LOX) (McLaughlin et al. 2006, Horiguchi et al. 2009, Yanagisawa and Davis 2010).

1.2.2.3 Cross-Linking

The LOX and LOX-like enzymes catalyze the oxidative deamination of the ε-amino group of lysine residues in peptide linkage to the highly reactive α-aminoadipic acid-δ-semialdehyde aldehyde, termed allysine. Most of tropoelastin's Lys residues (~80%) are involved in this enzymatic reaction (Kozel et al. 2003). These lysine residues are either located in the 10 KA domains, which are enriched in alanine, or in the five proline-containing KP domains (see Figure 1.1). After oxidation, intra- and intermolecular cross-links are spontaneously formed either by nonenzymatic condensation of two allysine residues via aldol condensation that produces allysine aldol or by reaction of an allysine residue with the ε-amino group of another lysine residue via Schiff base reaction that creates (dehydro)lysinonorleucine (Franzblau et al. 1969, Lent et al. 1969). Such reducible cross-links then further condense with each other—partly with participation of unmodified Lys residues or with other intermediates—to form the stable and nonreducible trifunctional cross-links dehydromerodesmosine, and cyclopentenosine (Francis et al. 1973, Nakamura et al. 1992, Akagawa et al. 1999), the tetrafunctional cross-links desmosine (DES), and its isomer isodesmosine (IDES) (Partridge et al. 1963, Akagawa and Suyama 2000). There is also evidence that pentafunctional cross-links such as allodesmosine and pentasine are formed to some extent (Nakamura and Suyama 1991, Akagawa and Suyama 2000). The structures and formation pathways of prominent elastin cross-links are shown in Figure 1.3.

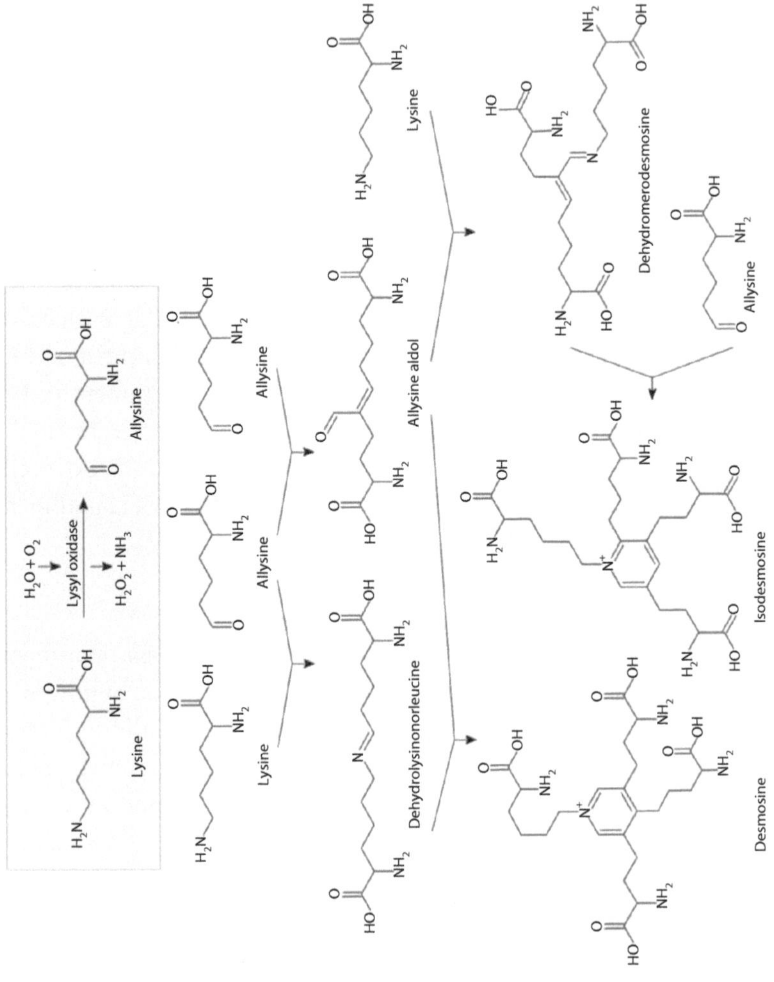

FIGURE 1.3 The formation of the major cross-links in elastin. Cross-linking is initiated by oxidative deamination of the side chains of lysine residues by the enzyme lysyl oxidase. The reaction produces a reactive aldehyde termed allysine under consumption of oxygen and the release of ammonia and hydrogen peroxide. The aldehyde groups subsequently condense spontaneously with another allysine residue by an aldol condensation forming allysine aldol, or with another lysine residue to form dehydrolysinonorleucine. These bifunctional cross-links can further condense with each other, or with other intermediates such as the trifunctional merodesmosine, to form the tetrafunctional cross-links desmosine and its isomer isodesmosine.

While for instance lysinonorleucine and allysine aldol are also present in collagen, DES and its isomer IDES are exclusively found in elastin (Rucker and Murray 1978, Eyre et al. 1984, Bedell-Hogan et al. 1993, Mithieux and Weiss 2005), and it is further assumed that DES/IDES formation involves the condensation of an allysine aldol formed between two allysine residues on one chain and an intramolecular dehydrolysinonorleucine on a second chain (Foster et al. 1974, Gerber and Anwar 1974, Gray 1977). It is worth mentioning that not all formed bifunctional cross-links such as allysine aldol and lysinonorleucine are incorporated into higher functional cross-links and that some bifunctional cross-links are likely to be formed intramolecularly (Schräder et al. 2016). The exact cross-linking pattern has not yet been elucidated. The only determined sites of cross-linking were elucidated by Brown-Augsburger et al. (1995) in a study using elastin derived from copper-deficient pigs. This copper deficiency resulted in a reduced LOX activity and consequently in an incomplete cross-linking and enhanced susceptibility of elastin to trypsin and chymotrypsin. The authors were able to identify a major cross-linking site that is formed through the association of three tropoelastin chains via one DES and two lysinonorleucine cross-links. The data further suggest that the DES cross-link is formed between the antiparallel arranged KA domains 19 and 25. These are the only two KA domains that contain three lysine residues that can participate in cross-linking (see Figure 1.1). The third available lysine residue in each domain joins with a lysine residue in the KP domain 10 of a third chain to form lysinonorleucine cross-links (Brown-Augsburger et al. 1995).

The conformation of the KA cross-linking domains is primarily α-helical, which results in the side chains of lysine residue pairs being on the same side of the helix and thus facilitating the formation of DES/IDES (Tamburro et al. 2006). Interestingly, this formation requires that one of the four lysine residues involved must retain its ε-amino group (Franzblau et al. 1977). This is probably ensured by the presence of a bulky hydrophobic residue such as tyrosine, phenylalanine, leucine, or isoleucine next to a lysine residue within a KA domain. The lysine residue is thus protected from oxidation by the amine oxidase (Gray et al. 1973, Foster et al. 1974). As shown in Figure 1.1, six of the ten KA domains in human tropoelastin have such a protected lysine residue and it can be assumed that DES/IDES is formed between two residues (lysine + allysine) of these domains and two further allysines of one of the four remaining KA domains. The proline residues in the KP domains impede the α-helical structure

(Muiznieks et al. 2014) and thus, it is thought that KP domains are not involved in DES/IDES formation, but are limited to bifunctional cross-links. This assumption is in contradiction to the finding that the DES/IDES contents of species such as frog or salamander, which are rich in KP domains, are approximately the same as in teleost elastins (Sage and Gray 1979), in which KA domains predominate (Keeley 2013). Thus, it remains to be further investigated whether DES/IDES exclusively are formed from KA domains.

1.2.2.4 Macromolecular Assembly

Over time, the cluster that is formed at the cell surface grows in size by the addition and cross-linking of newly secreted tropoelastin molecules. At some point, when enough tropoelastin is secreted and accumulated, the formed globules are released from the cell surface and move through the ECM. Fibulin-5 has the ability to interact with fibrillin and is thought to play a central role in controlling the deposition of the premature elastin aggregates onto the microfibril scaffold (Choudhury et al. 2009). The globules associate with fibrillin-containing microfibrils and readily coalesce into larger aggregates and eventually form a functional fiber. Another contributing protein is LTBP-4, which does not directly interact with tropoelastin but with the fibulin-5-tropoelastin complex and which is apparently required for the proper linear deposition on the microfibril network (Noda et al. 2013). The deposited elastin is further oxidized by LOX and/or condensation reactions take place until the elastin has been fully integrated into microfibrillar scaffold. Interestingly, this process seems to proceed rather slowly (Partridge et al. 1966).

1.2.2.5 Postneonatal Decrease in Elastin Synthesis

As mentioned above, elastogenesis is not a continuous process, but takes place over a relatively short period of time and is subject to dynamic regulation. Tropoelastin expression in most mammalian tissues begins in late fetal life, reaches high levels during early neonatal periods, and subsequently declines and ultimately ceases at maturity (Davis 1993, Holzenberger et al. 1993, Mecham 2008). The regulatory control varies with the cell type during the development of the tissue. In the lungs, for example, tropoelastin expression is downregulated after birth and later again upregulated during alveolarization before it is reattenuated

(Bruce and Honaker 1998). In the event of injury or diseases such as dermal elastosis or severe chronic obstructive pulmonary disease (COPD) tropoelastin expression can be reactivated, although this usually results not in functional elastic fibers (Bernstein and Uitto 1996, Deslee et al. 2009). It has been shown that elastin production is controlled through transcriptional and posttranscriptional mechanisms (Parks et al. 1993, Swee et al. 1995). Cytokines that influence this regulation can be classified into proelastogenic factors including transforming growth factor-β1 (TGFβ1) and insulin-like growth factor-I as well as anti-elastogenic factors such as basic fibroblast growth factor-2, heparin-binding EGF-like growth factor, EGF, platelet-derived growth factor-BB, TGF-α, tumor necrosis factor-alpha, interleukin-1β, and noncanonical TGFβ1 signaling (for review, see Sproul and Argraves 2013).

Although many positive and negative effectors have been identified in the past, elucidating the exact role of these cytokines as well as other messengers or autoregulatory processes in the elastic fiber formation remains difficult. It is likely that in vivo multiple factors simultaneously interact with elastogenic cells and thus contribute to the fine regulation of the complex and dynamic process of elastogenesis.

1.3 PROPERTIES OF ELASTIN

1.3.1 Durability and Proteolytic Resistance

Mature elastin is a completely insoluble and extremely resistant protein due to its extensive cross-linking. Under normal conditions, it is metabolically stable over the human lifespan. Elastin's half-life has been determined to be greater than 70 years using aspartic acid racemization analysis and measuring ^{14}C levels in postmortem tissues (Shapiro et al. 1991, Powell et al. 1992). One of the reasons for this outstanding durability is elastin's high resistance to proteolysis, which is mainly facilitated by its highly cross-linked nature and the extremely tight packing of the molecules. Mature elastin cannot be cleaved by trypsin as it contains very few arginines and most lysines are oxidized and incorporated in cross-links during maturation. However, among the many proteases in the human body are some that can hydrolyze elastin. The breakdown of elastic tissues is mainly caused by local degrading enzymes. Elastin-cleaving proteases are collectively termed elastases, although this description does not indicate that elastin degradation is a physiological function of the enzymes. Elastases may belong to at least three classes of families: serine (e.g., pancreatic elastase, cathepsin G, human leukocyte elastase) (Früh et al. 1996, Owen and Campbell 1999, Heinz et al. 2012, Schmelzer et al. 2012), metalloproteinases (e.g., MMP-9 and -12) (Senior et al. 1991, Gronski et al. 1997, Heinz et al. 2010), or cysteine proteinases (e.g., cathepsins K, L, and S) (Mason et al. 1986, Novinec et al. 2007). Elastases are produced by fibroblasts, platelets, macrophages, leukocytes, mesenchymal cells, or the pancreas (Shapiro 2002). In addition, many aggressive proteases that are capable of degrading elastin are of microbial origin (Morihara and Tsuzuki 1967). Despite the different catalytic mechanisms, all elastases are relatively nonspecific and have the common preference for cleaving at peptide bonds associated with hydrophobic or aromatic amino acids (Mecham et al. 1997). It is worth mentioning that the susceptibility of elastin depends on the intactness of the substrate. In vivo, the structural integrity of elastin can be weakened by enzymatic attack or other cause in the course of diseases or intrinsic aging. Indeed, when studying elastinolytic properties of proteases or the release of elastin peptides in vitro, the integrity of the substrate could have also been altered by the isolation procedure used for purification (Daamen et al. 2001). Hence, the isolation technique has to be chosen according to the requirements of the substrate and the specific study. Despite the classical isolation methods such as the hot alkali technique (Lansing et al. 1952) or the Starcher method (Starcher and Galione 1976), a few very gentle protocols have been introduced in the last decade, which result in intact fibers that lack the microfibrillar component but keep their regular fibrillar conformation (Daamen et al. 2005, Schmelzer et al. 2012). Methods for purification of insoluble elastin aim the removal of all other tissue components, of which some have to be degraded. The isolation techniques take advantage of elastin's remarkable properties such as insolubility, the absence of certain amino acids and the resistance to proteolysis, high temperatures, and extreme pH levels. The essential steps of such a rather gentle purification procedure are as follows: after reducing the tissue to small pieces—for instance by mincing or grinding to a fine powder in the frozen state—it is thoroughly washed with sodium chloride to remove soluble compounds. The sample is then rinsed with a series of organic solvents of increasing polarity (ethanol, chloroform, ether, and acetone, respectively) to remove lipids and other lipophilic components. This step is followed by treatment with cyanogen bromide that hydrolyzes peptide bonds at the carboxy termini of methionine residues. Methionine is present in almost all proteins but absent in elastin. Thus, a variety of tissue proteins including collagens are cleaved and solubilized. After further treatment with reducing (2-mercaptoethanol) and chaotropic agents (guanidine-HCl or urea) and another washing step, the sample is incubated with trypsin. This proteolysis step is important for the depletion of remnants of collagens and microfibrillar proteins. Further extraction and washing steps are the last steps of the isolation technique (Schmelzer et al. 2012).

Figure 1.4 shows such purified elastin fibers derived from human skin of two individuals of very different ages: 6 and 90 years. The fibers have diameters between 1 and 2 µm and appear to have smooth surfaces for the younger subject whereas the fibers of the old individual are fissured, porous, and show various cracks. It has been shown that the proteolytic resistance of elastin fibers having such damages is drastically reduced (Schmelzer et al. 2012). This indicates that elastic fibers lose their resistance against proteolytic degradation with increasing age, which may be an explanation for the accelerated disintegration of elastic fibers and their gradual functional loss in old age.

1.3.2 Biological Properties

The main biological function of elastin is to provide elasticity to tissues so that they withstand repetitive forces. However, elastin is not only a structural protein influencing the architecture and biomechanical properties of the ECM, but also plays a role in various physiological processes (Debelle and Tamburro 1999). Although elastin is an extremely durable ECM protein, it undergoes unwanted degradation throughout life,

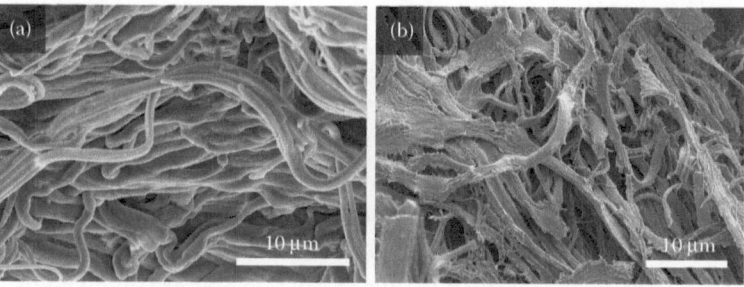

FIGURE 1.4 Scanning electron micrographs of fibrillar elastin (elastic fibers without the microfibrillar sheath) purified from human skin showing (a) fibers from the foreskin of a 6-year-old boy and (b) from a 90-year-old woman. The fibers have diameters of approximately 1–2 µm and appear with very different integrities.

especially during vascular aging or pathological and pathophysiological processes. Inflammatory diseases that involve elastin degradation with severe consequences include COPD (He et al. 2010, Maclay et al. 2012), atherosclerosis (Gayral et al. 2014), and aneurysm formation (Carmo et al. 2002). The decrease of elasticity in the respective organs is accompanied with the release of large amounts of elastin-derived peptides (EPs) that can enter the blood circulation and display a wide range of biological properties. EPs are also referred to as matrikines, that is, bioactive peptides that are released through degradation of ECM proteins.

At least three different receptors of EPs have been proposed (Toupance et al. 2012). The primary receptor is the ERC, which comprises EBP, PPCA, and Neu-1. EBP chaperones the newly synthesized tropoelastin to the plasma membrane in the course of elastogenesis but it can also bind to EPs. The latter interaction stimulates the Neu-1 sialidase activity that seems to be essential for the intracellular signal transduction leading to the activation of various signaling events that differ highly between different cell types (Duca et al. 2007). The peptides recognized by the receptor complex share the consensus sequence XGXXPG. This motif is known to favor the formation of a type VIII β-turn and this conformation is apparently required for binding to EBP (Floquet et al. 2004, Blanchevoye et al. 2013). Another receptor for EPs is galectin-3, a ~31 kDa laminin/elastin-binding protein that is expressed mainly in inflammatory cells and plays an important role in interactions between cells and the ECM (Ochieng et al. 2004). Integrin $\alpha_V\beta_3$ has also been reported to interact directly with elastin's precursor or with EPs (Rodgers and Weiss 2005, Bax et al. 2009) and could be responsible for some of the EP-induced effects.

EPs have been shown to modulate the cellular physiology of various cell lines including fibroblasts, smooth muscle cells, and leukocytes (for review, see Duca et al. 2004). Numerous in vitro and in vivo studies have shown that EPs exhibit a remarkable range of biological activities. It has been demonstrated in several studies that EPs are involved in cancer progression (Lapis and Timar 2002, Duca et al. 2004). Devy et al. (2010) have for instance reported from an in vivo study that EPs are involved in melanoma growth and invasion, and Blaise et al. (2013) demonstrated a possible link between EPs and the development of insulin resistance in mice. It has also been shown that EPs promote angiogenesis through upregulation of MT1-MMP (Robinet et al. 2005) and are further associated with the regulation of various cellular activities including adhesion, chemotaxis, proliferation, protease activation, or apoptosis (Fülöp et al. 1986, Jung et al. 1998, Maquart et al. 2004, 2005, Moroy et al. 2005, Antonicelli et al. 2007).

1.3.3 Structural Properties

On the macroscopic level, elastin appears as yellowish and amorphous mass. Ultrastructural investigations using electron microscopy and atomic force microscopy revealed that elastin has a fibrillar substructure composed of parallel-aligned 5-nm-thick filaments forming a three-dimensional network along the fiber (Pasquali-Ronchetti et al. 1979, 1998, Pasquali-Ronchetti and Baccarani-Contri 1997). The results of these and further studies suggest that the fine filaments are laterally connected and overall organized in an ordered array (Pasquali-Ronchetti et al. 1998). The extreme insolubility and high hydrophobicity of mature elastin make its structural characterization at the protein level difficult. One possibility to make elastin available for different analytical techniques—at least indirectly—is its solubilization either by chemicals or by elastases. Chemical solubilization is carried out by refluxing elastin either with oxalic acid or potassium hydroxide resulting in the so-called α-elastin and κ-elastin, respectively (Robert 2010). Numerous studies have been performed to characterize the secondary structures of purified elastin, solubilized elastin, synthetically produced elastin peptides, or full-length tropoelastin. Circular dichroism (CD) analysis of recombinantly produced human tropoelastin has shown a composition of 3% α-helix, 41% β-sheet, 21% β-turn, and 33% other structure (Vrhovski et al. 1997). Studies carried out by Debelle et al. (1998) on human elastin using Fourier transform infrared, near-infrared Fourier-transform Raman, and CD revealed secondary structures comprising 10% α-helix, 35% β-strand, and 55% undefined conformations. The α-helical structures are confined to the polyalanine motifs in the KA cross-link domains and might only be formed on coacervation. As mentioned in Section 1.2.2.3 these α-helices, which seem to be rather stable against temperature, are thought to be required for the formation of bifunctional intramolecular cross-links and thus facilitate the subsequent condensation to DES or IDES cross-links. From this, it can be concluded that α-helical structures must persist and are also present in mature elastin (Tamburro et al. 2006). No attempts in crystallizing either elastin or full-length tropoelastin have been successful. Both the structural flexibility of the molecule and the presence of concurrent conformations probably prevent the formation of a uniform crystal lattice. However, recently the three-dimensional shape of hydrated human tropoelastin has been determined using small angle X-ray and neutron scattering (Baldock et al. 2011). These data show that tropoelastin is an asymmetric protein with defined modular components responsible for elasticity (coil region), cell binding (C-terminus), and a highly exposed bridge region that links the other two regions and which might be involved in elastic fiber assembly (Yeo et al. 2012). The authors proposed an interesting head-to-tail model, by which tropoelastin monomers assemble in a tandem orientation to propagate elasticity. Besides the nanostructural data, this model is based on the only three cross-links that have been identified from incompletely cross-linked porcine elastin (Brown-Augsburger et al. 1995). Only three cross-link domains (10, 19, and 25) out of 15 present in tropoelastin are required for the formation of this string of monomers and thus the assembly would represent an intermediate in the formation of elastic fibers. The fine fibers might subsequently undergo lateral association with each other through hydrophobic interactions to form larger assemblies. Further cross-links involving the remaining KA and KP domains could stabilize this lateral extension. It remains to be verified whether such intermediate structures are formed in vivo.

1.3.4 Mechanical Properties

Elastic tissues such as lungs or elastic ligaments undergo continuous repetitive strain and deformation without rupture. The human heart, for instance, beats more than 3.5 billion times in an average lifetime without failure. These flexibilities are only possible because of elastin's remarkable mechanical properties. Unlike other ECM proteins such as collagens, which are relatively inelastic with a Young's modulus between 1 and 2 GPa in the hydrated state (Heim et al. 2006), elastic fibers can be linearly stretched to about 150% of their length before rupture occurs (Gosline et al. 2002). Young's modulus of single elastic fibers has been determined to lie between 0.3 and 1.5 MPa (Koenders et al. 2009) and thus elastic fibers yield easily to stretching and return virtually to their original length when tension is released. Elastin is very resilient (~90%), but has a low tensile strength of about 2 MPa (Aaron and Gosline 1981). These elastomeric properties are only available when the elastic fibers are hydrated (Partridge 1962). Dried elastin is a rigid, hard, and brittle material, but regains its elastic properties when rehydrated. The ability of elastin to contract after stretching is mainly driven by an increase in entropy and is closely related to disorder in the structure (Hoeve and Flory 1958, Gosline et al. 2002). The presence of the covalent cross-links that distribute the stress and strain throughout the biopolymer during deformation is essential. Stretching of the elastic fibers induces organization within the elastin core. When the strain is released, the system returns to maximum entropy. Several structural models for elastin that account for the maintenance of its flexibility have been proposed. They vary mainly in the contribution of ordered structures to the entropic properties of the molecule. The concept that the elasticity of elastin is an entropy-based property was first established by Hoeve and Flory (1958), who later introduced a simple isotropic model in which the elastic fiber has a random chain network (Hoeve and Flory 1974). However, the model cannot explain why elastin requires water for elasticity. Although elastin's precursor has many Gly (30%) and Pro (12%) residues, which prevent the formation of elongated secondary structures, several studies provided evidence for the presence of β-turns (types I, II, and VIII) and polyproline II helices (Tamburro et al. 2003). A number of anisotropic models account for the contribution of these rather short and labile structural features. Urry and Parker (2002) proposed a librational entropy model in which the elastin molecules fold into easily deformable β-spirals that consist of consecutive type II β-turns. However, there is no experimental evidence for such an anisotropic orientation, and molecular dynamics simulations by Li et al. also do not support this model (Li et al. 2001, Li and Daggett 2002). Another interesting model proposed by Tamburro et al. explains the entropy increase with the formation of labile β-turns and their sliding along the chain (Lelj et al. 1992, Tamburro et al. 2005). Overall, these and further models are supported by some experimental results, but none of them provides a complete explanation of elasticity and related observations such as the requirement of hydration. Recent molecular dynamics simulations of elastin-derived peptides but also solid-state NMR experiments with mature elastin suggest that hydrated elastin has a high degree of dynamic disorder in the relaxed state (Li and Daggett 2002, Pometun et al. 2004). Thus, it is becoming increasingly evident that the flexibility of elastin is rather based on distinct dynamics than on a fixed structure.

The comprehension of the precise mechanism behind elastin's flexibility requires further insights from structural investigations especially those aiming to elucidate the entire cross-linking pattern.

REFERENCES

Aaron, B. B. and J. M. Gosline. 1981. Elastin as a random-network elastomer—A mechanical and optical analysis of single elastin fibers. *Biopolymers* 20(6): 1247–1260.

Akagawa, M. and K. Suyama. 2000. Mechanism of formation of elastin cross-links. *Connect Tissue Res* 41(2): 131–141.

Akagawa, M., K. Yamazaki, and K. Suyama. 1999. Cyclopentenosine, major tri-functional crosslinking amino acid isolated from acid hydrolysate of elastin. *Arch Biochem Biophys* 372(1): 112–120.

Antonicelli, F., G. Bellon, L. Debelle, and W. Hornebeck. 2007. Elastin-elastases and inflamm-aging. *Curr Top Dev Biol* 79: 99–155.

Baldock, C., A. F. Oberhauser, L. Ma et al. 2011. Shape of tropoelastin, the highly extensible protein that controls human tissue elasticity. *Proc Natl Acad Sci USA* 108(11): 4322–4327.

Baldwin, A. K., A. Simpson, R. Steer, S. A. Cain, and C. M. Kielty. 2013. Elastic fibres in health and disease. *Expert Rev Mol Med* 15: e8.

Bashir, M. M., Z. Indik, H. Yeh et al. 1989. Characterization of the complete human elastin gene. Delineation of unusual features in the 5′-flanking region. *J Biol Chem* 264(15): 8887–8891.

Bax, D. V., Y. Mahalingam, S. Cain et al. 2007. Cell adhesion to fibrillin-1: Identification of an Arg-Gly-Asp-dependent synergy region and a heparin-binding site that regulates focal adhesion formation. *J Cell Sci* 120(Pt 8): 1383–1392.

Bax, D. V., U. R. Rodgers, M. M. Bilek, and A. S. Weiss. 2009. Cell adhesion to tropoelastin is mediated via the C-terminal GRKRK motif and integrin alphaVbeta3. *J Biol Chem* 284(42): 28616–28623.

Bedell-Hogan, D., P. Trackman, W. Abrams, J. Rosenbloom, and H. Kagan. 1993. Oxidation, cross-linking, and insolubilization of recombinant tropoelastin by purified lysyl oxidase. *J Biol Chem* 268(14): 10345–10350.

Bellingham, C. M., K. A. Woodhouse, P. Robson, S. J. Rothstein, and F. W. Keeley. 2001. Self-aggregation characteristics of recombinantly expressed human elastin polypeptides. *Biochim Biophys Acta* 1550(1): 6–19.

Bernstein, E. F. and J. Uitto. 1996. The effect of photodamage on dermal extracellular matrix. *Clin Dermatol* 14(2): 143–151.

Blaise, S., B. Romier, C. Kawecki et al. 2013. Elastin-derived peptides are new regulators of insulin resistance development in mice. *Diabetes* 62(11): 3807–3816.

Blanchevoye, C., N. Floquet, A. Scandolera et al. 2013. Interaction between the elastin peptide VGVAPG and human elastin binding protein. *J Biol Chem* 288(2): 1317–1328.

Bochicchio, B., A. Laurita, A. Heinz, C. E. H. Schmelzer, and A. Pepe. 2013. Investigating the role of (2S,4R)-4-hydroxyproline in elastin model peptides. *Biomacromolecules* 14 (12): 4278–4288.

Bressan, G. M., D. Daga-Gordini, A. Colombatti et al. 1993. Emilin, a component of elastic fibers preferentially located at the elastin-microfibrils interface. *J Cell Biol* 121(1): 201–212.

Broekelmann, T. J., B. A. Kozel, H. Ishibashi et al. 2005. Tropoelastin interacts with cell-surface glycosaminoglycans via its COOH-terminal domain. *J Biol Chem* 280(49): 40939–40947.

Brown-Augsburger, P., T. Broekelmann, J. Rosenbloom, and R. P. Mecham. 1996. Functional domains on elastin and microfibril-associated glycoprotein involved in elastic fibre assembly. *Biochem J* 318(Pt 1): 149–155.

Brown-Augsburger, P., C. Tisdale, T. Broekelmann, C. Sloan, and R. P. Mecham. 1995. Identification of an elastin cross-linking domain that joins three peptide chains. Possible role in nucleated assembly. *J Biol Chem* 270(30): 17778–17783.

Bruce, M. C. and C. E. Honaker. 1998. Transcriptional regulation of tropoelastin expression in rat lung fibroblasts: Changes with age and hyperoxia. *Am J Physiol* 274(6 Pt 1): L940–L950.

Carmo, M., L. Colombo, A. Bruno et al. 2002. Alteration of elastin, collagen and their cross-links in abdominal aortic aneurysms. *Eur J Vasc Endovasc Surg* 23(6): 543–549.

Charbonneau, N. L., E. J. Carlson, S. Tufa et al. 2010. In vivo studies of mutant fibrillin-1 microfibrils. *J Biol Chem* 285(32): 24943–24955.

Choudhury, R., A. McGovern, C. Ridley et al. 2009. Differential regulation of elastic fiber formation by fibulin-4 and -5. *J Biol Chem* 284(36): 24553–24567.

Chrzanowski, P., S. Keller, J. Cerreta, I. Mandl, and G. M. Turino. 1980. Elastin content of normal and emphysematous lung parenchyma. *Am J Med* 69(3): 351–359.

Clarke, A. W., E. C. Arnspang, S. M. Mithieux et al. 2006. Tropoelastin massively associates during coacervation to form quantized protein spheres. *Biochemistry* 45(33): 9989–9996.

Cloyd, J. M. and D. M. Elliott. 2007. Elastin content correlates with human disc degeneration in the anulus fibrosus and nucleus pulposus. *Spine (Phila Pa 1976)* 32(17): 1826–1831.

Corson, G. M., N. L. Charbonneau, D. R. Keene, and L. Y. Sakai. 2004. Differential expression of fibrillin-3 adds to microfibril variety in human and avian, but not rodent, connective tissues. *Genomics* 83(3): 461–472.

Daamen, W. F., T. Hafmans, J. H. Veerkamp, and T. H. Van Kuppevelt. 2001. Comparison of five procedures for the purification of insoluble elastin. *Biomaterials* 22(14): 1997–2005.

Daamen, W. F., T. Hafmans, J. H. Veerkamp, and T. H. Van Kuppevelt. 2005. Isolation of intact elastin fibers devoid of microfibrils. *Tissue Eng* 11(7–8): 1168–1176.

Damiano, V., A. Tsang, G. Weinbaum, P. Christner, and J. Rosenbloom. 1984. Secretion of elastin in the embryonic chick aorta as visualized by immuno-electron microscopy. *Coll Relat Res* 4(2): 153–164.

Davis, E. C. 1993. Stability of elastin in the developing mouse aorta: A quantitative radioautographic study. *Histochemistry* 100(1): 17–26.

Debelle, L., A. J. Alix, S. M. Wei et al. 1998. The secondary structure and architecture of human elastin. *Eur J Biochem* 258(2): 533–539.

Debelle, L. and A. M. Tamburro. 1999. Elastin: Molecular description and function. *Int J Biochem Cell Biol* 31(2): 261–272.

Deslee, G., J. C. Woods, C. M. Moore et al. 2009. Elastin expression in very severe human COPD. *Eur Respir J* 34(2): 324–331.

Devy, J., L. Duca, B. Cantarelli et al. 2010. Elastin-derived peptides enhance melanoma growth in vivo by upregulating the activation of Mcol-A (MMP-1) collagenase. *Br J Cancer* 103(10): 1562–1570.

Duca, L., C. Blanchevoye, B. Cantarelli et al. 2007. The elastin receptor complex transduces signals through the catalytic activity of its Neu-1 subunit. *J Biol Chem* 282(17): 12484–12491.

Duca, L., N. Floquet, A. J. Alix, B. Haye, and L. Debelle. 2004. Elastin as a matrikine. *Crit Rev Oncol Hematol* 49(3): 235–244.

Dyksterhuis, L. B., C. Baldock, D. Lammie, T. J. Wess, and A. S. Weiss. 2007. Domains 17–27 of tropoelastin contain key regions of contact for coacervation and contain an unusual turn-containing crosslinking domain. *Matrix Biol* 26(2): 125–135.

Eyre, D. R., M. A. Paz, and P. M. Gallop. 1984. Cross-linking in collagen and elastin. *Annu Rev Biochem* 53: 717–748.

Fazio, M. J., M. G. Mattei, E. Passage et al. 1991. Human elastin gene: New evidence for localization to the long arm of chromosome 7. *Am J Hum Genet* 48(4): 696–703.

Fernandes, R. J. and D. R. Eyre. 1999. The elastin-like protein matrix of lamprey branchial cartilage is cross-linked by lysyl pyridinoline. *Biochem Biophys Res Commun* 261(3): 635–640.

Floquet, N., S. Hery-Huynh, M. Dauchez et al. 2004. Structural characterization of VGVAPG, an elastin-derived peptide. *Biopolymers* 76(3): 266–280.

Foster, J. A., L. Rubin, H. M. Kagan et al. 1974. Isolation and characterization of crosslinked peptides from elastin. *J Biol Chem* 249(19): 6191–6196.

Francis, G., R. John, and J. Thomas. 1973. Biosynthetic pathway of desmosines in elastin. *Biochem J* 136(1): 45–55.

Franzblau, C., B. Faris, and R. Papaioannou. 1969. Lysinonorleucine. A new amino acid from hydrolysates of elastin. *Biochemistry* 8(7): 2833–2837.

Franzblau, C., J. A. Foster, and B. Faris. 1977. Role of crosslinking in fiber formation. *Adv Exp Med Biol* 79: 313–327.

Früh, H., G. Kostoulas, B. A. Michel, and A. Baici. 1996. Human myeloblastin (leukocyte proteinase 3): Reactions with substrates, inactivators and activators in comparison with leukocyte elastase. *Biol Chem* 377(9): 579–586.

Fülöp, T., Jr., M. P. Jacob, Z. Varga et al. 1986. Effect of elastin peptides on human monocytes: Ca²⁺ mobilization, stimulation of respiratory burst and enzyme secretion. *Biochem Biophys Res Commun* 141(1): 92–98.

Gayral, S., R. Garnotel, A. Castaing-Berthou et al. 2014. Elastin-derived peptides potentiate atherosclerosis through the immune Neu1-PI3Kgamma pathway. *Cardiovasc Res* 102(1): 118–127.

Gerber, G. E. and R. A. Anwar. 1974. Structural studies on cross-linked regions of elastin. *J Biol Chem* 249(16): 5200–5207.

Gibson, M. A., G. Hatzinikolas, J. S. Kumaratilake et al. 1996. Further characterization of proteins associated with elastic fiber microfibrils including the molecular cloning of MAGP-2 (MP25). *J Biol Chem* 271(2): 1096–1103.

Gibson, M. A., J. S. Kumaratilake, and E. G. Cleary. 1989. The protein components of the 12-nanometer microfibrils of elastic and nonelastic tissues. *J Biol Chem* 264(8): 4590–4598.

Gosline, J., M. Lillie, E. Carrington et al. 2002. Elastic proteins: Biological roles and mechanical properties. *Philos Trans R Soc Lond B Biol Sci* 357(1418): 121–132.

Gray, W. R. 1977. Some kinetic aspects of crosslink biosynthesis. *Adv Exp Med Biol* 79: 285–290.

Gray, W. R., L. B. Sandberg, and J. A. Foster. 1973. Molecular model for elastin structure and function. *Nature* 246(5434): 461–466.

Greenlee, T. K., Jr., R. Ross, and J. L. Hartman. 1966. The fine structure of elastic fibers. *J Cell Biol* 30(1): 59–71.

Gronski, T. J., Jr., R. L. Martin, D. K. Kobayashi et al. 1997. Hydrolysis of a broad spectrum of extracellular matrix proteins by human macrophage elastase. *J Biol Chem* 272(18): 12189–12194.

He, J., G. M. Turino, and Y. Y. Lin. 2010. Characterization of peptide fragments from lung elastin degradation in chronic obstructive pulmonary disease. *Exp Lung Res* 36(9): 548–557.

Heim, A. J., W. G. Matthews, and T. J. Koob. 2006. Determination of the elastic modulus of native collagen fibrils via radial indentation. *Appl Phys Lett* 89(18).

Heim, R. A., R. A. Pierce, S. B. Deak et al. 1991. Alternative splicing of rat tropoelastin mRNA is tissue-specific and developmentally regulated. *Matrix* 11(5): 359–366.

Heinz, A., M. C. Jung, L. Duca et al. 2010. Degradation of tropoelastin by matrix metalloproteinases—Cleavage site specificities and release of matrikines. *FEBS J* 277(8): 1939–1956.

Heinz, A., M. C. Jung, G. Jahreis et al. 2012. The action of neutrophil serine proteases on elastin and its precursor. *Biochimie* 94(1): 192–202.

Hinek, A., F. W. Keeley, and J. Callahan. 1995. Recycling of the 67-kDa elastin binding protein in arterial myocytes is imperative for secretion of tropoelastin. *Exp Cell Res* 220 (2): 312–324.

Hoeve, C. A. and P. J. Flory. 1974. The elastic properties of elastin. *Biopolymers* 13(4): 677–686.

Hoeve, C. A. J. and P. J. Flory. 1958. The elastic properties of elastin. *J Am Chem Soc* 80(24): 6523–6526.

Holzenberger, M., C. A. Lievre, and L. Robert. 1993. Tropoelastin gene expression in the developing vascular system of the chicken: An in situ hybridization study. *Anat Embryol (Berl)* 188(5): 481–492.

Horiguchi, M., T. Inoue, T. Ohbayashi et al. 2009. Fibulin-4 conducts proper elastogenesis via interaction with cross-linking enzyme lysyl oxidase. *Proc Natl Acad Sci USA* 106(45): 19029–19034.

Hsiao, H., P. J. Stone, P. Toselli et al. 1999. The role of the carboxy terminus of tropoelastin in its assembly into the elastic fiber. *Connect Tissue Res* 40(2): 83–95.

Hubmacher, D., E. I. El-Hallous, V. Nelea et al. 2008. Biogenesis of extracellular microfibrils: Multimerization of the fibrillin-1C terminus into bead-like structures enables self-assembly. *Proc Natl Acad Sci USA* 105(18): 6548–6553.

Isogai, Z., R. N. Ono, S. Ushiro et al. 2003. Latent transforming growth factor beta-binding protein 1 interacts with fibrillin and is a microfibril-associated protein. *J Biol Chem* 278 (4): 2750–2757.

Jensen, S. A., G. Aspinall, and P. A. Handford. 2014. C-terminal propeptide is required for fibrillin-1 secretion and blocks premature assembly through linkage to domains cbEGF41-43. *Proc Natl Acad Sci USA* 111(28): 10155–10160.

Jung, S., J. T. Rutka, and A. Hinek. 1998. Tropoelastin and elastin degradation products promote proliferation of human astrocytoma cell lines. *J Neuropathol Exp Neurol* 57(5): 439–448.

Kajiya, H., N. Tanaka, T. Inazumi et al. 1997. Cultured human keratinocytes express tropoelastin. *J Invest Dermatol* 109(5): 641–644.

Keeley, F. W. 1979. The synthesis of soluble and insoluble elastin in chicken aorta as a function of development and age. Effect of a high cholesterol diet. *Can J Biochem* 57(11): 1273–1280.

Keeley, F. W. 2013. The evolution of elastin. In *Evolution of Extracellular Matrix*, edited by F. W. Keeley and R. P. Mecham, pp. 73–119. Berlin/Heidelberg, Germany: Springer.

Koenders, M. M., L. Yang, R. G. Wismans et al. 2009. Microscale mechanical properties of single elastic fibers: The role of fibrillin-microfibrils. *Biomaterials* 30(13): 2425–2432.

Kozel, B. A., R. P. Mecham, and J. Rosenbloom. 2011. Elastin. In *The Extracellular Matrix: An Overview*, edited by R. P. Mecham, pp. 267–302. Berlin/Heidelberg, Germany: Springer.

Kozel, B. A., B. J. Rongish, A. Czirok et al. 2006. Elastic fiber formation: A dynamic view of extracellular matrix assembly using timer reporters. *J Cell Physiol* 207(1): 87–96.

Kozel, B. A., H. Wachi, E. C. Davis, and R. P. Mecham. 2003. Domains in tropoelastin that mediate elastin deposition in vitro and in vivo. *J Biol Chem* 278(20): 18491–18498.

Lansing, A. I., T. B. Rosenthal, M. Alex, and E. W. Dempsey. 1952. The structure and chemical characterization of elastic fibers as revealed by elastase and by electron microscopy. *Anat Rec* 114(4): 555–575.

Lapis, K. and J. Timar. 2002. Role of elastin-matrix interactions in tumor progression. *Semin Cancer Biol* 12(3): 209–217.

Lelj, F., A. M. Tamburro, V. Villani, P. Grimaldi, and V. Guantieri. 1992. Molecular dynamics study of the conformational behavior of a representative elastin building block: Boc-Gly-Val-Gly-Gly-Leu-OMe. *Biopolymers* 32(2): 161–172.

Lent, R. W., B. Smith, L. L. Salcedo, B. Faris, and C. Franzblau. 1969. Studies on the reduction of elastin. II. Evidence for the presence of alpha-aminoadipic acid delta-semialdehyde and its aldol condensation product. *Biochemistry* 8(7): 2837–2845.

Li, B., D. O. Alonso, B. J. Bennion, and V. Daggett. 2001. Hydrophobic hydration is an important source of elasticity in elastin-based biopolymers. *J Am Chem Soc* 123(48): 11991–11998.

Li, B. and V. Daggett. 2002. Molecular basis for the extensibility of elastin. *J Muscle Res Cell Motil* 23(5–6): 561–573.

Lin, G., K. Tiedemann, T. Vollbrandt et al. 2002. Homo- and heterotypic fibrillin-1 and -2 interactions constitute the basis for the assembly of microfibrils. *J Biol Chem* 277 (52): 50795–50804.

Maclay, J. D., D. A. McAllister, R. Rabinovich et al. 2012. Systemic elastin degradation in chronic obstructive pulmonary disease. *Thorax* 67(7): 606–612.

McLaughlin, P. J., Q. Chen, M. Horiguchi et al. 2006. Targeted disruption of fibulin-4 abolishes elastogenesis and causes perinatal lethality in mice. *Mol Cell Biol* 26(5): 1700–1709.

Maquart, F. X., G. Bellon, S. Pasco, and J. C. Monboisse. 2005. Matrikines in the regulation of extracellular matrix degradation. *Biochimie* 87(3–4): 353–360.

Maquart, F. X., S. Pasco, L. Ramont, W. Hornebeck, and J. C. Monboisse. 2004. An introduction to matrikines: Extracellular matrix-derived peptides which regulate cell activity. Implication in tumor invasion. *Crit Rev Oncol Hematol* 49(3): 199–202.

Marson, A., M. J. Rock, S. A. Cain et al. 2005. Homotypic fibrillin-1 interactions in microfibril assembly. *J Biol Chem* 280(6): 5013–5021.

Mason, R. W., D. A. Johnson, A. J. Barrett, and H. A. Chapman. 1986. Elastinolytic activity of human cathepsin L. *Biochem J* 233(3): 925–927.

Mecham, R. P. 2008. Methods in elastic tissue biology: Elastin isolation and purification. *Methods* 45(1): 32–41.

Mecham, R. P., T. J. Broekelmann, C. J. Fliszar et al. 1997. Elastin degradation by matrix metalloproteinases. Cleavage site specificity and mechanisms of elastolysis. *J Biol Chem* 272(29): 18071–18076.

Mecham, R. P. and M. A. Gibson. 2015. The microfibril-associated glycoproteins (MAGPs) and the microfibrillar niche. *Matrix Biol* 47: 13–33.

Mecham, R. P., B. D. Levy, S. L. Morris, J. G. Madaras, and D. S. Wrenn. 1985. Increased cyclic GMP levels lead to a stimulation of elastin production in ligament fibroblasts that is reversed by cyclic AMP. *J Biol Chem* 260(6): 3255–3258.

Mecham, R. P., J. Madaras, J. A. McDonald, and U. Ryan. 1983. Elastin production by cultured calf pulmonary artery endothelial cells. *J Cell Physiol* 116(3): 282–288.

Mikawa, Y., H. Hamagami, J. Shikata, and T. Yamamuro. 1986. Elastin in the human intervertebral disk. A histological and biochemical study comparing it with elastin in the human yellow ligament. *Arch Orthop Trauma Surg* 105(6): 343–349.

Milewicz, D. M., J. Grossfield, S. N. Cao et al. 1995. A mutation in FBN1 disrupts profibrillin processing and results in isolated skeletal features of the Marfan syndrome. *J Clin Invest* 95(5): 2373–2378.

Mithieux, S. M. and A. S. Weiss. 2005. Elastin. *Adv Protein Chem* 70: 437–461.

Morihara, K. and H. Tsuzuki. 1967. Elastolytic properties of various proteinases from microbial origin. *Arch Biochem Biophys* 120(1): 68–78.

Moroy, G., A. J. Alix, and S. Hery-Huynh. 2005. Structural characterization of human elastin derived peptides containing the GXXP sequence. *Biopolymers* 78(4): 206–220.

Muiznieks, L. D., J. T. Cirulis, A. van der Horst et al. 2014. Modulated growth, stability and interactions of liquid-like coacervate assemblies of elastin. *Matrix Biol* 36: 39–50.

Nakamura, F. and K. Suyama. 1991. Isolation and structural identification of a new cross-linking amino-acid, allodesmosine, from the acid hydrolysate of elastin. *Agric Biol Chem* 55(2): 547–554.

Nakamura, F., K. Yamazaki, and K. Suyama. 1992. Isolation and structural characterization of a new crosslinking amino acid, cyclopentenosine, from the acid hydrolysate of elastin. *Biochem Biophys Res Commun* 186(3): 1533–1538.

Narayanan, A. S., L. B. Sandberg, R. Ross, and D. L. Layman. 1976. The smooth muscle cell. III. Elastin synthesis in arterial smooth muscle cell culture. *J Cell Biol* 68(3): 411–419.

Noda, K., B. Dabovic, K. Takagi et al. 2013. Latent TGF-beta binding protein 4 promotes elastic fiber assembly by interacting with fibulin-5. *Proc Natl Acad Sci USA* 110(8): 2852–2857.

Novinec, M., R. N. Grass, W. J. Stark et al. 2007. Interaction between human cathepsins K, L, and S and elastins: Mechanism of elastinolysis and inhibition by macromolecular inhibitors. *J Biol Chem* 282(11): 7893–7902.

Ochieng, J., V. Furtak, and P. Lukyanov. 2004. Extracellular functions of galectin-3. *Glycoconj J* 19(7–9): 527–535.

Owen, C. A. and E. J. Campbell. 1999. The cell biology of leukocyte-mediated proteolysis. *J Leukoc Biol* 65(2): 137–150.

Parks, W. C. and S. B. Deak. 1990. Tropoelastin heterogeneity: Implications for protein function and disease. *Am J Respir Cell Mol Biol* 2(5): 399–406.

Parks, W. C., R. A. Pierce, K. A. Lee, and R. P. Mecham. 1993. Elastin. In *Advances in Molecular and Cell Biology*, edited by E. Edward Bittar, pp. 133–181. Greenwich, CT: JAI Press Inc.

Partridge, S. M. 1962. Elastin. *Adv Protein Chem* 17: 227–302.

Partridge, S. M., D. F. Elsden, and J. Thomas. 1963. Constitution of the cross-linkages in elastin. *Nature* 197: 1297–1298.

Partridge, S. M., D. F. Elsden, J. Thomas et al. 1966. Incorporation of labelled lysine into the desmosine cross-bridges in elastin. *Nature* 209(5021): 399–400.

Pasquali-Ronchetti, I., A. Alessandrini, M. Baccarani-Contri et al. 1998. Study of elastic fiber organization by scanning force microscopy. *Matrix Biol* 17(1): 75–83.

Pasquali-Ronchetti, I. and M. Baccarani-Contri. 1997. Elastic fiber during development and aging. *Microsc Res Tech* 38(4): 428–435.

Pasquali-Ronchetti, I., C. Fornieri, M. Baccarani-Contri, and D. Volpin. 1979. Ultrastructure of elastin revealed by freeze-fracture electron-microscopy. *Micron* 10(2): 89–99.

Peters, T. J. and I. S. Smillie. 1971. Studies on chemical composition of Menisci from human knee joint. *Proc R Soc Med London* 64(3): 261–262.

Piha-Gossack, A., W. Sossin, and D. P. Reinhardt. 2012. The evolution of extracellular fibrillins and their functional domains. *PLoS One* 7(3): e33560.

Pometun, M. S., E. Y. Chekmenev, and R. J. Wittebort. 2004. Quantitative observation of backbone disorder in native elastin. *J Biol Chem* 279(9): 7982–7987.

Powell, J. T., N. Vine, and M. Crossman. 1992. On the accumulation of D-aspartate in elastin and other proteins of the ageing aorta. *Atherosclerosis* 97(2–3): 201–208.

Privitera, S., C. A. Prody, J. W. Callahan, and A. Hinek. 1998. The 67-kDa enzymatically inactive alternatively spliced variant of beta-galactosidase is identical to the elastin/laminin-binding protein. *J Biol Chem* 273(11): 6319–6326.

Qian, R. Q. and R. W. Glanville. 1997. Alignment of fibrillin molecules in elastic microfibrils is defined by transglutaminase-derived cross-links. *Biochemistry* 36(50): 15841–15847.

Raghunath, M., E. A. Putnam, T. Ritty et al. 1999. Carboxy-terminal conversion of profibrillin to fibrillin at a basic site by PACE/furin-like activity required for incorporation in the matrix. *J Cell Sci* 112(Pt 7): 1093–1100.

Ramirez, F. 2000. Pathophysiology of the microfibril/elastic fiber system: Introduction. *Matrix Biol* 19(6): 455–456.

Ramirez, F. and D. B. Rifkin. 2009. Extracellular microfibrils: Contextual platforms for TGFbeta and BMP signaling. *Curr Opin Cell Biol* 21(5): 616–622.

Reber-Müller, S., T. Spissinger, P. Schuchert, J. Spring, and V. Schmid. 1995. An extracellular matrix protein of jellyfish homologous to mammalian fibrillins forms different fibrils depending on the life stage of the animal. *Dev Biol* 169(2): 662–672.

Reinhardt, D. P., J. E. Gambee, R. N. Ono, H. P. Bachinger, and L. Y. Sakai. 2000. Initial steps in assembly of microfibrils. Formation of disulfide-cross-linked multimers containing fibrillin-1. *J Biol Chem* 275(3): 2205–2210.

Reinhardt, D. P., D. R. Keene, G. M. Corson et al. 1996. Fibrillin-1: Organization in microfibrils and structural properties. *J Mol Biol* 258(1): 104–116.

Robert, L. 2010. The Saga of kappa-elastin or the promotion of elastin degradation products from "garbage" to receptor agonists and pharmacologically active principles. *Connect Tissue Res* 51(1): 8–13.

Robertson, I., S. Jensen, and P. Handford. 2011. TB domain proteins: Evolutionary insights into the multifaceted roles of fibrillins and LTBPs. *Biochem J* 433(2): 263–276.

Robinet, A., A. Fahem, J. H. Cauchard et al. 2005. Elastin-derived peptides enhance angiogenesis by promoting endothelial cell migration and tubulogenesis through upregulation of MT1-MMP. *J Cell Sci* 118(Pt 2): 343–356.

Robson, P., G. M. Wright, E. Sitarz et al. 1993. Characterization of lamprin, an unusual matrix protein from lamprey cartilage. Implications for evolution, structure, and assembly of elastin and other fibrillar proteins. *J Biol Chem* 268(2): 1440–1447.

Rodgers, U. R. and A. S. Weiss. 2005. Cellular interactions with elastin. *Pathol Biol (Paris)* 53 (7): 390–398.

Rucker, R. B. and M. A. Dubick. 1984. Elastin metabolism and chemistry: Potential roles in lung development and structure. *Environ Health Perspect* 55: 179–191.

Rucker, R. B. and J. Murray. 1978. Cross-linking amino acids in collagen and elastin. *Am J Clin Nutr* 31(7): 1221–1236.

Sabatier, L., J. Djokic, D. Hubmacher et al. 2014. Heparin/heparan sulfate controls fibrillin-1, -2 and -3 self-interactions in microfibril assembly. *FEBS Lett* 588(17): 2890–2897.

Sabatier, L., N. Miosge, D. Hubmacher et al. 2011. Fibrillin-3 expression in human development. *Matrix Biol* 30(1): 43–52.

Sage, H. and W. R. Gray. 1979. Studies on the evolution of elastin. 1. Phylogenetic distribution. *Comp Biochem Physiol Biochem Mol Biol* 64(4): 313–327.

Sakamoto, H., T. Broekelmann, D. A. Cheresh et al. 1996. Cell-type specific recognition of RGD- and non-RGD-containing cell binding domains in fibrillin-1. *J Biol Chem* 271(9): 4916–4922.

Sato, F., H. Wachi, M. Ishida et al. 2007. Distinct steps of cross-linking, self-association, and maturation of tropoelastin are necessary for elastic fiber formation. *J Mol Biol* 369(3): 841–851.

Scarselli, V. 1961. Increase in elastin content of the human aorta during growth. *Nature* 191: 710–711.

Schmelzer, C. E. H., M. C. Jung, J. Wohlrab, R. H. H. Neubert, and A. Heinz. 2012. Does human leukocyte elastase degrade intact skin elastin? *FEBS J* 279(22): 4191–4200.

Schräder, C. U., A. Heinz, and C. E. H. Schmelzer. 2016. Unpublished data.

Senior, R. M., G. L. Griffin, C. J. Fliszar et al. 1991. Human 92- and 72-kilodalton type IV collagenases are elastases. *J Biol Chem* 266(12): 7870–7875.

Shapiro, S. D. 2002. Neutrophil elastase: Path clearer, pathogen killer, or just pathologic? *Am J Respir Cell Mol Biol* 26(3): 266–268.

Shapiro, S. D., S. K. Endicott, M. A. Province, J. A. Pierce, and E. J. Campbell. 1991. Marked longevity of human lung parenchymal elastic fibers deduced from prevalence of D-aspartate and nuclear weapons-related radiocarbon. *J Clin Invest* 87(5): 1828–1834.

Sinha, S., A. M. Heagerty, C. A. Shuttleworth, and C. M. Kielty. 2002. Expression of latent TGF-beta binding proteins and association with TGF-beta 1 and fibrillin-1 following arterial injury. *Cardiovasc Res* 53(4): 971–9783.

Sinha, S., C. Nevett, C. A. Shuttleworth, and C. M. Kielty. 1998. Cellular and extracellular biology of the latent transforming growth factor-beta binding proteins. *Matrix Biol* 17(8–9): 529–545.

Spina, M., S. Garbisa, J. Hinnie, J. C. Hunter, and A. Serafini-Fracassini. 1983. Age-related changes in composition and mechanical properties of the tunica media of the upper thoracic human aorta. *Arteriosclerosis* 3(1): 64–76.

Sproul, E. P. and W. S. Argraves. 2013. A cytokine axis regulates elastin formation and degradation. *Matrix Biol* 32(2): 86–94.

Starcher, B. and S. Percival. 1985. Elastin turnover in the rat uterus. *Connect Tissue Res* 13(3): 207–215.

Starcher, B. C. 1977. Determination of the elastin content of tissues by measuring desmosine and isodesmosine. *Anal Biochem* 79(1–2): 11–15.

Starcher, B. C. and M. J. Galione. 1976. Purification and comparison of elastins from different animal species. *Anal Biochem* 74(2): 441–447.

Swee, M. H., W. C. Parks, and R. A. Pierce. 1995. Developmental regulation of elastin production. Expression of tropoelastin pre-mRNA persists after down-regulation of steady-state mRNA levels. *J Biol Chem* 270(25): 14899–14906.

Szabo, Z., S. A. Levi-Minzi, A. M. Christiano et al. 1999. Sequential loss of two neighboring exons of the tropoelastin gene during primate evolution. *J Mol Evol* 49(5): 664–671.

Tamburro, A. M., B. Bochicchio, and A. Pepe. 2003. Dissection of human tropoelastin: Exon-by-exon chemical synthesis and related conformational studies. *Biochemistry* 42(45): 13347–13362.

Tamburro, A. M., B. Bochicchio, and A. Pepe. 2005. The dissection of human tropoelastin: From the molecular structure to the self-assembly to the elasticity mechanism. *Pathol Biol (Paris)* 53(7): 383–389.

Tamburro, A. M., A. Pepe, and B. Bochicchio. 2006. Localizing alpha-helices in human tropoelastin: Assembly of the elastin "puzzle." *Biochemistry* 45(31): 9518–9530.

Toupance, S., B. Brassart, F. Rabenoelina et al. 2012. Elastin-derived peptides increase invasive capacities of lung cancer cells by post-transcriptional regulation of MMP-2 and uPA. *Clin Exp Metastasis* 29(5): 511–522.

Uitto, J. 1979. Biochemistry of the elastic fibers in normal connective tissues and its alterations in diseases. *J Invest Dermatol* 72(1): 1–10.

Urry, D. W. and T. M. Parker. 2002. Mechanics of elastin: Molecular mechanism of biological elasticity and its relationship to contraction. *J Muscle Res Cell Motil* 23(5–6): 543–559.

Urry, D. W., H. Sugano, K. U. Prasad, M. M. Long, and R. S. Bhatnagar. 1979. Prolyl hydroxylation of the polypentapeptide model of elastin impairs fiber formation. *Biochem Biophys Res Commun* 90(1): 194–198.

Vrhovski, B., S. Jensen, and A. S. Weiss. 1997. Coacervation characteristics of recombinant human tropoelastin. *Eur J Biochem* 250(1): 92–98.

Yanagisawa, H. and E. C. Davis. 2010. Unraveling the mechanism of elastic fiber assembly: The roles of short fibulins. *Int J Biochem Cell Biol* 42(7): 1084–1093.

Yeo, G. C., C. Baldock, A. Tuukkanen et al. 2012. Tropoelastin bridge region positions the cell-interactive C terminus and contributes to elastic fiber assembly. *Proc Natl Acad Sci USA* 109(8): 2878–2883.

Yeo, G. C., F. W. Keeley, and A. S. Weiss. 2011. Coacervation of tropoelastin. *Adv Colloid Interface Sci* 167(1–2): 94–103.

Zhang, H., S. D. Apfelroth, W. Hu et al. 1994. Structure and expression of fibrillin-2, a novel microfibrillar component preferentially located in elastic matrices. *J Cell Biol* 124(5): 855–863.

CHAPTER 2

Pathology of the Elastic Matrix

Beth A. Kozel and Dirk Hubmacher

CONTENTS

2.1 INTRODUCTION

Elastic matrices add resilience to tissues that undergo repetitive cycles of stretch and recoil. While collagen provides tensile strength, elastin (ELN) is necessary for resilience. ELN is one of the most highly expressed molecules in the extracellular matrix (ECM) of elastic tissues and is assembled into elastic fibers by the multimerization of the tropoelastin monomer in the extracellular space. In addition to cells, multiple accessory proteins, including fibrillins, fibulins, members of the lysyl oxidase (LOX) family, and latent TGFβ-binding proteins (LTBPs) are also required for the assembly, organization, or maintenance of elastic matrices in tissues.

Developmental elastic fiber diseases in humans occur as a result of mutations within several of these genes (Table 2.1), with evidence for both haploinsufficiency, that is, reduced amounts of the affected protein, and dominant negative effects, that is, formation of aberrant elastic matrices. In addition, several human conditions have been ascribed to the pathological activation of extracellular proteases that weaken or degrade elastic fibers, altering the biomechanical properties of the affected tissues, which ultimately leads to tissue failure. The most commonly affected organ systems are the aorta (resulting in altered arterial caliber and compliance), the lung (causing developmental or acquired emphysema), the skin (leading to alterations in skin mechanics and overly tight or loose skin), urogenital organs (contributing to pelvic organ prolapse or stress urinary incontinence), and joints (resulting in hyperextensible or stiff joints). For

TABLE 2.1 Human Monogenetic Disorders Associated with Alterations in Elastic Fibers

Gene	Genetic Disorder	MIM	Inheritance	Clinical Presentation	Elastic Fiber Appearance
ELN	Supravalvular aortic stenosis	185500	AD	Supravalvular aortic stenosis Pulmonary artery stenosis Hernia and joint laxity	Reduced elastin deposition
	ADCL	123700	AD	Loose skin folds Pulmonary emphysema Gastrointestinal diverticuli/hernia/genital prolapse Occasionally pulmonary artery stenosis /aortic root dilation	Disorganized/shortened elastic fibers Elastic fiber fragmentation
FBN1	Marfan syndrome	154700	AD	Aortic aneurysms/dissection/rupture Skin and joint laxity Ectopia lentis Long bone overgrowth Spontaneous pneumothorax	Fragmented elastic lamellae in tunica media Fragmented elastic fibers in dermis
	Stiff skin syndrome	184900	AD	Hard, thick skin Flexion contracture in joints Occasional focal lipodystrophy/muscle weakness	Abnormal presence of elastic fibers at dermal–epidermal junction Poorly assembled elastin core Accumulation of microfibrils
	Weill–Marchesani syndrome	608328	AD	Short stature/brachydactyly Thick skin/stiff joints Cardiac anomalies	Microfibril abnormalities in skin
FBLN4	ARCL1B	614437	AR	Redundant/inelastic skin Premature wrinkling Developmental pulmonary emphysema Arterial tortuosity/aortic aneurysm Pulmonary hypertension Bone fragility/joint laxity/arachnodactyly Diaphragmatic/inguinal hernias	Greatly reduced amounts of elastic fibers Decreased cross-linking Fragmented elastic lamellae Elastin aggregates with rod-like filaments

(Continued)

TABLE 2.1 (*Continued*) Human Monogenetic Disorders Associated with Alterations in Elastic Fibers

Gene	Genetic Disorder	MIM	Inheritance	Clinical Presentation	Elastic Fiber Appearance
FBLN5	ADCL2	614434	AD	Extensive folding and redundant skin, which improved in first decade of life Mitral valve regurgitation	n.d.
	ARCL1A	219100	AR	Redundant/inelastic skin Premature wrinkling Severe developmental pulmonary emphysema Supravalvular aortic stenosis Pulmonary artery stenosis Inguinal hernias	Impaired elastic fiber development Elastin poorly integrated into microfibril scaffold
LTBP4	ARCL1C	613177	AR	Redundant/inelastic skin Premature wrinkling Severe developmental emphysema Gastrointestinal diverticulosis/tortuosity/enlargement/stenosis Bladder diverticulosis Diaphragmatic and inguinal hernias	Abnormal morphology of elastic fibers Large elastin deposits with smooth, microfibril-free surface
ABCC6	PXE	264800	AR/AD	Small yellowish papules (early stage) Leathery inelastic skin (later stages) Angioid streaks/subretinal neovascularization/hemorrhage Coronary/peripheral vascular disease	Fragmentation of elastic fibers in dermis, retina, and peripheral vasculature Ectopic calcification of elastic fibers
	GACI	614473	AR	Arterial stenosis due to myointimal cell proliferation Severe/perinatal congestive heart failure Hypertension/myocardial ischemia	Calcification of internal elastic lamina

AD, autosomal dominant; ADCL, autosomal dominant cutis laxa; AR, autosomal recessive; ARCL, autosomal recessive cutis laxa; GACI, generalized arterial calcification of infancy; PXE, pseudoxanthema elasticum.

any given gene mutation or nongenetic insult, each tissue may be more or less severely affected, reflecting the relative quantity of the affected protein and its relative contribution to the proper function of the respective tissue.

In this chapter, we will describe the architecture and composition of the ECM in elastic tissues, focusing on the distribution of the elastic fiber system and illustrate how mutations in ECM components cause pathologies resulting in dysfunctional elastic matrices. In addition, we will present information on acquired pathologies of elastic matrices with currently no established genetic cause–effect relationship. The diseases discussed here are limited to the most relevant elastic fiber proteins. For connective tissue disorders caused by mutations in collagens, proteins related to vascular smooth muscle cell function, or components of the TGFβ signaling pathway, the reader is referred to several recent and comprehensive reviews (Byers and Murray 2014; Gillis et al. 2013; Humphrey et al. 2015; Jobling et al. 2014; Malfait and De Paepe 2014).

2.2 NORMAL ELASTIC FIBER DISTRIBUTION IN ELASTIC MATRICES OF SELECT TISSUES

2.2.1 Aorta: Structure and Elasticity of the Aortic Wall

The aorta is the largest artery in the body. It functions to carry oxygenated blood from the heart to the peripheral organs. Following cardiac systole, the aorta expands as it receives blood ejected from the left ventricle and then recoils to facilitate delivery of that blood further down the arterial tree ("Windkessel effect"). The aorta can be divided into two major segments, the thoracic aorta (including the aortic root, ascending aorta, aortic arch, and descending aorta) and the abdominal aorta (Figure 2.1a, left). Genetic and metabolic alterations can result in pathologies throughout the aorta (e.g., decreased vessel caliber and arterial stiffness) or can be restricted to specific arterial segments, for example, supravalvular aortic stenosis (SVAS), thoracic aortic aneurysms (TAA), or abdominal aortic aneurysms (AAA).

The aortic wall is composed of three distinct layers (Figure 2.1a, middle and right) (Wagenseil and Mecham 2009). The innermost layer, the tunica intima, which is in direct contact with the blood, is covered by the vascular endothelium that is anchored to an underlying basement membrane and supported by the internal elastic lamina (Davis 1993b). The ECM between the basement membrane and the internal elastic lamina contains fibrillin microfibrils, collagen, and other ECM components. However, the overall contribution of the tunica intima to the elasticity of the aortic wall is considered to be small. The tunica intima is followed by the tunica media,

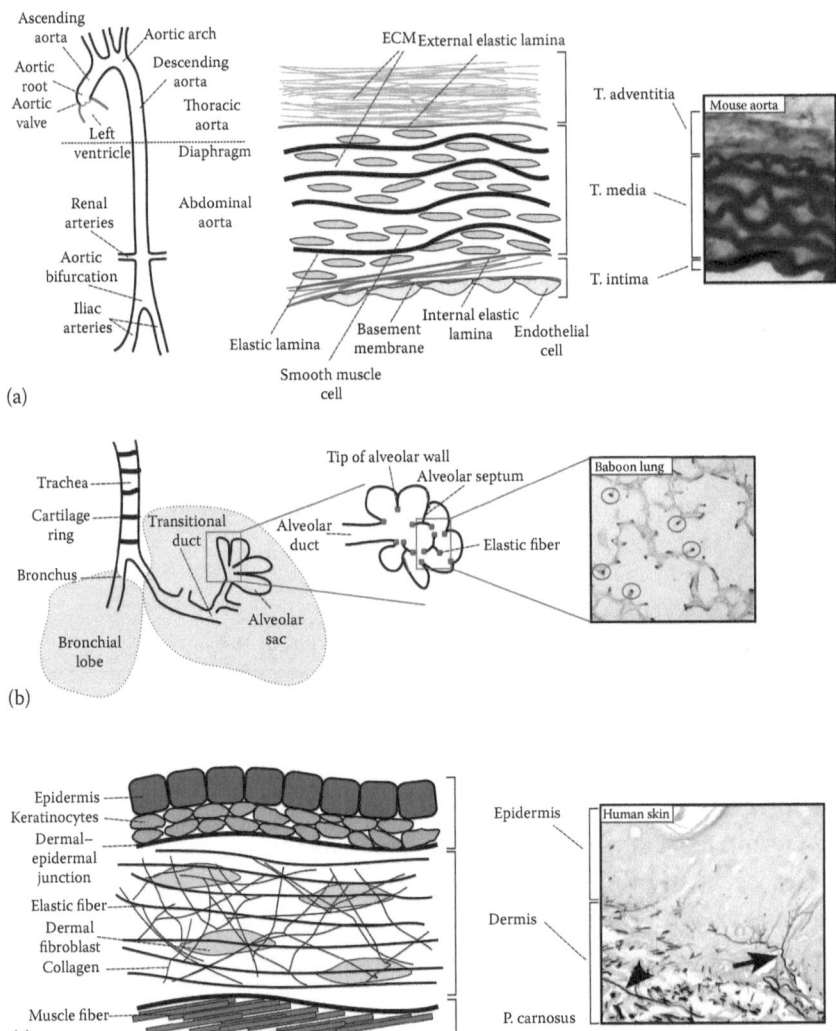

FIGURE 2.1 Anatomy and histology of elastic tissues. (a) The aorta consists of two major segments, the thoracic aorta and the abdominal aorta (left panel). The thoracic aorta includes the ascending aorta, the aortic arch, and the descending aorta. The abdominal aorta begins beneath the diaphragm and extends to the aortic bifurcation at the iliac arteries. The aortic wall is composed of three layers (from inside to outside): the tunica intima, the tunica media, and the tunica adventitia (middle panel). The tunica media shows circumferentially organized elastic fibers, the elastic lamellae. A cross section of mouse aorta stained with oxytalan is shown in the panel on the right (elastin is dark purple). T., tunica. (b) Segmental anatomy of the airways extending from the trachea, through the bronchus and transitional ducts to the alveoli (left panel). *(Continued)*

which provides the majority of the aortic wall thickness and defines the elastic properties of the artery. The tunica media is mainly composed of intercalated smooth muscle cells and elastic lamellae. These lamellae are organized as fenestrated sheets of ELN and are interconnected with each other as well as to the vascular smooth muscle cells by thin elastic fibers (Davis 1993a; Dingemans et al. 2000). Studies in model organisms showed that the absence of vascular smooth muscle cell function did not alter the overall mechanical properties of the aorta, suggesting a limited contribution of vascular smooth muscle cell contractility itself to the extension and recoil of the aorta (Berry et al. 1975). Interestingly, the number of elastic lamellae is proportionate to the tensile forces exerted on the aortic wall and becomes stable shortly after birth (Berry et al. 1993; Leung et al. 1977). The outermost layer of the aorta, adjacent to the external elastic lamina of the tunica media, is called the tunica adventitia (Figure 2.1a, middle and right). The tunica adventitia is rich in collagen and is thought to prevent the rupture of the aorta at extreme blood pressures (Burton 1954). More recently, the identification of abundant vascular wall progenitor cells in the tunica adventitia has suggested a novel role for the tunica adventitia as a niche for their storage and a processing compartment for these progenitor cells (Psaltis and Simari 2015; Stenmark et al. 2013). The vascular progenitor cells residing in this compartment appear to be involved in the pathogenesis of atherosclerosis and vascular inflammation (Hu et al. 2004; Psaltis et al. 2014).

FIGURE 2.1 (Continued)   The alveoli are saccular units at the end of each airway. Elastic fibers create rings at the entrance to each alveolus (middle panel, red). The right panel shows an image of baboon lung stained with Hart's elastic fiber stain (brown) and tartrazine (yellow). Elastic fibers at the alveolar tips are dark in color (circled). (Reprinted and modified by permission from Macmillan Publishers Ltd. Pierce, R.A. et al., 2007, Retinoids increase lung elastin expression but fail to alter morphology or angiogenesis genes in premature ventilated baboons. *Pediatr Res*, *61*, 703–709, Copyright 2007.) (c) The skin is divided into epidermis, dermis, and panniculus carnosus (left panel). The majority of the elastic fibers are present in the dermis and they are laid out in parallel to the skin surface. The right panel shows a section of human skin stained with Hart's elastin stain. Elastic fibers are shown in the dermal layer (arrowhead) and extending in the dermal–epidermal junction (arrow). P., panniculus. (Reprinted and modified from Urban, Z. et al., Mutations in LTBP4 cause a syndrome of impaired pulmonary, gastrointestinal, genitourinary, musculoskeletal, and dermal development. *Am J Hum Genet*, 85, 593–605, Copyright 2009, with permission from Elsevier.)

2.2.2 Lung: Structure and Elasticity of Bronchi and Alveoli

The functional units of the lungs are thin-walled alveoli, which constitute the lung parenchyma and are the sites for gas exchange during the breathing cycle. Alveoli are grouped in alveolar sacs, which are connected to the bronchial tree (Figure 2.1b, left). The bronchial tree is formed by branching events of the trachea into bronchi with a progressively smaller caliber ending in the alveolar sacs (Miura 2015). To avoid the collapse of alveoli, lung tissue has to be maintained under tensile strength ("pre-stressed"), which is achieved by generating a negative pressure in the thoracic cavity. During breathing, the alveoli become extended due to an increase in negative pressure caused by the contraction of the diaphragm with support from the intercostal muscles (Negrini and Moriondo 2013).

The major ECM components of the lung parenchyma are ELNs, collagens, and proteoglycans (Suki and Bates 2008). Cartilage rings further stabilize the trachea and the large conducting airways to avoid their collapse during the breathing cycle. The main site of gas exchange is the respiratory epithelium in the alveoli, which is separated from the underlying cell layers by a basement membrane. The major determinants of parenchymal elasticity are elastic fibers and collagen (predominantly types I and III), which are synthesized by lung fibroblasts residing in the alveolar wall (Foster and Curtiss 1990). The elastic fibers appear to form a continuous interconnected network of variable fiber thickness, extending from the pleural wall to the bronchioles and alveoli (Toshima et al. 2004). Around the respiratory bronchioles, the thicker circumferential elastic fibers are interconnected by thinner longitudinal elastic fibers. At the alveolar level, elastic fibers form a band around the entrance to the terminal alveoli and are further subdivided to form a coarse sac-like network around each alveolus (Figure 2.1b, middle and right). To facilitate gas exchange, elastic fibers are only sparsely distributed within the alveolar wall itself. In the mature lung, ELN is found in the alveoli, including the alveolar septae, the septal junctions, and the edges of the alveoli. In addition to the alveoli, elastic fibers are localized in the subepithelial layer of bronchi and the trachea as part of the basement membrane layer (Bock and Stockinger 1984). They are also found in the bronchial smooth muscle cell layer and at the junction of both (Bousquet et al. 1996).

2.2.3 Skin: Structure and Elasticity of the Dermis

The skin consists of two layers, the epidermis and the underlying dermis, which itself is divided into the thin upper papillary dermis and the thick lower reticular dermis (Figure 2.1c, left). Most of the elastic fibers are found in the reticular dermis and run parallel to the skin surface in humans. The reticular elastic fibers are connected to much thinner elaunin fibers, which are elastic fibers that stain with elaunin (Figure 2.1c, right) (Uitto et al. 2013). These elaunin fibers are connected to even thinner elastic fibers that terminate close to the dermal epidermal basement membrane. These thinnest fibers stain with oxytalan, which stains fibrillin microfibrils. As in other tissues, elastic fibers contribute resilience and elasticity to the skin, despite constituting only about 4% of the dry weight of the dermis (Hussain et al. 2013). The tensile strength of the skin is conferred by collagen type I and III fibers that constitute more than 80% of the dry weight of the dermis (Bernstein and Uitto 1996). The majority of the ECM in skin is deposited by dermal fibroblasts, which, together with vascular smooth muscle cells, are the prime research tools to study *in vitro* ECM assembly and turnover, and the effect of genetic mutations on elastic fiber formation.

2.3 PATHOLOGY OF MONOGENETIC GENETIC DISORDERS AFFECTING ELASTIC TISSUES

2.3.1 Elastin

ELN is generated through the multimerization and cross-linking of tropoelastin monomers in the extracellular space (see Chapter 1). Tropoelastin is encoded by the *ELN* gene and highly expressed in the latter half of pregnancy, and during infancy and early childhood (see Figure 2.2a for domain organization and location of disease-associated mutations). Relatively little ELN is laid down outside of this period. Once deposited, cross-linked ELN is very stable with an estimated half-life of 74 years (Shapiro et al. 1991). Consequently, diseases that alter the quantity or quality of ELN in tissues generally have dramatic and early onset phenotypes. No treatments have been identified to date that reliably increase deposition of functional ELN *in vivo.*

2.3.1.1 ELN Insufficiency (SVAS/Williams–Beuren Syndrome)

2.3.1.1.1 Aorta   Haploinsufficiency for ELN causes focal arterial stenosis, most typically affecting the supravalvular aorta and supravalvular pulmonary artery (SVAS and supravalvular pulmonary stenosis or SVPS, respectively), but any elastic artery may be affected (Pober et al. 2008) (Figure 2.2b). In addition, more global arterial findings such as reduced

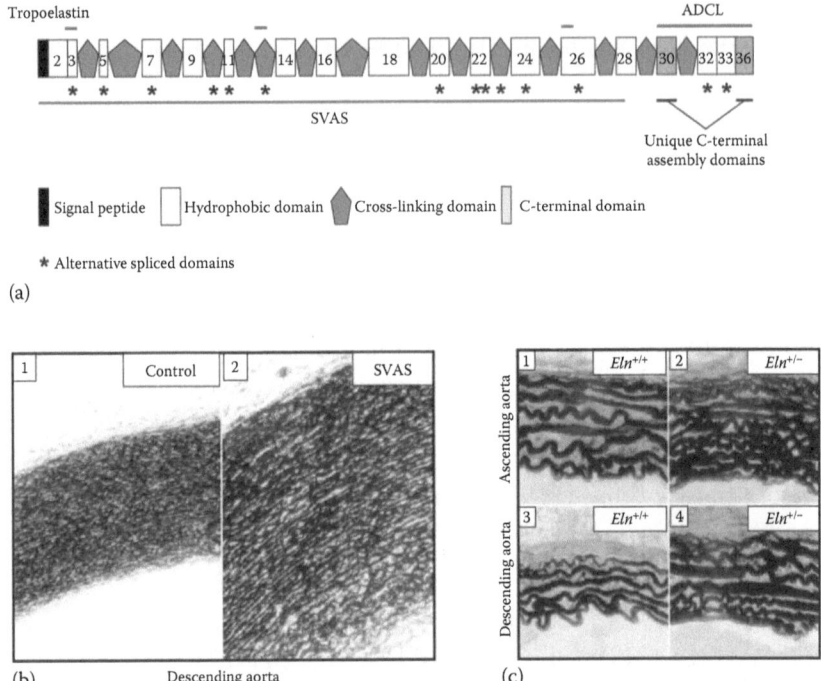

FIGURE 2.2 Elastin (*ELN*)-mediated disease. (a) Domain organization for elastin, which consists of repeated cross-linking (white rectangle, numbered) and hydrophobic (gray pentagon) domains. Exon 36 contains a charged domain including the molecule's only two cysteine residues and a terminal Arginine-Lysine-Arginine-Lysine (RKRK) domain. Mutations causing SVAS have been identified the N-terminal part of the molecule and result in elastin haploinsufficiency. The majority of mutations causing ADCL are located in the five most C-terminal exons with a few reported mutations existing outside of this region (denoted as lines above the molecule). Several exons may be alternatively spliced (asterisk). Exons 30 and 36 contain unique C-terminal assembly sites. (b) Humans with SVAS show a thickened arterial wall with an increased number of elastic lamellae compared with control biopsies. (Reprinted and modified from Li, D.Y. et al. 1998b. Novel arterial pathology in mice and humans hemizygous for elastin. *J Clin Invest* 102, 1783–1787, with permission from the publisher.) (c) Similarily, *Eln*⁺/⁻ mice have increased elastic lamellae compared with *Eln*⁺/⁺ mice in all segments of the thoracic aorta. (Reprinted and modified from Li et al. 1998b, with permission from the publisher.)

vascular caliber and arterial stiffness have also been extensively described in mice and humans (Kozel et al. 2011; Wagenseil et al. 2005). SVAS can be caused by mutations or deletions within the elastin gene (*ELN*) (Mendelian Inheritance in Man, MIM, #185500) or more commonly can present as part of a microdeletion disorder, Williams–Beuren syndrome (WBS; MIM #194050) in which *ELN* is deleted along with 25–27 additional genes on the q arm of chromosome 7 (Merla et al. 2012; Pober 2010).

Mouse models for ELN insufficiency show a dose dependency in the severity of the observed phenotypes. *Eln*$^{-/-}$ (knockout) mice die perinatally of stenosis of the aorta and other large conducting vessels due to enhanced vascular smooth muscle cell proliferation, indicating that ELN is required to control the number of vascular smooth muscle cells in the aortic wall (Li et al. 1998a). *Eln*$^{+/-}$ mice deposit 50%–60% of wild-type (WT) ELN. Like humans with ELN insufficiency, their conducting vessels have a narrower caliber and an increased length. Histology shows increased numbers of elastic lamellae throughout the aorta (Figure 2.2c) (Li et al. 1998b). Phenotypically, the *Eln*$^{+/-}$ mice have systolic hypertension with increased pulse pressure and increased arterial stiffness. They do not exhibit focal arterial stenosis and reportedly have a normal lifespan. *Eln*$^{-/-}$; *hELN BAC*+ mice express 35% of the normal amount of ELN (in this case, expressed from a transgene carrying the entire human *ELN* gene) and are viable, although with a shortened lifespan (Hirano et al. 2007). These mice have more significant hypertension and narrower vessel caliber compared with the *Eln*$^{+/-}$ mouse and the arrangement of the elastic lamellae is irregular and discontinuous.

Subsequent investigation in humans with ELN insufficiency confirms hypertension in up to 40% of individuals with WBS, with incidence increasing with age (Kozel et al. 2014b). In some instances, this finding is related to stenosis in the renal artery but hypertension often occurs independently. Approximately 70% of patients with WBS are known to have large artery stenosis while a smaller number of patients with WBS have intracardiac lesions that may or may not be related to ELN insufficiency (Pober et al. 2008). A recent study in a large cohort of individuals with WBS showed increased arterial stiffness, as measured by pulse wave velocity (PWV), an effect that was modified by chromosomal deletion size (larger deletions that removed the *NCF1a* gene in addition to *ELN* had decreased rate of hypertension and arterial stiffness) and use of antihypertension medications (use of these medications was associated with lower PWV) (Kozel et al. 2014b). Additional work in the *Eln*$^{+/-}$ mouse showed drug class independence for this effect (Halabi et al. 2015). As in the Marfan syndrome treatment paradigm (see Section 2.3.2 on Marfan syndrome), beta-blockers, calcium channel blockers, or angiotensin receptor blockers were unable to alter the biomechanical properties of the large arteries. Consequently, the effect of antihypertensive drugs in the context of WBS is to reduce blood pressure so that the vessel is exposed to a more compliant portion of the pressure diameter curve (Halabi et al. 2015).

2.3.1.1.2 Lungs   Patients with ELN insufficiency report a high rate of pulmonary symptoms including dyspnea, wheezing, and coughing, but measuring lung function by spirometry, the most common test to assess lung function, in a cohort of 16 individuals with WBS aged 15–27 years showed no obstructive changes (Wan et al. 2010). However, the missense mutation c2318 G>A (G773D) in the terminal exon of *ELN* is associated with early onset chronic obstructive pulmonary disease (COPD) in a large American pedigree (Kelleher et al. 2005).

Lung development in *Eln*$^{-/-}$ mice is arrested at the level of terminal airway branches due to reduced alveolar septation (Wendel et al. 2000). *Eln*$^{+/-}$ lungs contain ~50% less ELN compared with WT mice and have histologically normal alveoli but showed a reduced number of capillaries, while the transgenic expression of human ELN in an *Eln*$^{-/-}$ background (depositing 35% of WT quantities of ELN) caused congenital emphysema (Negrini and Moriondo 2013; Shifren et al. 2007). Emphysema was characterized by enlarged thoraxes and a significant increase in lung tissue volume, caused by histologically evident airspace enlargement. Together, these results suggest a dosage effect for ELN during lung development, with lower levels of ELN leading to increasingly more severe emphysema phenotypes, similar to what was observed in the vasculature. In addition, *Eln*$^{+/-}$ mice showed enhanced susceptibility to cigarette-smoke-induced lung injury, indicating that an aberrant elastic matrix in the lung predisposed these mice to a higher susceptibility for environmental insults (Shifren et al. 2007).

2.3.1.1.3 Skin   Individuals with decreased ELN deposition exhibit mild differences in the appearance and biomechanical properties of their skin. In a study by Urban et al. (2000), electron microscopy showed reduced and somewhat aberrant-appearing elastic fibers in the dermis from individuals with WBS. Recently, a large cohort study showed softer skin in patients with WBS with earlier onset of wrinkling and widening of some surgical scars, although the mechanism for these findings is not yet known (Kozel et al. 2014a). Biomechanical testing of skin elasticity in this same group showed that less force was required to lift the skin, but recoil time was normal. The biomechanical findings did not correlate with the presence of vascular stiffness, hypertension, or arterial stenosis in the same patient cohort. This variability among individuals with ELN insufficiency seems to be a general phenomenon, suggesting the presence of secondary genetic or environmental modifiers that influence the rate and severity of vascular, lung, and skin involvement in any given individual.

2.3.1.2 Disorders Related to ELN Overexpression (WBS Region Duplication)

The WBS region on chromosome 7 is flanked by low-copy-number repetitive regions of chromosomal DNA, rendering it susceptible to nonallelic homologous recombination and recurrent deletions cause WBS with a prevalence of ~1 in 8000 individuals as described above. On occasion, meiotic mispairing can lead to the duplication of this region rather than its deletion (WBS duplication, MIM #609757) (Merla et al. 2010). As a result, patients carry three copies of the *ELN* gene, potentially leading to increased ELN deposition. Individuals with *ELN* triplication are reported to have increased diameter of their ascending aortas (Guemann et al. 2015; Parrott et al. 2015; Zarate et al. 2014). A minority of the affected individuals reported to date have required surgical repair of the aortic aneurysm. Most of the patients presented in the three studies had Z-scores, a normalized measure for the aortic diameter in juveniles, of +2 to +4 standard deviations above age and gender means (mild aortic dilation) or diameters of less than 40 mm in adults (mild aortic dilation with no surgery recommended). However, long-term follow-up is needed to evaluate for aortic aneurysm progression. In a case report, where the gene duplication was apparently limited to the *ELN* and *LIMK1* genes (the precise boundaries were not mapped to confirm duplication of the entire *ELN* gene), aortic dilation was already evident prenatally in some family members (Zarate et al. 2014). In addition, failure of the closure of the ductus arteriosus has also been reported in individuals with the WBS duplication (Parrott et al. 2015). The ductus arteriosus is a transient embryonic blood vessel connecting the aortic and pulmonary vasculature that normally closes postnatally as a result of vascular smooth muscle cell proliferation and disruption of the elastic lamellae. Because the WBS duplication syndrome is a relatively newly described and rare disorder, there is currently no data published evaluating other elastic tissues in these patients.

2.3.1.3 Missense Mutations in ELN (Autosomal Dominant Cutis Laxa)

Missense mutations predominantly affecting the last five exons in the *ELN* gene, cause autosomal dominant cutis laxa (ADCL, MIM #123700) (Figure 2.2a) (Tassabehji et al. 1998). These changes result in an altered C-terminus of the ELN protein. Because the C-terminus is thought to be critical to elastic fiber formation, it is believed that these mutations cause disease due to aberrant elastic fiber assembly, either by affecting tropoelastin multimerization or its binding to other elastic fiber-associated proteins such as fibrillin, fibulin-4, fibulin-5, or LOX (Cirulis et al. 2008; Papke and Yanagisawa 2014; Urban and Davis 2014).

As the name of the syndrome implies, the characteristic features of ADCL are seen in the skin. Individuals with ADCL have loose, redundant, and prematurely wrinkled skin. Onset is often congenital but disease manifestations may appear as late as puberty. Electron micrographs of skin derived from affected individuals show abnormal branching and fragmentation of elastic fibers (Tassabehji et al. 1998). The quantity of ELN in the skin is also reduced but tissue healing is normal. Recent biomechanical testing on a group of patients with cutis laxa of multiple genotypes, including mutations in ELN, showed that a reduced force was required to lift patient skin and tissue recoil was markedly abnormal (Kozel et al. 2014c). Tissue-specific alternative splicing of mutated ELN alleles has been described in animal models that may at least partially explain the relative severity of the skin compared with vascular or lung findings for certain ADCL mutations (Sugitani et al. 2012). The finding of ultrastructurally abnormal elastic fibers in affected tissues supports the hypothesis that ELN mutations cause ADCL by a dominant negative mechanism.

Individuals with ADCL can also present with aortopathies ranging from relatively mild dilation to more severe aortic aneurysms and potentially aortic rupture (Szabo et al. 2006). Histological sections from these aortas displayed medial degeneration with decreased elastic fibers without apparent inflammation. Individuals with ADCL also have a high rate of cardiac valve abnormalities, leading to mitral valve prolapse and aortic regurgitation (Schrijver et al. 1999; Takeda et al. 2015).

Patients with ADCL develop severe pulmonary emphysema with an estimated incidence of about 35% (Callewaert et al. 2013; Hadj-Rabia et al. 2013; Urban et al. 2005). A transgenic mouse expressing human tropoelastin with a 25-nucleotide deletion in exon 30, described in a patient with ADCL, in addition to normal mouse ELN, developed pulmonary emphysema, suggesting a dominant negative mechanism for emphysema formation in ADCL (Hu et al. 2010). Mutant ELN copolymerized with endogenous mouse ELN and altered the mechanical properties of the lung tissue, reducing its stiffness.

Genitourinary prolapse was noted in several cutis laxa families (Choudhary et al. 2011; Damkier et al. 1991; Paladini et al. 2007; Urban et al. 2005). In most cases, molecular testing was not available at the time of publication to determine the specific cutis laxa subtype, but at least one individual with a mutation in *ELN* presenting with genitourinary prolapse was described (Urban et al. 2005). A biopsy taken from affected ligaments revealed decreased ELN and increased collagen type VI suggesting a role for ELN and other ECM components in genitourinary stability in these patients (Paladini et al. 2007).

2.3.2 Fibrillin-1 (FBN1) (Marfan Syndrome, Stiff Skin Syndrome, Weill–Marchesani Syndrome)

Fibrillins are the main components of extracellular microfibrils (Hubmacher and Reinhardt 2011). Microfibrils are found in association with elastic fibers and play a crucial role in the formation and homeostasis of elastic fibers. In ELN-free tissues, microfibrils fulfill a predominantly structural role; for example, in the ciliary zonule, which is a cell-free protein structure suspending the lens in the eye and mediating accommodation (Hubmacher et al. 2014; Wheatley et al. 1995). Fibrillin microfibrils are important regulators of extracellular TGFβ growth factor signaling. Fibrillin-1 binds to latent TGFβ via its interaction with LTBPs and confers latency to several bone morphogenetic proteins (BMPs) by directly binding to their prodomains (Dallas et al. 2000; Sengle et al. 2008; Zilberberg et al. 2012). Therefore, fibrillin microfibrils constitute a platform for the integration of TGFβ and BMP growth factors signaling in the ECM (Ramirez and Rifkin 2009).

Three fibrillin genes are present in the human genome (Corson et al. 2004). Mutations in fibrillin-1 (*FBN1*) cause Marfan syndrome, Weill–Marchesani syndrome (WMS), and other fibrillinopathies (Robinson et al. 2006). Human mutations in *FBN2* cause congenital contractural arachnodactyly (Beals–Hecht syndrome, MIM #121050), which presents with a marfanoid habitus, congenital joint contractures, and progressive scoliosis (Callewaert et al. 2009). Careful analysis of the Beals–Hecht syndrome patients' histories revealed the description of apparently nonprogressive aortic root dilation in 5 of 32 patients (Callewaert et al. 2011; Gupta et al. 2002, 2004). However, the formation of aortic aneurysms or aortic dissection in patients carrying *FBN2* mutations have been described only recently (Takeda et al. 2015). Mutations in *FBN2* can also cause early onset macular degeneration (MIM #616118) (Ratnapriya et al. 2014). So far, no human disease causing mutations in *FBN3* have been found, but a potential association of *FBN3* polymorphisms with polycystic ovary syndrome was proposed (Prodoehl et al. 2009; Urbanek et al. 2007).

2.3.2.1 Marfan Syndrome

2.3.2.1.1 Aorta Mutations in *FBN1* cause Marfan syndrome (MIM #154700), an autosomal dominant disorder predominantly affecting the vasculature, the skeletal system, the eyes, and several other organ systems. More than 3000 mutations in the *FBN1* gene have been described so far (www.umd.be/FBN1/). They are distributed throughout the entire gene and are predominantly missense mutations (~60%) and small deletions, insertions, or splice site mutations (~25%) (Figure 2.3a). The estimated prevalence for Marfan syndrome is 2–3 per 5000 newborns. The most severe complication in patients with Marfan syndrome is the progressive dilation of the ascending aortic, resulting in aortic aneurysms (Bolar et al. 2012). Aortic aneurysms are characterized by the widening of the diameter of the aorta, which can result in dissection (a separation of the layers of the aortic wall) and ultimately in the rupture of the aorta. Any segment of the aorta can be affected, but aneurysms in the thoracic aorta typically occur at younger ages and have a much stronger hereditary component (Davis et al. 2014). In Marfan syndrome, it is usually the aortic root that is affected. Consequently, the diameter of the aorta is carefully monitored in patients with Marfan syndrome by echocardiogram, and preventative replacement of the aortic root is considered if the diameter reaches 4.5–5 cm depending on a previous family history of aortic dissection or rupture (David 2010). The hallmark histological feature in aortic wall biopsies from patients with Marfan syndrome is cystic medial necrosis/degeneration (Figure 2.3b) (Summers et al. 2005). Cystic medial necrosis refers to the accumulation of mucopolysaccharides in the tunica media. In addition, the elastic fibers are also abnormal, ranging from thinning of the elastic lamina to breaks and the complete absence of elastic fibers in areas proximal to the lumen of the aortic wall. On a molecular level, mutations in FBN1 can affect its secretion and deposition in the ECM or increase its

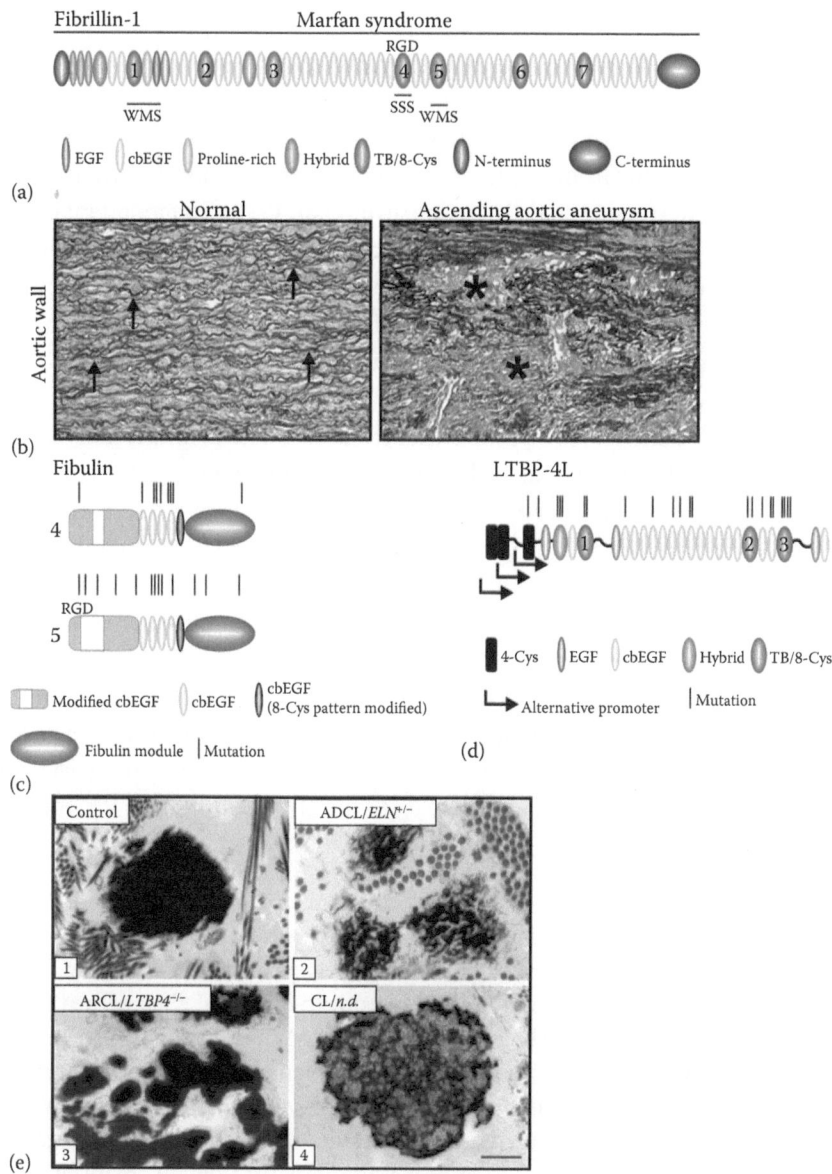

FIGURE 2.3 Fibrillin, fibulins, and LTBPs. (a) Domain organization for fibrillin-1, which mainly consists of calcium-binding EGF domains (light gray ovals), interspersed with TB/8-cysteine domains (red ovals, numbered) and a unique N- and C-terminal region (dark gray ovals). Marfan syndrome mutations are spread throughout the entire length of the molecule, while Weill–Marchesani syndrome and stiff skin syndrome mutations are found in specific domains of the molecule (indicated below the respective domains). *(Continued)*

proteolytic susceptibility and affect protein stability (Booms et al. 1997; Kielty et al. 1994; Kielty and Shuttleworth 1994; Kirschner et al. 2011; Vollbrandt et al. 2004). In addition, certain missense mutations may also exert a dominant negative effect, where the mutant protein is incorporated into microfibrils alongside the WT protein and modifies their function (Hilhorst-Hofstee et al. 2011; Schrijver et al. 1999). Independent of the exact mechanism, pathological TGFβ activation was described in mouse models of Marfan syndrome and human patients and interference with TGFβ signaling rescued the formation of aortic root aneurysms in Marfan syndrome mice (Franken et al. 2013; Habashi et al. 2006; Matt et al. 2009; Neptune et al. 2003).

Two mouse models are predominantly used to study molecular mechanisms of FBN1-related disorders and to evaluate potential treatment options. An *Fbn1* hypomorphic mouse model (*Fbn1*$^{mgR/mgR}$) results in ~80% reduction of normal fibrillin microfibrils in the ECM (Pereira et al. 1999). Alternatively, a knock-in mouse harboring a mutation described in patients with Marfan syndrome (*Fbn1*$^{C1039G/+}$) deposits equal amounts of normal and mutant fibrillin microfibrils (Judge et al. 2004). The *Fbn1*$^{C1039G/+}$ mice develop aortic root aneurysms with an incidence of 90% after six months of age, but only 5% subsequently die due to the rupture of the aortic aneurysm. In contrast, in *Fbn1*$^{mgR/mgR}$ mice, rupture of the aortic aneurysms is fully penetrant, causing mortality of virtually all animals before 12 months

FIGURE 2.3 (Continued) (b) Pathology of an ascending aortic aneurysm. Aortic cross sections were stained with orcein, showing the elastic lamellae in the normal aortic wall (left). Note the continuous elastic fibers (arrows) in the normal specimen and the central medial necrosis (asterisks) with disrupted fibers shown in the aneurysmal section (right). (Reprinted and modified from de Figueiredo Borges, L. et al., Collagen is reduced and disrupted in human aneurysms and dissections of ascending aorta. *Hum Pathol*, 39, 437–443, Copyright 2008, with permission from Elsevier.) (c) Domain organization for fibulin-4 and -5 with the localization of mutations causing dominant or recessive cutis laxa. (d) Domain organization of LTBP4-L with localization of mutations causing recessive cutis laxa. (e) Elastic fibers in skin from control patient (1) and patients with ADCL (2), ARCL (3), and from cutis laxa with an unidentified underlying genetic mutation (4). Elastic fiber structures vary according to the specific cutis laxa subtype. (Reprinted and modified from Urban, Z. and Davis, E.C., Cutis laxa: Intersection of elastic fiber biogenesis, TGFbeta signaling, the secretory pathway and metabolism. *Matrix Biol*, 33, 16–22, Copyright 2014, with permission from Elsevier.)

of age. Data obtained with the $Fbn1^{C1039G/+}$ model showed that elevated canonical and noncanonical TGFβ signaling was responsible for aortic root dilation and aneurysm formation (Habashi et al. 2006). Consequently, the pharmacological inhibition of the angiotensin II type-1 receptor with Losartan or the neutralization of active TGFβ with a pan-specific TGFβ neutralizing antibody could prevent the formation of aortic aneurysms in the $Fbn1^{C1039G/+}$ mouse model (Habashi et al. 2006). Recently, it was described that early stages of aortic root dilation in the $Fbn1^{mgR/mgR}$ mice, as early as postnatal day 16, were characterized by enhanced phosphorylation of Erk1/2 (Cook et al. 2015). At this stage, Smad2/3 phosphorylation, a typical readout for canonical TGFβ signaling, did not differ between $Fbn1^{mgR/mgR}$ and WT mice. However, at postnatal day 60, Erk1/2 phosphorylation was less prominent, but now phosphorylation of Smad2/3 was significantly enhanced in aortic aneurysms of $Fbn1^{mgR/mgR}$ mice. Based on this biphasic response, a carefully timed treatment protocol for Losartan and TGFβ neutralization was developed, consisting of early administration of Losartan followed by a combination of Losartan and TGFβ neutralizing antibody at later stages. This treatment regimen was most effective in preventing the formation of aortic aneurysms.

Because the formation of aortic aneurysms is the most dangerous complication in Marfan syndrome, pharmacological interventions in patients aim to prevent the dilation of the aortic root or slow the growth of the aortic aneurysm. The current pharmacological treatment is based on the administration of beta-blockers to reduce hemodynamic stress on the aortic wall. This treatment strategy was implemented after a small randomized trial using the beta-blocker propranolol showed beneficial effects on the aortic aneurysm pathology in patients with Marfan (Shores et al. 1994). Based on the prominent role of TGFβ signaling in the pathogenesis of aortic aneurysm in several mouse models of Marfan syndrome and the efficiency of Losartan, an FDA-approved drug, in preventing the formation of aortic aneurysms in those mice, clinical trials were initiated. Three initial studies showed beneficial effects of Losartan on attenuating the progression of aortic root dilation in patients with Marfan (Chiu et al. 2013; Groenink et al. 2013; Pees et al. 2013). However, two recent randomized multicenter trials (608 and 303 participants, respectively) failed to show a beneficial effect of Losartan on the growth of the aortic root in patients with Marfan compared with beta-blocker therapy (Lacro et al. 2014; Milleron et al. 2015).

2.3.2.1.2 Lung   In Marfan syndrome, pneumothorax is frequently reported (Suzuki et al. 2010; Viveiro et al. 2013). Pneumothorax most commonly occurs secondary to the enlargement and subsequent rupture of pulmonary airspaces, allowing air to escape into the pleural space and resulting in the collapse of the ruptured lung. Other case reports of Marfan syndrome described congenital lobar anomalies, honeycombing, apical fibrosis, and emphysema (Bolande and Tucker 1964; Lipton et al. 1971; Teoh 1977). Histologically, the presence of distal acinar emphysema was recently described in five cases of Marfan syndrome (Dyhdalo and Farver 2011).

In a mouse model of fibrillin deficiency, progressive postnatal enlargement of the pulmonary airspaces was attributed to an impairment of secondary alveolar septation (Neptune et al. 2003). In the absence of impaired cell differentiation or ELN deposition, an elevated level of active TGFβ was found in FBN1-deficient lungs. The administration of a TGFβ neutralizing antibody rescued the enlargement of the airspaces in a dose-dependent manner, indicating a role for aberrant TGFβ signaling in emphysema formation.

2.3.2.1.3 Other Tissue Involvement in Marfan Syndrome   In the skeletal system, disproportional long bone overgrowth of the limbs is the most prominent external sign of Marfan syndrome. In addition, scoliosis and chest deformation are prevalent. The potential molecular mechanisms are not entirely resolved. However, in mice, microfibrils differentially regulate the bioavailability of TGFβ and BMP in bones, modulating the differentiation of osteoblasts and the formation of osteoclasts (Nistala et al. 2010a,b). According to the revised Ghent nosology for the diagnosis of Marfan syndrome, skin striae (atrophicae) are considered a minor sign (Loeys et al. 2010a). A recent case control study showed the good diagnostic value of skin striae, especially, when lesions were present in unusual areas, such as back, breast, shoulders, or hips (Ledoux et al. 2011). An earlier study indicated the presence of mild-to-moderate skin hyperextensibility in about two-thirds of patients (Grahame and Pyeritz 1995).

2.3.2.2 Stiff Skin Syndrome
Mutations in the fourth TB domain of *FBN1*, which contains the sole integrin-binding RGD motif cause stiff skin syndrome (MIM #184900), a congenital form of scleroderma (Figure 2.3a) (Loeys et al. 2010b). More than 50 cases have been reported and patients present with hard and thick

skin covering the entire body surface. The fibrotic skin severely limits joint mobility. In addition, small stature was noted in some patients. Histologically, microfibrils appear stubby and more abundant at the dermal epidermal junction, and the elastic fibers appear abnormal. Interestingly, in the dermis of patients with stiff skin syndrome an accumulation of LTBP4 was observed, concomitant with an increase in SMAD2 phosphorylation, suggesting pathologically elevated canonical TGFβ signaling.

Human mutations directly affecting the RGD-integrin-binding motif have not been described so far. However, a knock-in mouse model was generated mutating the RGD sequence to RGE ($Fbn1^{RGD/RGE}$), which abolishes integrin binding, and its phenotype was compared with a knock-in of a stiff skin syndrome mutation ($Fbn1^{W1570C}$) (Gerber et al. 2013). Both mouse models phenocopied the histological features of stiff skin syndrome in the heterozygous state. While the $Fbn1^{RGD/RGE}$ mouse died during early embryonic development, the homozygous $Fbn1^{W1570C}$ knock-in showed even more accelerated skin fibrosis when compared with $Fbn1^{W1570C/+}$ or the WT. In the same study, several therapeutic approaches were assessed using an integrin-β3 activating antibody or a TGFβ neutralizing antibody. Both treatment regimens resulted in the prevention and/or full reversal of the stiff skin phenotype. A mouse model harboring an internal in-frame duplication in the $Fbn1$ gene, the tight skin mouse ($Fbn1^{Tsk}$) also develops extended skin fibrosis (Green et al. 1976). It is assumed, that in stiff skin syndrome as well as in the $Fbn1^{Tsk}$ mouse model, an accumulation of altered fibrillin microfibrils results in the pathological accumulation and/or activation of latent TGFβ, which in turn is a major driver of the fibrotic response (Gayraud et al. 2000; Kielty et al. 1998).

2.3.2.3 Weill–Marchesani Syndrome

Dominant mutations in $FBN1$ (MIM #608328) and recessive mutation in $ADAMTS10$ and $ADAMTS17$ cause WMS (MIM #277600) or WMS-like syndrome (MIM #613195), respectively (Faivre et al. 2003; Morales et al. 2009; Shah et al. 2014). Like individuals with Marfan syndrome, those with WMS have a high rate of ectopia lentis. Unlike patients with Marfan syndrome, however, individuals with WMS have short stature and short, broad digits (brachydactyly). Patients with WMS present with muscular build and cardiac abnormalities including cardiac valve defects and patent ductus arteriosus. The skin is thick, and joint limitations are common. Mutations causing WMS have been identified in the heparin-binding domains of the fibrillin molecule (Cain et al. 2012). A recent paper by Cecchi et al. (2013) describes WMS mutations in exons 41 and 42 of *FBN1* that have features of both Marfan syndrome and WMS.

2.3.3 Fibulins (FBLN) (Cutis Laxa)

Fibulin-4 and -5 are mutated in autosomal recessive cutis laxa 1B (ARCL1B, MIM #614437) and ARCL1A (MIM #219100), respectively (Callewaert et al. 2013; Loeys et al. 2002). Some mutations in fibulin-5 can also cause ADCL (MIM #614434 (Figure 2.3c,e). Fibulin-4 binds fibrillin-1, tropoelastin, and LTBP1. It is able to form a complex with tropoelastin, and LOX and is thought to support the LOX-mediated cross-linking of monomeric tropoelastin during the biogenesis of elastic fibers (Choudhury et al. 2009; Horiguchi et al. 2009). Consequently, biopsies from patients and mice with fibulin-4 deficiency show reduced elastic fibers and a disorganized elastic fiber structure (Hucthagowder et al. 2006). This is in contrast to what is observed in patients and mice where fibulin-5 is mutated. Fibulin-5 binds to LOX-like 1, -2, and -4; fibrillin-1; tropoelastin; and LTBP2 and -4 (reviewed in Papke and Yanagisawa 2014). Fibulin-5 harbors an integrin-binding RGD motif, the role of which remains elusive. Although fibulin-5 binds to integrins ($\alpha5\beta1$, $\alpha v\beta3$, and $\alpha v\beta5$) *in vitro*, knock-in mice, containing a fibulin-5 RGD to RGE mutation exhibit normal elastic fibers in their aortas, lungs, skin, and urogenital systems (Budatha et al. 2011; Lomas et al. 2007; Nakamura et al. 2002). Biallelic mutations in fibulin-5 result in disorganized elastic fibers. Knockout mouse studies show the accumulation of large deposits of ELN globules that are not well integrated with the microfibril scaffold, suggesting that fibulin-5 may regulate the size of the tropoelastin aggregates during normal elastic fiber assembly or that it may assist in its deposition on the elastic fiber network (Nakamura et al. 2002; Yanagisawa et al. 2002). Interestingly, higher levels of fibulin-5 than fibulin-4 are detected in the ECM of most elastic tissues, but null mutations for fibulin-4 cause more severe disease (Kobayashi et al. 2007; Papke and Yanagisawa 2014). Perinatal death occurs in *Fbln4$^{-/-}$*, while *Fbln5$^{-/-}$* mice often survive until adulthood with progressive disease in multiple elastic tissues (Horiguchi et al. 2009; Huang et al. 2010; McLaughlin et al. 2006; Nakamura et al. 2002; Yanagisawa et al. 2002).

2.3.3.1 Fibulin 4 (EFEMP2) (ARCL)

Biallelic mutations in *FBLN4* (EFEMP2) are associated with ARCL1B (MIM #614437). In addition to loose skin, individuals with mutations in *FBLN4* have significant vascular disease (Hucthagowder et al. 2006). Vascular features include arterial tortuosity and aneurysm formation, vascular fragility leading to bleeding, and frank stenosis (Dasouki et al. 2007; Hoyer et al. 2009; Hucthagowder et al. 2006). Two studies analyzing a large cohort of Indian patients with homozygous mutations in exon 7 of *FBLN4* (c.608A > C; p. Asp203Ala), located in a conserved calcium-binding EGF (cbEGF) sequence, showed high rates of mortality related to vascular complications (Kappanayil et al. 2012; Rajeshkannan et al. 2014). The majority of *FBLN4* mutations published to date localize to these cbEGF domains and are expected to cause misfolding of the protein and poor calcium binding and, similar to fibrillin-1 mutations in these domains, may alter proteolytic susceptibility and protein–protein interactions (Al-Hassnan et al. 2012; Djokic et al. 2013; Erickson et al. 2012; Hayward et al. 1997; Iascone et al. 2012; Kirschner et al. 2011; Sawyer et al. 2013; Vollbrandt et al. 2004).

Fbln4$^{-/-}$ mice show degenerative changes in the aortic wall and display reduced gene expression of contractile genes in vascular smooth muscle cells. Vascular smooth muscle cells remain immature in nature and proliferate excessively (Huang et al. 2010). Histological sections of aortic tissue from these mice show focal degeneration of the medial wall, and decreased elastic fibers. Apoptosis of multiple cell types are seen in the aneurysmal wall with aneurysm developing primarily in the ascending aorta. Notably, treatment with angiotensin type II receptor blockers prevents aneurysm development but does not improve the arterial stiffness seen in these mice (Huang et al. 2013). Multiple reports show evidence of lung dysfunction, most notably emphysema and abnormalities of the diaphragm (Hucthagowder et al. 2006; Iascone et al. 2012). Diaphragm herniation and rupture have also been described in the *Fbln4*$^{-/-}$ mouse (Horiguchi et al. 2009). Patients with ARCL1B have a skin presentation that is similar to that of ADCL. The skin is loose and redundant with reduced elasticity. In addition, Hucthagowder et al. (2006) describe the skin in their patient cohort as soft, velvety, and transparent with vascular tortuosity notable on the skin surface.

2.3.3.2 Fibulin-5 (Autosomal Recessive/Dominant Cutis Laxa)

Mutations in *FBLN5* have been associated with both ARCL (MIM #219100) and ADCL (MIM #614434). Individuals with ARCL have a vasculopathy consisting of arterial stenosis (most commonly SVAS and SVPS) without vascular tortuosity or ascending aortic aneurysms (Callewaert et al. 2013;

Elahi et al. 2006; Loeys et al. 2002). For the recessive condition, both missense and nonsense mutations have been reported. One patient with a 22-kb tandem duplication of the FBLN5 genomic sequence between intron 4 and exon 9 is described as the only dominant case of FBLN5-mediated ADCL (Markova et al. 2003). This insertion leads to an internal 483-nucleotide duplication on the mRNA level. In addition to cutis laxa, this patient had mitral valve regurgitation, but otherwise normal vasculature. *Fbln5*$^{-/-}$ mice exhibit disorganized elastic fibers with vascular abnormalities including arterial tortuosity and decreased arterial compliance (Nakamura et al. 2002; Yanagisawa et al. 2002). The *Fbln5*$^{-/-}$ mutant mice do not develop aortic aneurysms.

Pulmonary disease, predominantly emphysema, in individuals with recessive mutations in *FBLN5* is particularly devastating. The disease is often lethal in childhood, due to the development of emphysema and subsequent respiratory distress (Callewaert et al. 2013; Elahi et al. 2006). In the family presented by Loeys et al. (2002), the lung phenotype was also pronounced. Several of the children had recurrent lung infections in infancy with emphysema detected as early as 6 months of age. In one case, bronchoscopy revealed an easily collapsible trachea and small airways. In *Fbln5*$^{-/-}$ mice, elastic fibers were noted to deteriorate with age in multiple tissues, including the lungs suggesting a possible role in maintenance of elastic fibers (Drewes et al. 2007; Yanagisawa et al. 2002).

Similar to *FBLN4*-associated disease, patients with *FBLN5* mutations have loose skin with sagging facial appearance. Histological skin sections from affected patients show disorganized elastic fibers with a granular appearance (Loeys et al. 2002). Pelvic organ prolapse is also seen in mouse models of the condition but is a late onset phenotype (Drewes et al. 2007; Yanagisawa et al. 2002). Urogenital prolapse is not described in human patients with ARCL1A, but variants in the *FBLN5* gene and differences in fibulin-5 mRNA expression in pelvic ligaments are associated with pelvic organ prolapse in otherwise healthy individuals (Jung et al. 2009; Khadzhieva et al. 2014).

2.3.4 LTBP

LTBPs, together with fibrillins, constitute a family of ECM proteins that is distinguished by the presence of a unique TGFβ-binding/8-cysteine domain (TB) (Robertson et al. 2010). LTBPs bind the latency-associated peptide of TGFβ and are responsible for ECM storage of latent TGFβ, in a form to be ready for activation by proteolysis, integrin-mediated mechanical force, and other mechanisms (Todorovic and Rifkin 2012). LTBP1 and LTBP3 bind strongly to all three TGFβ isoforms, while LTBP4 binds only weakly to the latency-associated peptide of TGFβ1 (Gleizes et al. 1996; Saharinen et al. 1996). LTBP2 as well as the fibrillin isoforms are incapable of binding directly to latent TGFβ, due to the absence of a crucial two amino acid insertion between the sixth and seventh cysteine residue of the third TB domain of the TGFβ-binding LTBPs, LTBP1, -3, and -4. So far, human mutations were described in the genes coding for *LTBP2*, *LTBP3*, and *LTBP4*. Mutations in *LTBP2* cause congenital primary glaucoma (MIM #613086), microspherophakia and/or megalocornea with ectopia lentis (MIM #250750), or WMS (MIM #614819) and mutations in *LTBP3* cause oligodontia, short stature, and mitral valve prolapse (MIM #613097) (Desir et al. 2010; Dugan et al. 2015; Haji-Seyed-Javadi et al. 2012; Narooie-Nejad et al. 2009).

2.3.4.1 LTBP4 (ARCL)

Mutations in *LTBP4* cause ARCL type 1C (ARCL1C, MIM #613177) (Figure 2.3d,e) (Callewaert et al. 2013; Urban et al. 2009). Patients present with lax and redundant skin, severe developmental emphysema, pulmonary stenosis, arterial tortuosity, severe diverticulosis, tortuosity, enlargement and stenosis of the gastrointestinal tract, and diaphragmatic and inguinal hernias. Developmental emphysema can cause respiratory failure and can result in premature death. Skin biopsies from patients with LTBP4 mutations show an altered elastic fiber ultrastructure, where ELN is found as large globular deposits and fibrillin microfibrils are poorly integrated (Figure 2.3e) (Urban et al. 2009). The surface of elastic fibers appeared smooth whereas in controls, microfibrils form a coat around elastic fibers.

LTBP4 binds to fibulin-5 and was shown to facilitate the incorporation of tropoelastin around fibrillin microfibrils in cell culture (Isogai et al. 2003; Noda et al. 2013). Because LTBP4 cannot bind to tropoelastin directly, it was proposed that LTBP4 promotes the linear integration of tropoelastin onto microfibrils. In the absence of LTBP4 in cell culture, tropoelastin accumulates as globular aggregates on the microfibrils, similar to what was observed in patient biopsies. The three human LTBP4 isoforms, LTBP4S and two LTBP4L isoforms, respectively, are generated by alternative promoters and are differentially expressed in tissues (Figure 2.3d). Mice with a deficiency of the short isoform of LTBP4 (*Ltbp4S*$^{-/-}$) develop pulmonary emphysema due to a defect in alveolar septation (Dabovic et al. 2009; Sterner-Kock et al. 2002). The emphysema could be rescued by reducing the amount of TGFβ2, despite the fact that LTBP4 binds exclusively to latent TGFβ1. However, the abnormal elastic fiber appearance in rescued *Ltbp4S*$^{-/-}$ lungs persisted. These findings indicated two independent roles for LTBP4S in lung tissue, one in modulating TGFβ signaling and one in facilitating the assembly of elastic fibers, respectively. Interestingly, a recent study using skin fibroblasts from patients with ARCL1C described a role for LTBP4 in modulating the endocytosis of TGFβ receptor-2 by forming a molecular complex and stabilizing TGFβ receptor-2 complex at the cell surface (Su et al. 2015). This could explain the paradox, that despite elevated amounts of active TGFβ, the downstream signaling was reduced in patient-derived dermal fibroblasts. Recently, a complete LTBP4 knockout was generated by deleting *Ltbp4L* in an *Ltbp4S*$^{-/-}$ background (Bultmann-Mellin et al. 2015). The lungs of these mice showed disorganized lobular architecture and a more severe air space enlargement compared with *Ltbp4S*$^{-/-}$ lungs. In addition, the aortic wall in *Ltbp4*$^{-/-}$ mice was thicker and the dermal thickness was reduced, when compared with the controls. The ultrastructure of the elastic fibers showed distinct pathologies in the lung tissue from *Ltbp4S*$^{-/-}$, where elastic fibers were short and fragmented, compared with *Ltbp4*$^{-/-}$ mice, where no elastic fibers were found and ELN was deposited in scattered patches. On a mechanistic level, it was demonstrated that the absence of both LTBP4 isoforms correlated with a reduction in fibulin-5 mRNA in tissue and primary skin fibroblasts cultured from the different knockout mice strains. In addition, the N-terminus of recombinant LTBP4L bound stronger to recombinant fibulin-4 and -5 compared with the N-terminus of the LTBP4S. Because mutations in LTBP4 in patients with ARCL1C affect both LTBP4 isoforms, the *Ltbp4*$^{-/-}$ mouse may provide a useful animal model for this syndrome and could help understanding pathophysiological mechanisms.

2.3.5 ABCC6 (Pseudoxanthoma Elasticum)

The gene ATP-binding cassette subfamily C, member 6 (*ABCC6*) encodes a transmembrane efflux transporter, which is part of the multidrug resistance protein family. ABCC6 is expressed predominantly in the liver and proximal tubules of the kidneys. A substrate has not been identified. Biallelic human mutations in ABCC6 cause pseudoxanthoma elasticum (PXE,

MIM #264800) (Li and Uitto 2012). The hallmark clinical finding of PXE is leathery, inelastic skin. However, in addition to skin involvement, PXE can cause ocular and vascular symptoms; both are related to ectopic mineralization in these tissues (Georgalas et al. 2011; Leftheriotis et al. 2013). In histological sections of the skin, elastic fibers in the mid-dermis appear fragmented and show abundant mineral deposits, indicating ectopic mineralization (Hosen et al. 2012). In young individuals, electron microscopy studies showed ectopic mineralization on otherwise normal elastic fibers at early stages of PXE (Lebwohl et al. 1993). This indicates that the fragmentation of the elastic fibers in PXE is a consequence of inappropriate mineralization. In the eye, mineralized elastic fibers were found in Bruch's membrane of the retina and in the heart elastic fibers were mineralized in the myocardium, pericardium, and in small-to-medium caliber arteries. Analysis of key mineralization inhibitors in the plasma indicated lower levels of fetuin-A, osteocalcin, and matrix-associated Gla protein (Hosen et al. 2012). However, in skin immunohistology, the mid-dermis of patients with PXE showed abundant staining for these molecules. Interestingly, the elastic fiber alterations in the blood vessel walls found in PXE resembled those of two other ectopic calcification disorders. The mild calcification disorder of the tunica media, Moenckeberg-type arteriosclerosis, is frequently associated with type-2 diabetes and end-stage renal disease (Couri et al. 2005). In contrast, the severe idiopathic type of generalized arterial calcification in infancy (IACI, MIM #208000), leads to perinatal lethality in humans due to calcified arteries (Karthikeyan 2013). Interestingly, *ABCC6* mutations have been found in patients with IACI and mutations in *ENPP1*, causing IACI, have been described in patients with PXE (Li et al. 2014; Nitschke et al. 2012; Nitschke and Rutsch 2012).

Defining the pathophysiology underlying PXE is hampered by the elusive physiological role of ABCC6, because no substrate for the transporter has been identified so far. Two hypotheses for PXE pathophysiology are currently under investigation. The metabolic hypothesis states that ABCC6 deficiency leads to a systemic alteration of one or more substrates in blood plasma triggering ectopic elastic fiber mineralization (Uitto et al. 2001). The cellular hypothesis is based on the observation that fibroblasts from patients with PXE are producing more reactive oxygen species and less antioxidants and therefore are constantly exposed to oxidative stress (Pasquali-Ronchetti et al. 2006). How the cellular hypothesis is related to ectopic calcification in skin is not clear. In a mouse model of ABCC6 deficiency, ectopic elastic fiber calcification in Bruch's membrane and in blood vessels was readily observed, but the dermal ECM appeared normal (Gorgels et al. 2005). In an independently developed mouse model, ABCC6-deficient mice showed a similar pattern of ectopic elastic fiber calcification, including the involvement of dermal elastic fibers (Klement et al. 2005). The observed differences in dermal involvement could be mouse strain specific.

2.4 NONGENETIC, ACQUIRED, AND ENVIRONMENTAL DISEASES AFFECTING ELASTIC MATRICES

2.4.1 Abdominal Aortic Aneurysms

The main risk factors for developing AAA are male gender, smoking, and hypercholesterolemia (Kent et al. 2010). Despite evidence suggesting a strong genetic component in the formation of AAAs, no single mutation in a human gene has so far been described in families with a history of AAA (Saratzis and Bown 2014). However, several gene loci have been linked to AAA by candidate gene analysis and genome wide association studies, including LRP1, LDL-receptor, DAB2IP, AAA-1, and AAA-2.

The histological analysis of specimens dissected from patients with AAA shows an infiltration with leukocytes and degradation of ECM in conjunction with a reduced number of vascular smooth muscle cells. This is in contrast to the cystic medial necrosis, found in cross sections of the aortic wall from patients with Marfan syndrome and other TAA. To understand the molecular mechanisms leading to the formation of AAAs, three rodent models are used. AAA formation can be induced by (i) calcium chloride exposure of the adventitia of the abdominal aorta; (ii) transient perfusion of the infrarenal aorta with elastase (an ELN-degrading protease), or (iii) chronic subcutaneous angiotensin II infusion, using implanted minipumps (Manning et al. 2002; Thompson et al. 2006; Wang et al. 2013a). Combining the results from these different models suggest that the events, which initiate AAA formation, are mediated by local inflammation in the aortic wall, which then triggers the release of various cytokines and ECM-degrading proteases. These early events ultimately result in the degradation of the ECM and apoptosis of vascular smooth muscle cells as observed in biopsies dissected from patients with advanced AAA (Lopez-Candales et al. 1997; Shimizu et al. 2006). Macrophages play an important role in the response to the inflammatory phase of AAA formation. Macrophages secrete a suite of proteases, including matrix metalloproteinase-2 (MMP2) and MMP9 that are implicated in the degradation of ELN and collagen. These proteases are major players in the destruction of the aortic wall ultimately resulting in the dilation of the aorta. Genetic depletion of MMP2 or MMP9 had a protective effect on AAA formation in the elastase and calcium chloride model (Longo et al. 2002). Doxycycline, a broad-spectrum MMP inhibitor is considered as a potential drug to prevent the formation of AAAs (Kurosawa et al. 2013). Doxycycline was effective in preventing AAA initiation in the elastase and calcium chloride models, but conflicting data exist about its effectiveness in the angiotensin II AAA model (Bartoli et al. 2006; Xie et al. 2012). Therefore, the development of more specific MMP inhibitors, selectively targeting MMP2 or MMP9, will be crucial in exploring MMPs as pharmacological targets in stabilizing pre-existing AAAs in humans.

TGFβ plays a prominent role among the cytokines implicated in AAA formation (Wang et al. 2013b). In AAAs, elevated TGFβ appears to be protective. For example, it was shown that systemic blockade of TGFβ signaling enhanced AAA formation in the angiotensin II model (Wang et al. 2010). Further, local adenovirus-mediated TGFβ overexpression stabilized established AAAs in a rat model and drugs like cyclosporine, which induce TGFβ expression, resulted in a protective effect in AAA formation in an experimental rat and mouse model (Dai et al. 2005). This is in contrast to TAA, where elevated TGFβ signaling seems to be a central feature and genetic or pharmacological reduction of TGFβ signaling prevented the formation of ascending aortic aneurysms in mice. To resolve the role of TGFβ in AAA formation, future research is needed to address the timeline of TGFβ signaling during the formation and progression of AAAs. It is conceivable, that TGFβ plays a biphasic role, for example, protective versus harmful, in the formation and/or progression of AAAs as well.

2.4.2 Solar Elastosis

Solar elastosis is the main presentation of photoaged skin. Photoaging is a process in which cumulative exposure to sunlight or UV radiation causes histological alterations of the skin (Han et al. 2014). As a consequence, the skin is characterized by dryness, rough texture, thickening, deep creases, and fine wrinkles (Gilchrest 1989). Most of the alterations are found within the dermis and include aberrant distribution of melanocytes, a thickening of the basement membrane and the stratum corneum. The hallmark histological finding in solar elastosis, however, is the accumulation of so-called elastolytic material, that is, abnormal extracellular material, derived from the degradation of dermal elastic fibers (Braverman and Fonferko 1982; Matsuta et al. 1987; Tsuji 1984). Two distinct alterations of elastic fibers are observed in histological sections. Areas of thickened and tangled elastic fibers, the fibrous areas, are interspersed with areas of granular and more homogeneous elastolytic material. The latter areas are thought to arise from the degradation of the elastic fibers in the fibrous areas.

Mechanistically, the role of enhanced oxidative stress, neutrophil influx, and an imbalance in the production of ECM proteases has been implicated (Rijken and Bruijnzeel 2009; Sander et al. 2002). UV exposure enhances the production of reactive oxygen species and overwhelms the natural antioxidant defense system in the skin. These reactive oxygen species can either directly damage components of the ECM or can promote the influx of inflammatory cells, including neutrophils. The UV-induced secretion of MMP1, MMP3, and MMP9 has been shown in photoaged skin (Fisher et al. 1996, 1997). However, there is some debate about the cell types responsible for this increase in MMP activity. Some reports propose keratinocytes and others dermal fibroblasts as the major sources of these MMPs. In the case of keratinocytes-derived MMPs, it would require that the proteases cross the basement membrane, because the elastolytic material is observed in the upper and middle dermis. Alternatively, several reports propose neutrophils as the major source of elevated MMP activity in solar elastosis (Rijken and Bruijnzeel 2009). Among other proteases, neutrophils can produce MMP1, MMP8, MMP9, and MMP12 and neutrophil elastase, which is a potent protease capable of degrading ELN and collagen. The most convincing evidence for the active role of elastases derived from neutrophils came from mouse studies, showing that mice, genetically depleted of neutrophil elastase, did not develop solar elastosis on prolonged UV exposure, when compared with WT mice (Starcher and Conrad 1995).

2.4.3 Aging Processes in Skin and Lung

Changes in the skin due to intrinsic or natural aging are different from the changes described in solar elastosis (Kadoya et al. 2005; Watson et al. 1999). However, the biomechanical outcome and the appearance of the skin may be similar. Histologically, intrinsic skin aging is characterized by (i) a loss in dermal thickness, accompanied by a reduced cell number, loss of collagen fibers, and a reduced number of blood vessels; (ii) degeneration of dermal elastic fibers; and (iii) loss of hydration, attributed to an alteration in the composition or amount of proteoglycans/glycoproteins ("ground substance") (Bernstein and Uitto 1996). The skin appears to retain its extensibility up to 70 years of age, but loses its elasticity earlier (Hussain et al. 2013). Therefore, the intrinsic aging process of skin can be described as a gradual depletion of functional ECM components, concomitant with a reduced capability of dermal cells to assemble new ECM. Therefore, the ECM turnover balance is shifted toward gradual ECM degradation.

Similar to the skin, the lung is exposed to environmental insults with every breathing cycle. Therefore, dissecting intrinsic aging processes from extrinsically triggered events is challenging. The reduced elasticity of aged pulmonary tissue is related to the development of emphysema, which causes a reduction in parameters of lung capacity (Escolar et al. 1994; Fredberg and Kamm 2006). On a histological level, aged lung tissue from humans and rodents presents with dilated alveoli and increased thickness of the alveolar wall. The content of collagen type I and elastic fiber in the lung changed inconsistently with age, with increased, decreased, and unchanged values reported depending on the specific study (reviewed in Sherratt 2009). These conflicting reports may point to a more important role of ECM organization relative to quantitative changes as a driver of age-related decline in lung compliance. In rats, it was shown, that the diameter of elastic fibers increased with age. In addition, proteolytic and, more specifically, elastolytic enzymes are present in normal lung that contribute to the progressive turnover of ECM components (Lagente and Boichot 2010). Finally, other age-related changes, like the formation of advanced glycation end products, reactive oxygen species, or low-grade chronic inflammation may contribute to the progressive stiffening of lung tissue with age (Bellmunt et al. 1995a,b).

2.4.4 Age-Related Arterial Stiffening

Intrinsic aging processes also affect the vasculature, which typically leads to the stiffening of arteries and the subsequent reduction of arterial compliance (arteriosclerosis) (Mitchell 2008). Arterial stiffening is correlated with elevated blood pressure and represents a major risk factor for developing heart failure and stroke. However, the cause and consequence relationship between arterial stiffness and elevated blood pressure is still unclear. While it is clear that the stiffness of arteries increases with age, the contribution of individual ECM components toward age-related increased arterial stiffness is less well defined. For example, conflicting reports show an increase or no change in collagen with age (Hosoda et al. 1984). The absolute amount of ELN decreases in aging blood vessels, but one report suggested that the concentration of ELN in relation to other components of the vascular wall actually increases with age due to its exceptionally long half-life (Hosoda et al. 1984; Suzuki et al. 2010; Viveiro et al. 2013). However, similar to lung tissue, several studies point toward a relative importance of ECM organization over quantitative changes as determinants of arterial stiffness (Avolio et al. 1998; Bruel and Oxlund 1996). For example, it was demonstrated that the collagen/ELN ratio is an unreliable predictor of biomechanical properties of tissues (Cox 1981). Transesophageal echocardiography or PWV measurements may be used to assess the degree of arterial stiffening (O'Rourke et al. 1968; Pearson et al. 1994). In addition, the organization of elastic lamellae in the aorta becomes increasingly disrupted with age. Further evidence for the importance of ECM organization comes from the fact that nonenzymatic cross-linking processes mediated by glucose and its metabolites via the Maillard reactions and the formation of advanced glycation end products, contribute to age-related arterial stiffening (Bailey 2001).

2.4.5 Pulmonary Emphysema due to ELN Degradation by Neutrophil Elastase and MMPs

Pulmonary emphysema can be caused by matrix-degrading enzymes, including several MMPs and neutrophil elastase. COPD is the third leading cause of death in the United States, and emphysema is one of the major contributors (Hoyert and Xu 2012). Neutrophil elastase and several MMPs are induced or activated by chronic exposure to cigarette smoke, silica dust, and potentially other environmental hazards. The biological function of neutrophil elastase may be to facilitate the infiltration of tissues by neutrophils in response to inflammatory stimuli. Patients with a mutation in the natural inhibitor of neutrophil elastase, α-1 antitrypsin (AAT) (MIM #613490), develop emphysema and COPD due to the degradation of ELN (Turino et al. 1969). Genetic AAT deficiency can be corrected by intravenous administration of purified AAT, the so-called augmentation therapy (Wewers and Crystal 2013).

The most prominent MMP responsible for ELN degradation in emphysema is MMP12 (McGarry Houghton 2015). MMP12 is predominantly found in macrophages and is typically inactive at baseline. MMP12 activity increased after exposure of lung tissue to cigarette smoke via multiple activation mechanisms on a protein and gene expression level (Raza et al. 2000). In a crucial experiment, Hautamaki et al. (1997) showed that MMP12-deficient mice were protected from cigarette-smoke-induced emphysema concomitant with a decrease in lung-resident macrophages. The failure to recruit macrophages was attributed to the absence of

MMP12-mediated generation of chemotactic ELN peptides, which act as matrikines (ECM-derived chemokines), in the recruitment of macrophages in the WT mice. In patients with COPD, MMP12 expression is strongly induced by cigarette smoke and a single nucleotide polymorphism in *MMP12* was associated with a higher prevalence of COPD (Hunninghake et al. 2009). Treatment strategies to inhibit MMP12 and MMP9 or to interfere with macrophage recruitment by blocking ELN-derived peptides are currently evaluated (Churg et al. 2007; Le Quement et al. 2008).

The contribution of other MMPs, including MMP2, MMP3, MMP7, MMP9, and MMP10 to the development of emphysema is less well understood. All of these MMPs can degrade ELN, at least *in vitro* (Sternlicht and Werb 2001). MMP9, for example, does not degrade elastic fibers in cigarette-smoke-induced lung injury, but does degrade elastic fibers in mouse models for AAA (Atkinson et al. 2011; Longo et al. 2002). However, MMP9 may contribute to emphysema formation by degrading collagen and by triggering the release of chemoattractants for neutrophils and the subsequent degradation of elastic fibers by neutrophil elastase.

2.5 SUMMARY AND OUTLOOK

Elastic matrices are important components contributing to the stability and physiological function of several tissues. The identification of genetic causes for several human disorders of elastic matrices in combination with targeted genetic experiments in mice identified possible underlying molecular pathomechanisms for many of these disorders (Figure 2.4). For example, novel roles for components of elastic tissues in TGFβ and BMP signaling have emerged. The following principles seem to apply broadly to several disease conditions of elastic matrices.

First, the formation of elastic matrices relies on multiple players, best exemplified in the multistep process of cell-mediated elastic fiber assembly, which can be affected by mutations in tropoelastin, fibrillin-1, fibulin-4/5, and LTBP4, in addition to other proteins not discussed here and to be discovered. This has implications for tissue engineering approaches in that focusing on the interaction of isolated components of elastic fibers in the absence of cells may not be sufficient to regenerate fully functional elastic fibers. In addition, post-translational modifications like N- and O-linked glycosylation, disulfide-bond formation, or enzyme-mediated cross-linking maybe essential to produce fully functional and biologically active elastic matrices.

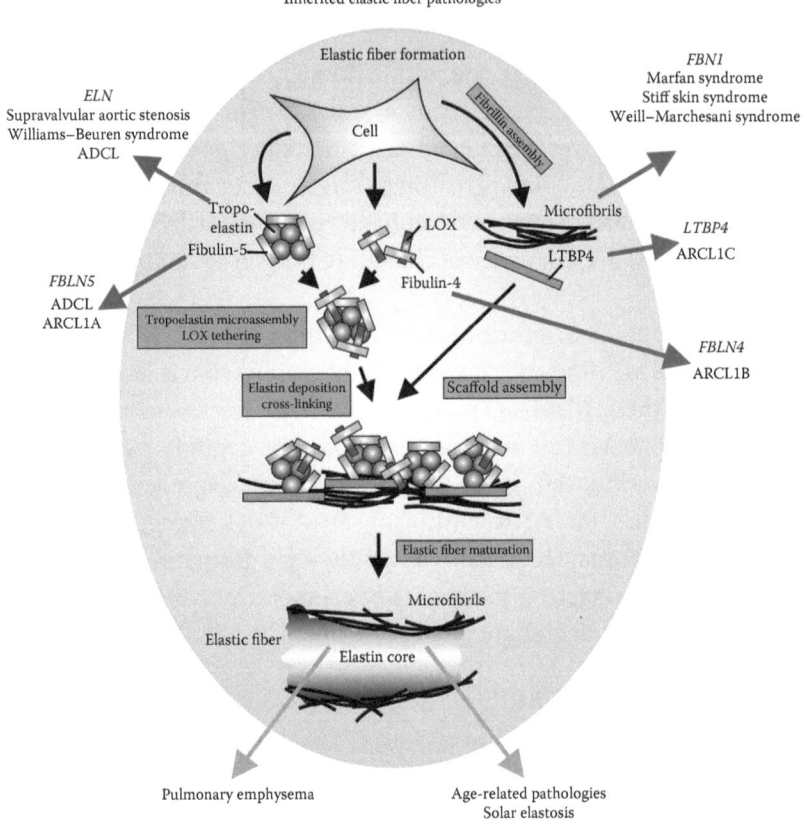

FIGURE 2.4 Pathology of elastic fibers. Depiction of the elastic fiber assembly process with the proposed roles for molecules mutated in disorders of elastic matrices. Inherited elastic fiber pathologies are indicated with red arrows, while acquired elastic fiber pathologies are depicted with green arrows.

Second, most, if not all, monogenetic disorders of elastic matrices involve pathological alteration of TGFβ and BMP signaling. This raises the question how mutations in various ECM proteins all seem to converge in the activation of TGFβ. One hypothesis that was recently proposed states that tissue-resident cells sense a defective matrix and, independent of its molecular cause, attempt to repair the ECM with a default repair response (Horiguchi et al. 2012). One central part of this response is the activation of TGFβ, which may subsequently coordinate the expression of tissue-specific sets of ECM repair genes. Alternatively, pathological TGFβ activation could be caused by the absence or impaired function of proteins, which maintain latency of extracellular TGFβ and BMP growth factors. From a therapeutic perspective, the aberrant activation of canonical and noncanonical TGFβ signaling pathways represent potential drug targets for pathologies of elastic matrices, as currently explored in Marfan syndrome and other hereditary forms of TAA, where clinical studies have been already completed or are underway.

Third, ELN-degrading proteases, including members of the MMP family and other elastases, play an important role in the pathology of several genetic and acquired disorders of elastic matrices. Fragmentation and degradation of elastic fibers is observed in multiple tissues in several disease conditions. MMPs are potential targets for small molecule inhibitors. However, the high homology of MMPs and their essential physiological functions require the development of isoform-specific MMP inhibitors (Fields 2015).

Lastly, elastic matrices and their components like ELN and fibrillin microfibrils are typically long-lived. That implies, for example, that humans need to rely on the proper function of the elastic fibers with which they were initially endowed. With time, elastic matrices are altered by the accumulation of advanced glycation end products, by the constant exposure to oxidative stress, UV radiation from sun rays, or other environmental insults. With an aging population, it is conceivable that pathological alterations of elastic matrices will become a relevant source of concern for the elderly and their physicians. Interestingly, some researchers have already proposed that aging and subsequent failing of elastic matrices especially in the aorta may limit the human lifespan to 100–120 years (Robert et al. 2008).

Going forward, elastic matrices can no longer be thought of as merely biomechanical support structures. Instead, scientists and physicians need to perceive elastic matrices as platforms for the integration of extracellular growth factor signaling and substrates that are able to determine and modulate the identity of cells and their behavior. Based on this expanded view of elastic matrices, scientists may identify new mechanisms on which to institute new rationally designed treatment strategies and to develop novel biomaterials.

ACKNOWLEDGMENTS

This work was in part supported by the NIH (K08 HL109076 to BAK) and the Marfan Foundation (Early Investigator Grant to DH).

REFERENCES

Al-Hassnan, Z.N., Almesned, A.R., Tulbah, S. et al. 2012. Recessively inherited severe aortic aneurysm caused by mutated EFEMP2. *Am J Cardiol 109*, 1677–1680.

Atkinson, J.J., Lutey, B.A., Suzuki, Y. et al. 2011. The role of matrix metalloproteinase-9 in cigarette smoke-induced emphysema. *Am J Respir Crit Care Med 183*, 876–884.

Avolio, A., Jones, D., and Tafazzoli-Shadpour, M. 1998. Quantification of alterations in structure and function of elastin in the arterial media. *Hypertension 32*, 170–175.

Bailey, A.J. 2001. Molecular mechanisms of ageing in connective tissues. *Mech Ageing Dev 122*, 735–755.

Bartoli, M.A., Parodi, F.E., Chu, J. et al. 2006. Localized administration of doxycycline suppresses aortic dilatation in an experimental mouse model of abdominal aortic aneurysm. *Ann Vasc Surg 20*, 228–236.

Bellmunt, M.J., Portero, M., Pamplona, R., Cosso, L., Odetti, P., and Prat, J. 1995a. Evidence for the Maillard reaction in rat lung collagen and its relationship with solubility and age. *Biochim Biophys Acta 1272*, 53–60.

Bellmunt, M.J., Portero, M., Pamplona, R., Muntaner, M., and Prat, J. 1995b. Age-related fluorescence in rat lung collagen. *Lung 173*, 177–185.

Bernstein, E.F. and Uitto, J. 1996. The effect of photodamage on dermal extracellular matrix. *Clin Dermatol 14*, 143–151.

Berry, C.L., Greenwald, S.E., and Rivett, J.F. 1975. Static mechanical properties of the developing and mature rat aorta. *Cardiovasc Res 9*, 669–678.

Berry, C.L., Sosa-Melgarejo, J.A., and Greenwald, S.E. 1993. The relationship between wall tension, lamellar thickness, and intercellular junctions in the fetal and adult aorta: Its relevance to the pathology of dissecting aneurysm. *J Pathol 169*, 15–20.

Bock, P. and Stockinger, L. 1984. Light and electron microscopic identification of elastic, elaunin and oxytalan fibers in human tracheal and bronchial mucosa. *Anat Embryol (Berl) 170*, 145–153.

Bolande, R.P. and Tucker, A.S. 1964. Pulmonary emphysema and other cardiorespiratory lesions as part of the marfan abiotrophy. *Pediatrics 33*, 356–366.

Bolar, N., Van Laer, L., and Loeys, B.L. 2012. Marfan syndrome: From gene to therapy. *Curr Opin Pediatr 24*, 498–504.

Booms, P., Withers, A.P., Boxer, M. et al. 1997. A novel de novo mutation in exon 14 of the fibrillin-1 gene associated with delayed secretion of fibrillin in a patient with a mild Marfan phenotype. *Hum Genet 100*, 195–200.

Bousquet, J., Lacoste, J.Y., Chanez, P., Vic, P., Godard, P., and Michel, F.B. 1996. Bronchial elastic fibers in normal subjects and asthmatic patients. *Am J Respir Crit Care Med 153*, 1648–1654.

Braverman, I.M. and Fonferko, E. 1982. Studies in cutaneous aging: I. The elastic fiber network. *J Invest Dermatol 78*, 434–443.

Bruel, A. and Oxlund, H. 1996. Changes in biomechanical properties, composition of collagen and elastin, and advanced glycation endproducts of the rat aorta in relation to age. *Atherosclerosis 127*, 155–165.

Budatha, M., Roshanravan, S., Zheng, Q. et al. 2011. Extracellular matrix proteases contribute to progression of pelvic organ prolapse in mice and humans. *J Clin Invest 121*, 2048–2059.

Bultmann-Mellin, I., Conradi, A., Maul, A.C. et al. 2015. Modeling autosomal recessive cutis laxa type 1C (ARCL1C) in mice reveals distinct functions of Ltbp-4 isoforms. *Dis Model Mech 8*, 403–415.

Burton, A.C. 1954. Relation of structure to function of the tissues of the wall of blood vessels. *Physiol Rev 34*, 619–642.

Byers, P.H. and Murray, M.L. 2014. Ehlers-Danlos syndrome: A showcase of conditions that lead to understanding matrix biology. *Matrix Biol 33*, 10–15.

Cain, S.A., McGovern, A., Baldwin, A.K., Baldock, C., and Kielty, C.M. 2012. Fibrillin-1 mutations causing Weill-Marchesani syndrome and acromicric and geleophysic dysplasias disrupt heparan sulfate interactions. *PLoS one 7*, e48634.

Callewaert, B., Renard, M., Hucthagowder, V. et al. 2011. New insights into the pathogenesis of autosomal-dominant cutis laxa with report of five ELN mutations. *Hum Mutat 32*, 445–455.

Callewaert, B., Su, C.T., Van Damme, T. et al. 2013. Comprehensive clinical and molecular analysis of 12 families with type 1 recessive cutis laxa. *Hum Mutat 34*, 111–121.

Callewaert, B.L., Loeys, B.L., Ficcadenti, A. et al. 2009. Comprehensive clinical and molecular assessment of 32 probands with congenital contractural arachnodactyly: Report of 14 novel mutations and review of the literature. *Hum Mutat 30*, 334–341.

Cecchi, A., Ogawa, N., Martinez, H.R. et al. 2013. Missense mutations in FBN1 exons 41 and 42 cause Weill-Marchesani syndrome with thoracic aortic disease and Marfan syndrome. *Am J Med Genet A 161A*, 2305–2310.

Chiu, H.H., Wu, M.H., Wang, J.K. et al. 2013. Losartan added to beta-blockade therapy for aortic root dilation in Marfan syndrome: A randomized, open-label pilot study. *Mayo Clin Proc 88*, 271–276.

Choudhary, S.V., Bisati, S., and Koley, S. 2011. Congenital cutis laxa with rectal and uterovaginal prolapse. *Indian J Dermatol Venereol Leprol 77*, 321–324.

Choudhury, R., McGovern, A., Ridley, C. et al. 2009. Differential regulation of elastic fiber formation by fibulin-4 and -5. *J Biol Chem 284*, 24553–24567.

Churg, A., Wang, R., Wang, X., Onnervik, P.O., Thim, K., and Wright, J.L. 2007. Effect of an MMP-9/MMP-12 inhibitor on smoke-induced emphysema and airway remodelling in guinea pigs. *Thorax 62*, 706–713.

Cirulis, J.T., Bellingham, C.M., Davis, E.C. et al. 2008. Fibrillins, fibulins, and matrix-associated glycoprotein modulate the kinetics and morphology of in vitro self-assembly of a recombinant elastin-like polypeptide. *Biochemistry 47*, 12601–12613.

Cook, J.R., Clayton, N.P., Carta, L. et al. 2015. Dimorphic effects of transforming growth factor-beta signaling during aortic aneurysm progression in mice suggest a combinatorial therapy for Marfan syndrome. *Arterioscler Thromb Vasc Biol 35*, 911–917.

Corson, G.M., Charbonneau, N.L., Keene, D.R., and Sakai, L.Y. 2004. Differential expression of fibrillin-3 adds to microfibril variety in human and avian, but not rodent, connective tissues. *Genomics 83*, 461–472.

Couri, C.E., da Silva, G.A., Martinez, J.A., Pereira Fde, A., and de Paula, F.J. 2005. Monckeberg's sclerosis—Is the artery the only target of calcification? *BMC Cardiovasc Disord 5*, 34.

Cox, R.H. 1981. Basis for the altered arterial wall mechanics in the spontaneously hypertensive rat. *Hypertension 3*, 485–495.

Dabovic, B., Chen, Y., Choi, J. et al. 2009. Dual functions for LTBP in lung development: LTBP-4 independently modulates elastogenesis and TGF-beta activity. *J Cell Physiol 219*, 14–22.

Dai, J., Losy, F., Guinault, A.M. et al. 2005. Overexpression of transforming growth factor-beta1 stabilizes already-formed aortic aneurysms: A first approach to induction of functional healing by endovascular gene therapy. *Circulation 112*, 1008–1015.

Dallas, S.L., Keene, D.R., Bruder, S.P. et al. 2000. Role of the latent transforming growth factor beta binding protein 1 in fibrillin-containing microfibrils in bone cells in vitro and in vivo. *J Bone Miner Res 15*, 68–81.

Damkier, A., Brandrup, F., and Starklint, H. 1991. Cutis laxa: Autosomal dominant inheritance in five generations. *Clin Genet 39*, 321–329.

Dasouki, M., Markova, D., Garola, R. et al. 2007. Compound heterozygous mutations in fibulin-4 causing neonatal lethal pulmonary artery occlusion, aortic aneurysm, arachnodactyly, and mild cutis laxa. *Am J Med Genet A 143A*, 2635–2641.

David, T.E. 2010. Surgical treatment of ascending aorta and aortic root aneurysms. *Prog Cardiovasc Dis 52*, 438–444.

Davis, E.C. 1993a. Endothelial cell connecting filaments anchor endothelial cells to the subjacent elastic lamina in the developing aortic intima of the mouse. *Cell Tissue Res 272*, 211–219.

Davis, E.C. 1993b. Smooth muscle cell to elastic lamina connections in developing mouse aorta. Role in aortic medial organization. *Lab Invest 68*, 89–99.

Davis, F.M., Rateri, D.L., and Daugherty, A. 2014. Mechanisms of aortic aneurysm formation: Translating preclinical studies into clinical therapies. *Heart 100*, 1498–1505.

de Figueiredo Borges, L., Jaldin, R.G., Dias, R.R., Stolf, N.A., Michel, J.B., and Gutierrez, P.S. 2008. Collagen is reduced and disrupted in human aneurysms and dissections of ascending aorta. *Hum Pathol 39*, 437–443.

Desir, J., Sznajer, Y., Depasse, F. et al. 2010. LTBP2 null mutations in an autosomal recessive ocular syndrome with megalocornea, spherophakia, and secondary glaucoma. *Eur J Hum Genet 18*, 761–767.

Dingemans, K.P., Teeling, P., Lagendijk, J.H., and Becker, A.E. 2000. Extracellular matrix of the human aortic media: An ultrastructural histochemical and immunohistochemical study of the adult aortic media. *Anat Rec 258*, 1–14.

Djokic, J., Fagotto-Kaufmann, C., Bartels, R., Nelea, V., and Reinhardt, D.P. 2013. Fibulin-3, -4, and -5 are highly susceptible to proteolysis, interact with cells and heparin, and form multimers. *J Biol Chem 288*, 22821–22835.

Drewes, P.G., Yanagisawa, H., Starcher, B. et al. 2007. Pelvic organ prolapse in fibulin-5 knockout mice: Pregnancy-induced changes in elastic fiber homeostasis in mouse vagina. *Am J Pathol 170*, 578–589.

Dugan, S.L., Temme, R.T., Olson, R.A. et al. 2015. New recessive truncating mutation in LTBP3 in a family with oligodontia, short stature, and mitral valve prolapse. *Am J Med Genet A 167*, 1396–1399.

Dyhdalo, K. and Farver, C. 2011. Pulmonary histologic changes in Marfan syndrome: A case series and literature review. *Am J Clin Pathol 136*, 857–863.

Elahi, E., Kalhor, R., Banihosseini, S.S. et al. 2006. Homozygous missense mutation in fibulin-5 in an Iranian autosomal recessive cutis laxa pedigree and associated haplotype. *J Invest Dermatol 126*, 1506–1509.

Erickson, L.K., Opitz, J.M., and Zhou, H. 2012. Lethal osteogenesis imperfecta-like condition with cutis laxa and arterial tortuosity in MZ twins due to a homozygous fibulin-4 mutation. *Pediatr Dev Pathol 15*, 137–141.

Escolar, J.D., Gallego, B., Tejero, C., and Escolar, M.A. 1994. Changes occurring with increasing age in the rat lung: Morphometrical study. *Anat Rec 239*, 287–296.

Faivre, L., Gorlin, R.J., Wirtz, M.K. et al. 2003. In frame fibrillin-1 gene deletion in autosomal dominant Weill-Marchesani syndrome. *J Med Genet 40*, 34–36.

Fields, G.B. 2015. New strategies for targeting matrix metalloproteinases. *Matrix Biol 44–46C*, 239–246.

Fisher, G.J., Datta, S.C., Talwar, H.S. et al. 1996. Molecular basis of sun-induced premature skin ageing and retinoid antagonism. *Nature 379*, 335–339.

Fisher, G.J., Wang, Z.Q., Datta, S.C., Varani, J., Kang, S., and Voorhees, J.J. 1997. Pathophysiology of premature skin aging induced by ultraviolet light. *N Engl J Med 337*, 1419–1428.

Foster, J.A. and Curtiss, S.W. 1990. The regulation of lung elastin synthesis. *Am J Physiol 259*, L13–L23.

Franken, R., den Hartog, A.W., de Waard, V. et al. 2013. Circulating transforming growth factor-beta as a prognostic biomarker in Marfan syndrome. *Int J Cardiol 168*, 2441–2446.

Fredberg, J.J. and Kamm, R.D. 2006. Stress transmission in the lung: Pathways from organ to molecule. *Annu Rev Physiol 68*, 507–541.

Gayraud, B., Keene, D.R., Sakai, L.Y., and Ramirez, F. 2000. New insights into the assembly of extracellular microfibrils from the analysis of the fibrillin 1 mutation in the tight skin mouse. *J Cell Biol 150*, 667–680.

Georgalas, I., Tservakis, I., Papaconstaninou, D., Kardara, M., Koutsandrea, C., and Ladas, I. 2011. Pseudoxanthoma elasticum, ocular manifestations, complications and treatment. *Clin Exp Optom 94*, 169–180.

Gerber, E.E., Gallo, E.M., Fontana, S.C. et al. 2013. Integrin-modulating therapy prevents fibrosis and autoimmunity in mouse models of scleroderma. *Nature 503*, 126–130.

Gilchrest, B.A. 1989. Skin aging and photoaging: An overview. *J Am Acad Dermatol 21*, 610–613.

Gillis, E., Van Laer, L., and Loeys, B.L. 2013. Genetics of thoracic aortic aneurysm: At the crossroad of transforming growth factor-beta signaling and vascular smooth muscle cell contractility. *Circ Res 113*, 327–340.

Gleizes, P.E., Beavis, R.C., Mazzieri, R., Shen, B., and Rifkin, D.B. 1996. Identification and characterization of an eight-cysteine repeat of the latent transforming growth factor-beta binding protein-1 that mediates bonding to the latent transforming growth factor-beta1. *J Biol Chem 271*, 29891–29896.

Gorgels, T.G., Hu, X., Scheffer, G.L. et al. 2005. Disruption of Abcc6 in the mouse: Novel insight in the pathogenesis of pseudoxanthoma elasticum. *Hum Mol Genet 14*, 1763–1773.

Grahame, R. and Pyeritz, R.E. 1995. The Marfan syndrome: Joint and skin manifestations are prevalent and correlated. *Br J Rheumatol 34*, 126–131.

Green, M.C., Sweet, H.O., and Bunker, L.E. 1976. Tight-skin, a new mutation of the mouse causing excessive growth of connective tissue and skeleton. *Am J Pathol 82*, 493–512.

Groenink, M., den Hartog, A.W., Franken, R. et al. 2013. Losartan reduces aortic dilatation rate in adults with Marfan syndrome: A randomized controlled trial. *Eur Heart J 34*, 3491–3500.

Guemann, A.S., Andrieux, J., Petit, F. et al. 2015. ELN gene triplication responsible for familial supravalvular aortic aneurysm. *Cardiol Young 25*, 712–717.

Gupta, P.A., Putnam, E.A., Carmical, S.G. et al. 2002. Ten novel FBN2 mutations in congenital contractural arachnodactyly: Delineation of the molecular pathogenesis and clinical phenotype. *Hum Mutat 19*, 39–48.

Gupta, P.A., Wallis, D.D., Chin, T.O. et al. 2004. FBN2 mutation associated with manifestations of Marfan syndrome and congenital contractural arachnodactyly. *J Med Genet 41*, e56.

Habashi, J.P., Judge, D.P., Holm, T.M. et al. 2006. Losartan, an AT1 antagonist, prevents aortic aneurysm in a mouse model of Marfan syndrome. *Science 312*, 117–121.

Hadj-Rabia, S., Callewaert, B.L., Bourrat, E. et al. 2013. Twenty patients including 7 probands with autosomal dominant cutis laxa confirm clinical and molecular homogeneity. *Orphanet J Rare Dis 8*, 36.

Haji-Seyed-Javadi, R., Jelodari-Mamaghani, S., Paylakhi, S.H. et al. 2012. LTBP2 mutations cause Weill-Marchesani and Weill-Marchesani-like syndrome and affect disruptions in the extracellular matrix. *Hum Mutat 33*, 1182–1187.

Halabi, C.M., Broekelmann, T.J., Knutsen R.H. et al. 2015. Chronic antihypertensive treatment improves pulse pressure but not large artery mechanics in a mouse model of congenital vascular stiffness. *Am J Physiol Heart Circ Physiol 309*, H1008–H1016.

Han, A., Chien, A.L., and Kang, S. 2014. Photoaging. *Dermatol Clin 32*, 291–299, vii.

Hautamaki, R.D., Kobayashi, D.K., Senior, R.M., and Shapiro, S.D. 1997. Requirement for macrophage elastase for cigarette smoke-induced emphysema in mice. *Science 277*, 2002–2004.

Hayward, C., Porteous, M.E., and Brock, D.J. 1997. Mutation screening of all 65 exons of the fibrillin-1 gene in 60 patients with Marfan syndrome: Report of 12 novel mutations. *Hum Mutat 10*, 280–289.

Hilhorst-Hofstee, Y., Hamel, B.C., Verheij, J.B. et al. 2011. The clinical spectrum of complete FBN1 allele deletions. *Eur J Hum Genet 19*, 247–252.

Hirano, E., Knutsen, R.H., Sugitani, H., Ciliberto, C.H., and Mecham, R.P. 2007. Functional rescue of elastin insufficiency in mice by the human elastin gene: Implications for mouse models of human disease. *Circ Res 101*, 523–531.

Horiguchi, M., Inoue, T., Ohbayashi, T. et al. 2009. Fibulin-4 conducts proper elastogenesis via interaction with cross-linking enzyme lysyl oxidase. *Proc Natl Acad Sci USA 106*, 19029–19034.

Horiguchi, M., Ota, M., and Rifkin, D.B. 2012. Matrix control of transforming growth factor-beta function. *J Biochem 152*, 321–329.

Hosen, M.J., Lamoen, A., De Paepe, A., and Vanakker, O.M. 2012. Histopathology of pseudoxanthoma elasticum and related disorders: Histological hallmarks and diagnostic clues. *Scientifica 2012*, 598262.

Hosoda, Y., Kawano, K., Yamasawa, F., Ishii, T., Shibata, T., and Inayama, S. 1984. Age-dependent changes of collagen and elastin content in human aorta and pulmonary artery. *Angiology 35*, 615–621.

Hoyer, J., Kraus, C., Hammersen, G., Geppert, J.P., and Rauch, A. 2009. Lethal cutis laxa with contractural arachnodactyly, overgrowth and soft tissue bleeding due to a novel homozygous fibulin-4 gene mutation. *Clin Genet 76*, 276–281.

Hoyert, D.L. and Xu, J. 2012. Deaths: Preliminary data for 2011. *Natl Vital Stat Rep 61*, 1–51.

Hu, Q., Shifren, A., Sens, C. et al. 2010. Mechanisms of emphysema in autosomal dominant cutis laxa. *Matrix Biol 29*, 621–628.

Hu, Y., Zhang, Z., Torsney, E. et al. 2004. Abundant progenitor cells in the adventitia contribute to atherosclerosis of vein grafts in ApoE-deficient mice. *J Clin Invest 113*, 1258–1265.

Huang, J., Davis, E.C., Chapman, S.L. et al. 2010. Fibulin-4 deficiency results in ascending aortic aneurysms: A potential link between abnormal smooth muscle cell phenotype and aneurysm progression. *Circ Res 106*, 583–592.

Huang, J., Yamashiro, Y., Papke, C.L. et al. 2013. Angiotensin-converting enzyme-induced activation of local angiotensin signaling is required for ascending aortic aneurysms in fibulin-4-deficient mice. *Sci Transl Med 5*, 183ra158, 1–11.

Hubmacher, D. and Reinhardt, D. 2011. Microfibrils and fibrillin. In *The Extracellular Matrix: An Overview*, R.P. Mecham, ed. (Berlin/Heidelberg, Germany: Springer), pp. 233–265.

Hubmacher, D., Reinhardt, D.P., Plesec, T., Schenke-Layland, K., and Apte, S.S. 2014. Human eye development is characterized by coordinated expression of fibrillin isoforms. *Invest Ophthalmol Vis Sci 55*, 7934–7944.

Hucthagowder, V., Sausgruber, N., Kim, K.H., Angle, B., Marmorstein, L.Y., and Urban, Z. 2006. Fibulin-4: A novel gene for an autosomal recessive cutis laxa syndrome. *Am J Hum Genet 78*, 1075–1080.

Humphrey, J.D., Schwartz, M.A., Tellides, G., and Milewicz, D.M. 2015. Role of mechanotransduction in vascular biology: Focus on thoracic aortic aneurysms and dissections. *Circ Res 116*, 1448–1461.

Hunninghake, G.M., Cho, M.H., Tesfaigzi, Y. et al. 2009. MMP12, lung function, and COPD in high-risk populations. *N Engl J Med 361*, 2599–2608.

Hussain, S.H., Limthongkul, B., and Humphreys, T.R. 2013. The biomechanical properties of the skin. *Dermatol Surg 39*, 193–203.

Iascone, M., Sana, M.E., Pezzoli, L. et al. 2012. Extensive arterial tortuosity and severe aortic dilation in a newborn with an EFEMP2 mutation. *Circulation 126*, 2764–2768.

Isogai, Z., Ono, R.N., Ushiro, S. et al. 2003. Latent transforming growth factor beta-binding protein 1 interacts with fibrillin and is a microfibril-associated protein. *J Biol Chem 278*, 2750–2757.

Jobling, R., D'Souza, R., Baker, N. et al. 2014. The collagenopathies: Review of clinical phenotypes and molecular correlations. *Curr Rheumatolo Rep 16*, 394.

Judge, D.P., Biery, N.J., Keene, D.R. et al. 2004. Evidence for a critical contribution of haploinsufficiency in the complex pathogenesis of Marfan syndrome. *J Clin Invest 114*, 172–181.

Jung, H.J., Jeon, M.J., Yim, G.W., Kim, S.K., Choi, J.R., and Bai, S.W. 2009. Changes in expression of fibulin-5 and lysyl oxidase-like 1 associated with pelvic organ prolapse. *Eur J Obstet Gynecol Reprod Biol 145*, 117–122.

Kadoya, K., Sasaki, T., Kostka, G. et al. 2005. Fibulin-5 deposition in human skin: Decrease with ageing and ultraviolet B exposure and increase in solar elastosis. *Br J Dermatol 153*, 607–612.

Kappanayil, M., Nampoothiri, S., Kannan, R. et al. 2012. Characterization of a distinct lethal arteriopathy syndrome in twenty-two infants associated with an identical, novel mutation in FBLN4 gene, confirms fibulin-4 as a critical determinant of human vascular elastogenesis. *Orphanet J Rare Dis 7*, 61.

Karthikeyan, G. 2013. Generalized arterial calcification of infancy. *J Pediatr 162*, 1074 e1071.

Kelleher, C.M., Silverman, E.K., Broekelmann, T. et al. 2005. A functional mutation in the terminal exon of elastin in severe, early-onset chronic obstructive pulmonary disease. *Am J Respir Cell Mol Biol 33*, 355–362.

Kent, K.C., Zwolak, R.M., Egorova, N.N. et al. 2010. Analysis of risk factors for abdominal aortic aneurysm in a cohort of more than 3 million individuals. *J Vasc Surg 52*, 539–548.

Khadzhieva, M.B., Kamoeva, S.V., Chumachenko, A.G. et al. 2014. Fibulin-5 (FBLN5) gene polymorphism is associated with pelvic organ prolapse. *Maturitas 78*, 287–292.

Kielty, C.M., Phillips, J.E., Child, A.H., Pope, F.M., and Shuttleworth, C.A. 1994. Fibrillin secretion and microfibril assembly by Marfan dermal fibroblasts. *Matrix Biol 14*, 191–199.

Kielty, C.M., Raghunath, M., Siracusa, L.D. et al. 1998. The Tight skin mouse: Demonstration of mutant fibrillin-1 production and assembly into abnormal microfibrils. *J Cell Biol 140*, 1159–1166.

Kielty, C.M. and Shuttleworth, C.A. 1994. Abnormal fibrillin assembly by dermal fibroblasts from two patients with Marfan syndrome. *J Cell Biol 124*, 997–1004.

Kirschner, R., Hubmacher, D., Iyengar, G. et al. 2011. Classical and neonatal Marfan syndrome mutations in fibrillin-1 cause differential protease susceptibilities and protein function. *J Biol Chem 286*, 32810–32823.

Klement, J.F., Matsuzaki, Y., Jiang, Q.J. et al. 2005. Targeted ablation of the abcc6 gene results in ectopic mineralization of connective tissues. *Mol Cell Biol 25*, 8299–8310.

Kobayashi, N., Kostka, G., Garbe, J.H. et al. 2007. A comparative analysis of the fibulin protein family. Biochemical characterization, binding interactions, and tissue localization. *J Biol Chem 282*, 11805–11816.

Kozel, B.A., Bayliss, S.J., Berk, D.R. et al. 2014a. Skin findings in Williams syndrome. *Am J Med Genet A 164A*, 2217–2225.

Kozel, B.A., Danback, J.R., Waxler, J.L. et al. 2014b. Williams syndrome predisposes to vascular stiffness modified by antihypertensive use and copy number changes in NCF1. *Hypertension 63*, 74–79.

Kozel, B.A., Knutsen, R.H., Ye, L., Ciliberto, C.H., Broekelmann, T.J., and Mecham, R.P. 2011. Genetic modifiers of cardiovascular phenotype caused by elastin haploinsufficiency act by extrinsic noncomplementation. *J Biol Chem 286*, 44926–44936.

Kozel, B.A., Su, C.T., Danback, J.R. et al. 2014c. Biomechanical properties of the skin in cutis laxa. *J Invest Dermatol 134*, 2836–2838.

Kurosawa, K., Matsumura, J.S., and Yamanouchi, D. 2013. Current status of medical treatment for abdominal aortic aneurysm. *Circ J 77*, 2860–2866.

Lacro, R.V., Dietz, H.C., Sleeper, L.A. et al. 2014. Atenolol versus losartan in children and young adults with Marfan's syndrome. *N Engl J Med 371*, 2061–2071.

Lagente, V. and Boichot, E. 2010. Role of matrix metalloproteinases in the inflammatory process of respiratory diseases. *J Mol Cell Cardiol 48*, 440–444.

Lebwohl, M., Schwartz, E., Lemlich, G., Lovelace, O., Shaikh-Bahai, F., and Fleischmajer, R. 1993. Abnormalities of connective tissue components in lesional and non-lesional tissue of patients with pseudoxanthoma elasticum. *Arch Dermatol Res 285*, 121–126.

Ledoux, M., Beauchet, A., Fermanian, C., Boileau, C., Jondeau, G., and Saiag, P. 2011. A case-control study of cutaneous signs in adult patients with Marfan disease: Diagnostic value of striae. *J Am Acad Dermatol 64*, 290–295.

Leftheriotis, G., Omarjee, L., Le Saux, O. et al. 2013. The vascular phenotype in Pseudoxanthoma elasticum and related disorders: Contribution of a genetic disease to the understanding of vascular calcification. *Front Genet 4*, 4.

Le Quement, C., Guenon, I., Gillon, J.Y. et al. 2008. The selective MMP-12 inhibitor, AS111793 reduces airway inflammation in mice exposed to cigarette smoke. *Br J Pharmacol 154*, 1206–1215.

Leung, D.Y., Glagov, S., and Mathews, M.B. 1977. Elastin and collagen accumulation in rabbit ascending aorta and pulmonary trunk during postnatal growth. Correlation of cellular synthetic response with medial tension. *Circ Res 41*, 316–323.

Li, D.Y., Brooke, B., Davis, E.C. et al. 1998a. Elastin is an essential determinant of arterial morphogenesis. *Nature 393*, 276–280.

Li, D.Y., Faury, G., Taylor, D.G. et al. 1998b. Novel arterial pathology in mice and humans hemizygous for elastin. *J Clin Invest 102*, 1783–1787.

Li, Q., Brodsky, J.L., Conlin, L.K. et al. 2014. Mutations in the ABCC6 gene as a cause of generalized arterial calcification of infancy: Genotypic overlap with pseudoxanthoma elasticum. *J Invest Dermatol 134*, 658–665.

Li, Q. and Uitto, J. 2012. Heritable ectopic mineralization disorders: The paradigm of pseudoxanthoma elasticum. *J Invest Dermatol 132*, E15–E19.

Lipton, R.A., Greenwald, R.A., and Seriff, N.S. 1971. Pneumothorax and bilateral honeycombed lung in Marfan syndrome. Report of a case and review of the pulmonary abnormalities in this disorder. *Am Rev Respir Dis 104*, 924–928.

Loeys, B., Van Maldergem, L., Mortier, G. et al. 2002. Homozygosity for a missense mutation in fibulin-5 (FBLN5) results in a severe form of cutis laxa. *Hum Mol Genet 11*, 2113–2118.

Loeys, B.L., Dietz, H.C., Braverman, A.C. et al. 2010a. The revised Ghent nosology for the Marfan syndrome. *J Med Genet 47*, 476–485.

Loeys, B.L., Gerber, E.E., Riegert-Johnson, D. et al. 2010b. Mutations in fibrillin-1 cause congenital scleroderma: Stiff skin syndrome. *Sci Transl Med 2*, 23ra20.

Lomas, A.C., Mellody, K.T., Freeman, L.J., Bax, D.V., Shuttleworth, C.A., and Kielty, C.M. 2007. Fibulin-5 binds human smooth-muscle cells through alpha5beta1 and alpha4beta1 integrins, but does not support receptor activation. *Biochem J 405*, 417–428.

Longo, G.M., Xiong, W., Greiner, T.C., Zhao, Y., Fiotti, N., and Baxter, B.T. 2002. Matrix metalloproteinases 2 and 9 work in concert to produce aortic aneurysms. *J Clin Invest 110*, 625–632.

Lopez-Candales, A., Holmes, D.R., Liao, S., Scott, M.J., Wickline, S.A., and Thompson, R.W. 1997. Decreased vascular smooth muscle cell density in medial degeneration of human abdominal aortic aneurysms. *Am J Pathol 150*, 993–1007.

McGarry Houghton, A. 2015. Matrix metalloproteinases in destructive lung disease. *Matrix Biol 44–46C*, 167–174.

McLaughlin, P.J., Chen, Q., Horiguchi, M. et al. 2006. Targeted disruption of fibulin-4 abolishes elastogenesis and causes perinatal lethality in mice. *Mol Cell Biol 26*, 1700–1709.

Malfait, F. and De Paepe, A. 2014. The Ehlers-Danlos syndrome. *Adv Exp Med Biol 802*, 129–143.

Manning, M.W., Cassi, L.A., Huang, J., Szilvassy, S.J., and Daugherty, A. 2002. Abdominal aortic aneurysms: Fresh insights from a novel animal model of the disease. *Vasc Med 7*, 45–54.

Markova, D., Zou, Y., Ringpfeil, F. et al. 2003. Genetic heterogeneity of cutis laxa: A heterozygous tandem duplication within the fibulin-5 (FBLN5) gene. *Am J Hum Genet 72*, 998–1004.

Matsuta, M., Izaki, S., Ide, C., and Izaki, M. 1987. Light and electron microscopic immunohistochemistry of solar elastosis: A study with cutis rhomboidalis nuchae. *J Dermatol 14*, 364–374.

Matt, P., Schoenhoff, F., Habashi, J. et al. 2009. Circulating transforming growth factor-beta in Marfan syndrome. *Circulation 120*, 526–532.

Merla, G., Brunetti-Pierri, N., Micale, L., and Fusco, C. 2010. Copy number variants at Williams-Beuren syndrome 7q11.23 region. *Hum Genet 128*, 3–26.

Merla, G., Brunetti-Pierri, N., Piccolo, P., Micale, L., and Loviglio, M.N. 2012. Supravalvular aortic stenosis: Elastin arteriopathy. *Circ Cardiovasc Genet 5*, 692–696.

Milleron, O., Arnoult, F., Ropers, J. et al. 2015. Marfan Sartan: A randomized, double-blind, placebo-controlled trial. *Eur Heart J 36*, 2160–2166.

Mitchell, G.F. 2008. Effects of central arterial aging on the structure and function of the peripheral vasculature: Implications for end-organ damage. *J Appl Physiol* (1985) *105*, 1652–1660.

Miura, T. 2015. Models of lung branching morphogenesis. *J Biochem 157*, 121–127.

Morales, J., Al-Sharif, L., Khalil, D.S. et al. 2009. Homozygous mutations in ADAMTS10 and ADAMTS17 cause lenticular myopia, ectopia lentis, glaucoma, spherophakia, and short stature. *Am J Hum Genet 85*, 558–568.

Nakamura, T., Lozano, P.R., Ikeda, Y. et al. 2002. Fibulin-5/DANCE is essential for elastogenesis in vivo. *Nature 415*, 171–175.

Narooie-Nejad, M., Paylakhi, S.H., Shojaee, S. et al. 2009. Loss of function mutations in the gene encoding latent transforming growth factor beta binding protein 2, LTBP2, cause primary congenital glaucoma. *Hum Mol Genet 18*, 3969–3977.

Negrini, D. and Moriondo, A. 2013. Pleural function and lymphatics. *Acta Physiol 207*, 244–259.

Neptune, E.R., Frischmeyer, P.A., Arking, D.E. et al. 2003. Dysregulation of TGF-beta activation contributes to pathogenesis in Marfan syndrome. *Nat Genet 33*, 407–411.

Nistala, H., Lee-Arteaga, S., Smaldone, S. et al. 2010a. Fibrillin-1 and -2 differentially modulate endogenous TGF-beta and BMP bioavailability during bone formation. *J Cell Biol 190*, 1107–1121.

Nistala, H., Lee-Arteaga, S., Smaldone, S., Siciliano, G., and Ramirez, F. 2010b. Extracellular microfibrils control osteoblast-supported osteoclastogenesis by restricting TGF{beta} stimulation of RANKL production. *J Biol Chem 285*, 34126–34133.

Nitschke, Y., Baujat, G., Botschen, U. et al. 2012. Generalized arterial calcification of infancy and pseudoxanthoma elasticum can be caused by mutations in either ENPP1 or ABCC6. *Am J Hum Genet 90*, 25–39.

Nitschke, Y. and Rutsch, F. 2012. Generalized arterial calcification of infancy and pseudoxanthoma elasticum: Two sides of the same coin. *Front Genet 3*, 302.

Noda, K., Dabovic, B., Takagi, K. et al. 2013. Latent TGF-beta binding protein 4 promotes elastic fiber assembly by interacting with fibulin-5. *Proc Natl Acad Sci USA 110*, 2852–2857.

O'Rourke, M.F., Blazek, J.V., Morreels, C.L., Jr., and Krovetz, L.J. 1968. Pressure wave transmission along the human aorta. Changes with age and in arterial degenerative disease. *Circ Res 23*, 567–579.

Paladini, D., Di Spiezio Sardo, A., Mandato, V.D. et al. 2007. Association of cutis laxa and genital prolapse: A case report. *Int Urogynecol J Pelvic Floor Dysfunct 18*, 1367–1370.

Papke, C.L. and Yanagisawa, H. 2014. Fibulin-4 and fibulin-5 in elastogenesis and beyond: Insights from mouse and human studies. *Matrix Biol 37*, 142–149.

Parrott, A., James, J., Goldenberg, P. et al. 2015. Aortopathy in the 7q11.23 microduplication syndrome. *Am J Med Genet A 167A*, 363–370.

Pasquali-Ronchetti, I., Garcia-Fernandez, M.I., Boraldi, F. et al. 2006. Oxidative stress in fibroblasts from patients with pseudoxanthoma elasticum: Possible role in the pathogenesis of clinical manifestations. *J Pathol 208*, 54–61.

Pearson, A.C., Guo, R., Orsinelli, D.A., Binkley, P.F., and Pasierski, T.J. 1994. Transesophageal echocardiographic assessment of the effects of age, gender, and hypertension on thoracic aortic wall size, thickness, and stiffness. *Am Heart J 128*, 344–351.

Pees, C., Laccone, F., Hagl, M., Debrauwer, V., Moser, E., and Michel-Behnke, I. 2013. Usefulness of losartan on the size of the ascending aorta in an unselected cohort of children, adolescents, and young adults with Marfan syndrome. *Am J Cardiol 112*, 1477–1483.

Pereira, L., Lee, S.Y., Gayraud, B. et al. 1999. Pathogenetic sequence for aneurysm revealed in mice underexpressing fibrillin-1. *Proc Natl Acad Sci USA 96*, 3819–3823.

Pierce, R.A., Joyce, B., Officer, S. et al. 2007. Retinoids increase lung elastin expression but fail to alter morphology or angiogenesis genes in premature ventilated baboons. *Pediatr Res 61*, 703–709.

Pober, B.R. 2010. Williams-Beuren syndrome. *N Engl J Med 362*, 239–252.

Pober, B.R., Johnson, M., and Urban, Z. 2008. Mechanisms and treatment of cardiovascular disease in Williams-Beuren syndrome. *J Clin Invest 118*, 1606–1615.

Prodoehl, M.J., Hatzirodos, N., Irving-Rodgers, H.F. et al. 2009. Genetic and gene expression analyses of the polycystic ovary syndrome candidate gene fibrillin-3 and other fibrillin family members in human ovaries. *Mol Hum Reprod 15*, 829–841.

Psaltis, P.J., Puranik, A.S., Spoon, D.B. et al. 2014. Characterization of a resident population of adventitial macrophage progenitor cells in postnatal vasculature. *Circ Res 115*, 364–375.

Psaltis, P.J. and Simari, R.D. 2015. Vascular wall progenitor cells in health and disease. *Circ Res 116*, 1392–1412.

Rajeshkannan, R., Kulkarni, C., Kappanayil, M. et al. 2014. Imaging findings in a distinct lethal inherited arteriopathy syndrome associated with a novel mutation in the FBLN4 gene. *Eur Radiol 24*, 1742–1748.

Ramirez, F. and Rifkin, D.B. 2009. Extracellular microfibrils: Contextual platforms for TGFbeta and BMP signaling. *Curr Opin Cell Biol 21*, 616–622.

Ratnapriya, R., Zhan, X., Fariss, R.N. et al. 2014. Rare and common variants in extracellular matrix gene Fibrillin 2 (FBN2) are associated with macular degeneration. *Hum Mol Genet 23*, 5827–5837.

Raza, S.L., Nehring, L.C., Shapiro, S.D., and Cornelius, L.A. 2000. Proteinase-activated receptor-1 regulation of macrophage elastase (MMP-12) secretion by serine proteinases. *J Biol Chem 275*, 41243–41250.

Rijken, F. and Bruijnzeel, P.L. 2009. The pathogenesis of photoaging: The role of neutrophils and neutrophil-derived enzymes. *J Investig Dermatol Symp Proc 14*, 67–72.

Robert, L., Robert, A.M., and Fulop, T. 2008. Rapid increase in human life expectancy: Will it soon be limited by the aging of elastin? *Biogerontology 9*, 119–133.

Robertson, I., Jensen, S., and Handford, P. 2010. TB domain proteins: Evolutionary insights into the multifaceted roles of fibrillins and LTBPs. *Biochem J 433*, 263–276.

Robinson, P.N., Arteaga-Solis, E., Baldock, C. et al. 2006. The molecular genetics of Marfan syndrome and related disorders. *J Med Genet 43*, 769–787.

Saharinen, J., Taipale, J., and Keski-Oja, J. 1996. Association of the small latent transforming growth factor-beta with an eight cysteine repeat of its binding protein LTBP-1. *EMBO J 15*, 245–253.

Sander, C.S., Chang, H., Salzmann, S. et al. 2002. Photoaging is associated with protein oxidation in human skin in vivo. *J Invest Dermatol 118*, 618–625.

Saratzis, A. and Bown, M.J. 2014. The genetic basis for aortic aneurysmal disease. *Heart 100*, 916–922.

Sawyer, S.L., Dicke, F., Kirton, A. et al. 2013. Longer term survival of a child with autosomal recessive cutis laxa due to a mutation in FBLN4. *Am J Med Genet A 161A*, 1148–1153.

Schrijver, I., Liu, W., Brenn, T., Furthmayr, H., and Francke, U. 1999. Cysteine substitutions in epidermal growth factor-like domains of fibrillin-1: Distinct effects on biochemical and clinical phenotypes. *Am J Hum Genet 65*, 1007–1020.

Sengle, G., Charbonneau, N.L., Ono, R.N. et al. 2008. Targeting of bone morphogenetic protein growth factor complexes to fibrillin. *J Biol Chem 283*, 13874–13888.

Shah, M.H., Bhat, V., Shetty, J.S., and Kumar, A. 2014. Whole exome sequencing identifies a novel splice-site mutation in ADAMTS17 in an Indian family with Weill-Marchesani syndrome. *Mol Vis 20*, 790–796.

Shapiro, S.D., Endicott, S.K., Province, M.A., Pierce, J.A., and Campbell, E.J. 1991. Marked longevity of human lung parenchymal elastic fibers deduced from prevalence of D-aspartate and nuclear weapons-related radiocarbon. *J Clin Invest 87*, 1828–1834.

Sherratt, M.J. 2009. Tissue elasticity and the ageing elastic fibre. *Age 31*, 305–325.

Shifren, A., Durmowicz, A.G., Knutsen, R.H., Hirano, E., and Mecham, R.P. 2007. Elastin protein levels are a vital modifier affecting normal lung development and susceptibility to emphysema. *Am J Physiol Lung Cell Mol Physiol 292*, L778–L787.

Shimizu, K., Mitchell, R.N., and Libby, P. 2006. Inflammation and cellular immune responses in abdominal aortic aneurysms. *Arterioscler Thromb Vasc Biol 26*, 987–994.

Shores, J., Berger, K.R., Murphy, E.A., and Pyeritz, R.E. 1994. Progression of aortic dilatation and the benefit of long-term beta-adrenergic blockade in Marfan's syndrome. *N Engl J Med 330*, 1335–1341.

Starcher, B. and Conrad, M. 1995. A role for neutrophil elastase in the progression of solar elastosis. *Connect Tissue Res 31*, 133–140.

Stenmark, K.R., Yeager, M.E., El Kasmi, K.C. et al. 2013. The adventitia: Essential regulator of vascular wall structure and function. *Annu Rev Physiol 75*, 23–47.

Sterner-Kock, A., Thorey, I.S., Koli, K. et al. 2002. Disruption of the gene encoding the latent transforming growth factor-beta binding protein 4 (LTBP-4) causes abnormal lung development, cardiomyopathy, and colorectal cancer. *Genes Dev 16*, 2264–2273.

Sternlicht, M.D. and Werb, Z. 2001. How matrix metalloproteinases regulate cell behavior. *Annu Rev Cell Dev Biol 17*, 463–516.

Su, C.T., Huang, J.W., Chiang, C.K. et al. 2015. Latent transforming growth factor binding protein 4 regulates transforming growth factor beta receptor stability. *Hum Mol Genet 24*, 4024–4036.

Sugitani, H., Hirano, E., Knutsen, R.H. et al. 2012. Alternative splicing and tissue-specific elastin misassembly act as biological modifiers of human elastin gene frameshift mutations associated with dominant cutis laxa. *J Biol Chem 287*, 22055–22067.

Suki, B. and Bates, J.H. 2008. Extracellular matrix mechanics in lung parenchymal diseases. *Respir Physiol Neurobiol 163*, 33–43.

Summers, K.M., Nataatmadja, M., Xu, D. et al. 2005. Histopathology and fibrillin-1 distribution in severe early onset Marfan syndrome. *American J Med Genet A 139*, 2–8.

Suzuki, T., Akiba, T., Miyake, R., Marushima, H., and Morikawa, T. 2010. Familial spontaneous pneumothorax in two adult siblings with Marfan syndrome. *Ann Thorac Cardiovasc Surg 16*, 362–364.

Szabo, Z., Crepeau, M.W., Mitchell, A.L. et al. 2006. Aortic aneurysmal disease and cutis laxa caused by defects in the elastin gene. *J Med Genet 43*, 255–258.

Takeda, N., Morita, H., Fujita, D. et al. 2015. Congenital contractural arachnodactyly complicated with aortic dilatation and dissection: Case report and review of literature. *Am J Med Genet A 167*, 2382–2387.

Tassabehji, M., Metcalfe, K., Hurst, J. et al. 1998. An elastin gene mutation producing abnormal tropoelastin and abnormal elastic fibres in a patient with autosomal dominant cutis laxa. *Hum Mol Genet 7*, 1021–1028.

Teoh, P.C. 1977. Bronchiectasis and spontaneous pneumothorax in Marfan's syndrome. *Chest 72*, 672–673.

Thompson, R.W., Curci, J.A., Ennis, T.L., Mao, D., Pagano, M.B., and Pham, C.T. 2006. Pathophysiology of abdominal aortic aneurysms: Insights from the elastase-induced model in mice with different genetic backgrounds. *Ann N Y Acad Sci 1085*, 59–73.

Todorovic, V. and Rifkin, D.B. 2012. LTBPs, more than just an escort service. *J Cell Biochem 113*, 410–418.

Toshima, M., Ohtani, Y., and Ohtani, O. 2004. Three-dimensional architecture of elastin and collagen fiber networks in the human and rat lung. *Arch Histol Cytol 67*, 31–40.

Tsuji, T. 1984. The surface structural alterations of elastic fibers and elastotic material in solar elastosis: A scanning electron microscopic study. *J Cutan Pathol 11*, 300–308.

Turino, G.M., Seniorrm, Garg, B.D., Keller, S., Levi, M.M., and Mandl, I. 1969. Serum elastase inhibitor deficiency and alpha 1-antitrypsin deficiency in patients with obstructive emphysema. *Science 165*, 709–711.

Uitto, J., Li, Q., and Urban, Z. 2013. The complexity of elastic fibre biogenesis in the skin—A perspective to the clinical heterogeneity of cutis laxa. *Exp Dermatol 22*, 88–92.

Uitto, J., Pulkkinen, L., and Ringpfeil, F. 2001. Molecular genetics of pseudoxanthoma elasticum: A metabolic disorder at the environment-genome interface? *Trends Mol Med 7*, 13–17.

Urban, Z. and Davis, E.C. 2014. Cutis laxa: Intersection of elastic fiber biogenesis, TGFbeta signaling, the secretory pathway and metabolism. *Matrix Biol 33*, 16–22.

Urban, Z., Gao, J., Pope, F.M., and Davis, E.C. 2005. Autosomal dominant cutis laxa with severe lung disease: Synthesis and matrix deposition of mutant tropoelastin. *J Invest Dermatol 124*, 1193–1199.

Urban, Z., Hucthagowder, V., Schurmann, N. et al. 2009. Mutations in LTBP4 cause a syndrome of impaired pulmonary, gastrointestinal, genitourinary, musculoskeletal, and dermal development. *Am J Hum Genet 85*, 593–605.

Urban, Z., Peyrol, S., Plauchu, H. et al. 2000. Elastin gene deletions in Williams syndrome patients result in altered deposition of elastic fibers in skin and a subclinical dermal phenotype. *Pediatr Dermatol 17*, 12–20.

Urbanek, M., Sam, S., Legro, R.S., and Dunaif, A. 2007. Identification of a polycystic ovary syndrome susceptibility variant in fibrillin-3 and association with a metabolic phenotype. *J Clin Endocrinol Metab 92*, 4191–4198.

Viveiro, C., Rocha, P., Carvalho, C., and Zarcos, M.M. 2013. Spontaneous pneumothorax as manifestation of Marfan syndrome. *BMJ Case Rep. 2013.*

Vollbrandt, T., Tiedemann, K., El-Hallous, E. et al. 2004. Consequences of cysteine mutations in calcium-binding epidermal growth factor modules of fibrillin-1. *J Biol Chem 279*, 32924–32931.

Wagenseil, J.E. and Mecham, R.P. 2009. Vascular extracellular matrix and arterial mechanics. *Physiol Rev 89*, 957–989.

Wagenseil, J.E., Nerurkar, N.L., Knutsen, R.H., Okamoto, R.J., Li, D.Y., and Mecham, R.P. 2005. Effects of elastin haploinsufficiency on the mechanical behavior of mouse arteries. *Am J Physiol Heart Circ Physiol 289*, H1209–H1217.

Wan, E.S., Pober, B.R., Washko, G.R., Raby, B.A., and Silverman, E.K. 2010. Pulmonary function and emphysema in Williams-Beuren syndrome. *Am J Med Genet A 152A*, 653–656.

Wang, Y., Ait-Oufella, H., Herbin, O. et al. 2010. TGF-beta activity protects against inflammatory aortic aneurysm progression and complications in angiotensin II-infused mice. *J Clin Invest 120*, 422–432.

Wang, Y., Krishna, S., and Golledge, J. 2013a. The calcium chloride-induced rodent model of abdominal aortic aneurysm. *Atherosclerosis 226*, 29–39.

Wang, Y., Krishna, S., Walker, P.J., Norman, P., and Golledge, J. 2013b. Transforming growth factor-beta and abdominal aortic aneurysms. *Cardiovasc Pathol 22*, 126–132.

Watson, R.E., Griffiths, C.E., Craven, N.M., Shuttleworth, C.A., and Kielty, C.M. 1999. Fibrillin-rich microfibrils are reduced in photoaged skin. Distribution at the dermal-epidermal junction. *J Invest Dermatol 112*, 782–787.

Wendel, D.P., Taylor, D.G., Albertine, K.H., Keating, M.T., and Li, D.Y. 2000. Impaired distal airway development in mice lacking elastin. *Am J Respir Cell Mol Biol 23*, 320–326.

Wewers, M.D. and Crystal, R.G. 2013. Alpha-1 antitrypsin augmentation therapy. *COPD 10(Suppl 1)*, 64–67.

Wheatley, H.M., Traboulsi, E.I., Flowers, B.E. et al. 1995. Immunohistochemical localization of fibrillin in human ocular tissues. Relevance to the Marfan syndrome. *Arch Ophthalmol 113*, 103–109.

Xie, X., Lu, H., Moorleghen, J.J. et al. 2012. Doxycycline does not influence established abdominal aortic aneurysms in angiotensin II-infused mice. *PLoS one 7*, e46411.

Yanagisawa, H., Davis, E.C., Starcher, B.C. et al. 2002. Fibulin-5 is an elastin-binding protein essential for elastic fibre development in vivo. *Nature 415*, 168–171.

Zarate, Y.A., Lepard, T., Sellars, E. et al. 2014. Cardiovascular and genitourinary anomalies in patients with duplications within the Williams syndrome critical region: Phenotypic expansion and review of the literature. *Am J Med Genet A 164A*, 1998–2002.

Zilberberg, L., Todorovic, V., Dabovic, B. et al. 2012. Specificity of latent TGF-beta binding protein (LTBP) incorporation into matrix: Role of fibrillins and fibronectin. *J Cell Physiol 227*, 3828–3836.

CHAPTER 3

Synthetic-Elastin Systems

Richard Wang, Suzanne M. Mithieux,
Jazmin Ozsvar, and Anthony S. Weiss

CONTENTS

3.1 INTRODUCTION

The mammalian extracellular matrix (ECM) constitutes a complex array of different proteins, proteoglycans, and glycosaminoglycans (GAGs). Of these, perhaps the most durable element is the mature elastic fiber. Elastin is found in various tissues, including the vasculature, skin, and lungs (Giro et al. 1985, McGowan et al. 1997, Uitto et al. 1976), and is essential for providing elasticity and resilience to biological tissues. Moreover, among many other proteins that constitute the immediate environment surrounding cells, elastin plays important signaling roles that modulate cell activity.

In terms of tissue regeneration, elastin and elastin-derived materials have shown great potential in emulating ECM structure and function, incorporating important properties into biologically interfacing constructs such as elasticity or cell adhesion sites. In particular, when combined with integrative design strategies, elastin-based materials can offer new avenues of tailored constructs specific for contextual applications.

This chapter offers a brief introduction to natural and synthetic elastin, and then focuses on the engineering and application of different synthetic-elastin-based biomaterials for tissue regeneration and repair.

3.2 STRUCTURE OF ELASTIN AND TROPOELASTIN

Elastin is an insoluble biopolymer composed of the soluble monomer tropoelastin that is expressed as an ~60–70 kDa protein by elastogenic cells, including smooth muscle cells, endothelial cells, and fibroblasts (Debelle and Tamburro 1999, Pasquali-Ronchetti et al. 1993). Elastic fiber synthesis is the highest during early development, especially in the late fetal and early neonatal stages (Parks et al. 1988, Swee et al. 1995), and is almost completely repressed in adulthood; elevation of elastin synthesis in adults generally follows tissue injury where elastin fragments released by damaged ECM signals the upregulation of tropoelastin production (Duca et al. 2004).

A distinguishing feature of the tropoelastin amino acid sequence is alternating hydrophobic and hydrophilic domains (Indik et al. 1987) with hydrophobic residues accounting for over 80% of the primary sequence (Debelle et al. 1998). The hydrophobic domains constitute nonpolar amino acids such as glycine, valine, proline, and leucine (Rodrıguez-Cabello et al. 1999), and the hydrophilic domains are rich in lysine and alanine residues, of which lysine is essential for cross-linking (Wise et al. 2005).

Structurally, tropoelastin is an asymmetric protein monomer with distinct functional domains separated by a mechanically coupling bridge region (Baldock et al. 2011) (Figure 3.1). The bridge and hinge regions contribute to conformational flexibility and structural alignment during assembly (Muiznieks et al. 2003, Wise et al. 2014). A coil region accounts for the majority of the elasticity of tropoelastin (Holst et al. 2010); stretch and relaxation profiles of tropoelastin exhibit ideal elastic behavior with minimal energy loss (Baldock et al. 2011). The N-terminus is also thought to contribute to tropoelastin cross-linking and fiber assembly (Wise et al. 2014).

One of the most functionally significant regions is the C-terminus. This region terminates with a positively charged Arginine-Lysine-Arginine-Lysine (RKRK) sequence and contains the only two cysteine residues in the entire molecule that form an intramolecular disulfide bond (Brown et al. 1992). Both of these regions have functional significance; removal

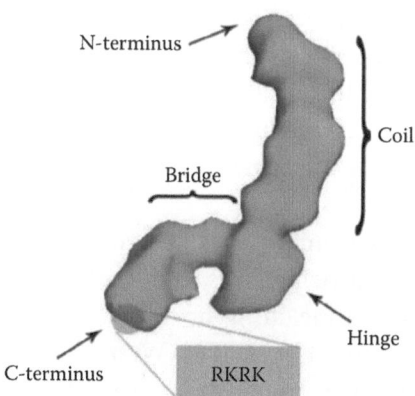

FIGURE 3.1   Schematic representation of a tropoelastin monomer depicting the most important functional regions of the structure. The N-terminus may play important roles in tropoelastin cross-linking and elastin assembly. The Coil region accounts for the majority of tropoelastin's elasticity with the Bridge and Hinge regions contributing to structural conformational flexibility. The C-terminus, particularly the terminal RKRK sequence, is essential for cell interactions. (Adapted with permission from Wise, S.G. et al., *Acta Biomater.*, 10, 1532, 2004.)

of the C-terminus or disruption of the disulfide bond severely debilitates tropoelastin from essential assembling processes, such as deposition onto the ECM or incorporation into fibers, presumably due to loss of integrin and/or GAG interactions (Brown et al. 1992, Kozel et al. 2003).

3.3 TYPES OF SYNTHETIC-ELASTIN SYSTEMS

As elastin is insoluble in a range of solvents, it is very difficult to extract from biological systems. Similarly, the isolation of tropoelastin is inherently difficult due to the rapidity at which elastogenesis occurs (in the order of hours), consequently limiting the opportunity to extract it before it is incorporated into the growing insoluble elastic fiber (Clarke et al. 2006, Vrhovski and Weiss 1998). Therefore, using synthetic alternatives to human elastin have been explored. The two main categories of synthetic-elastin-based systems discussed in this context include solubilized animal-derived elastin and recombinant human tropoelastin.

3.3.1 Animal-Derived Elastin

The human elastin amino acid sequence exhibits more than 70% similarity (Figure 3.2) to a variety of vertebrate mammals including baboon (*Papio hamadryas*), cat (*Felis catus*), dog (*Canis familiaris*), and pig (*Sus scrofa*) (Piontkivska et al. 2004). However, the most important functional features, such as the RKRK sequence in the C-terminus, are strictly conserved in classical tropoelastin across different species (Chung et al. 2006). Because of this interspecies conservation of important functional structures, animal sources of solubilized elastin have been used to address the difficulty in attaining adequate quantities of human tropoelastin for study and research.

Multiple isoforms of animal-derived tropoelastin have been identified from a variety of elastin-rich tissues, such as ligaments or the aorta, in different animal sources including bovine, ovine, porcine, and equine (Davidson et al. 1984, Foster et al. 1981, Wrenn et al. 1987). Isolating the animal-derived tropoelastin protein monomer, however, generally requires inhibiting the natural cross-linking process involving lysyl oxidase (LOX), which requires copper ions for correct function (Lucero and Kagan 2006). This is often achieved through administering a copper-deficient diet to animals (Mecham and Foster 1979) or using a chemical inhibitor; however, both methods are highly inefficient and ethically questionable.

Other research has explored the chemical treatment of animal-derived elastin to form synthetic soluble elastin. This class of materials includes

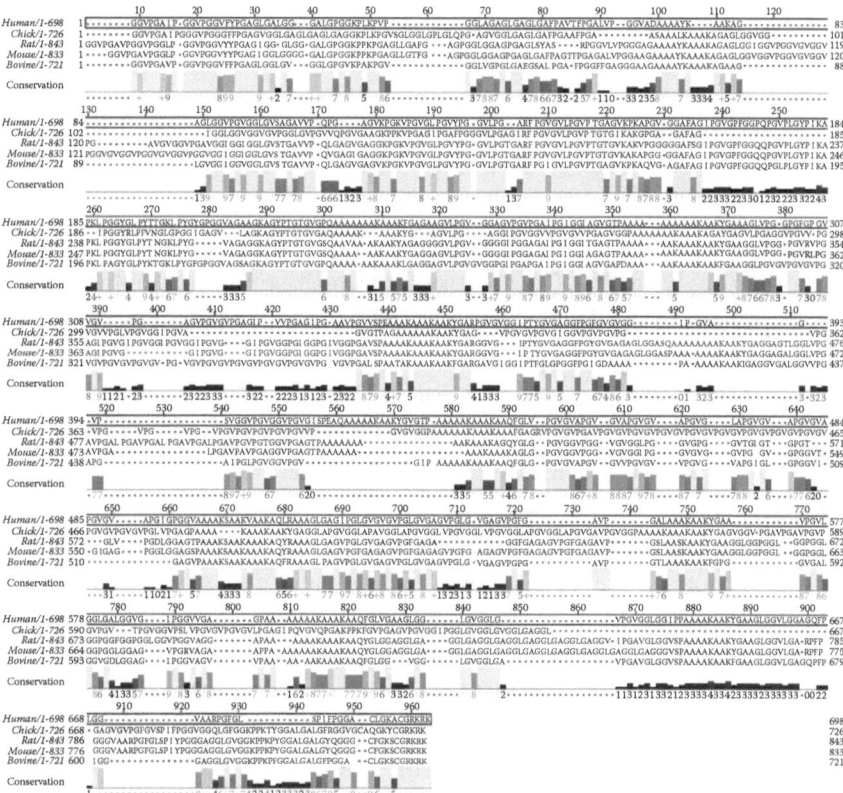

FIGURE 3.2 Alignment and comparison of elastin protein (ELN gene) amino acid sequence across five mammalian species: human (*Homo sapiens*, accession AAC98394), cow (*Bos taurus*, isoform 1, accession P04985-1), mouse (*Mus musculus*, accession P54320), rat (*Rattus norvegicus*, isoform 1, accession Q99372-1), and chick (*Gallus gallus*, isoform 1, accession P07916-1). Sequences were retrieved from GenBank and UniProt searches and aligned using Clustal Omega. The amount of conservation across all species is displayed below each amino acid. The signal sequence was removed from all sequences as it is not present in the final form of the functional protein. Numbers represent quantitative alignment annotations calculated based on the Analysis of Multiply Aligned Sequences (AMAS) method of multiple sequence alignment analysis (Livingstone and Barton 1993). * indicates conserved columns with default amino acid property grouping: score of 11. + indicates columns with mutations where all properties are conserved: score of 10.

α-elastin (an oxalic-acid-solubilized derivative of elastin) and κ-elastin (animal-derived elastin that is solubilized with potassium hydroxide) that demonstrate functional similarities to the free monomer tropoelastin, such as the ability to coacervate (Cox et al. 1973, Debelle et al. 1995, 1998).

However, there are still remaining drawbacks, for example, α-elastin inherently contains a low number of lysine residues that impact amine-based cross-linking and, subsequently, the mechanical properties of α-elastin-based scaffolds (Annabi et al. 2009b).

3.3.2 Recombinant Human Tropoelastin

An alternative substitute for native tropoelastin has been generated through expressing the human DNA sequence for tropoelastin in recombinant bacterial systems such as *Escherichia coli* (Indik et al. 1990). Despite the high-purity end product resulting from this manufacturing procedure, the initial average yield of 2–4 mg/L of bacterial culture was ultimately a limitation. Codon optimization, by employing a highly expressing synthetic recombinant counterpart of the human tropoelastin gene in *E. coli*, improved fermentation and drastically increased yields of highly purified recombinant tropoelastin (more than 30 mg/L of bacterial culture) (Martin et al. 1995).

This recombinant tropoelastin is functionally and structurally similar to native tropoelastin in that it can be incorporated into elastic fibers by mammalian cells (Stone et al. 2001) and cross-linked both enzymatically and chemically *in vitro* (Mithieux et al. 2005, Wise et al. 2005). The increased access to tropoelastin has helped to improve our understanding of the protein's structural, functional, and assembly properties. Furthermore, this monomeric form of elastin provides newfound opportunities to build biomimics of natural elastic tissues.

3.4 SYNTHETIC-ELASTIN BIOMATERIALS

The availability and usage of natural tropoelastin analogs has given rise to exciting new classes of materials especially in the biomedical and clinical context. Moreover, the fabrication of hybrid synthetic-elastin-based systems has also become more achievable: in this context, *hybrid* represents any biomaterial composed of more than one base material. The following sections particularly emphasize the three main domains of synthetic-elastin-based biomaterial research, namely hydrogels, electrospinning, and material coatings.

3.4.1 Synthetic-Elastin Hydrogels

3.4.1.1 *Principles*

Hydrogels are classically described as water-saturated polymeric networks comprising cross-linked hydrophilic monomers. Modulating the polymer concentration and methods of synthesis allows tuning of specific hydrogel properties such as porosity, stiffness, swelling behavior, and biodegradability. This flexibility has led to increasing interest in utilizing hydrogels for biological applications, ranging from drug delivery to supporting tissue regeneration and remodeling (Gauvin et al. 2012). Hydrogel scaffolds can additionally be preseeded with cells or bioactive molecules, such as growth factors and drugs, to facilitate cellular activity and signaling within biological systems.

In designing materials and scaffolds for the purposes of ECM regeneration, it is intuitive to consider proteins that are native to the *in vivo* tissue matrix as a construction material. Although there has been much research on developing ECM substitutes from synthetic polymers, the purification and production of recombinant human tropoelastin particularly advocates synthetic-elastin-based systems that are more comparable to native ECM.

3.4.1.2 Synthetic-Elastin-Based Hydrogels and Cross-Linking Options

Hydrogel synthesis is partly analogous to elastogenesis in that both require cross-linking of monomers; in the case of elastogenesis, this involves LOX-driven cross-linking of tropoelastin (Figure 3.3). However, for the purposes of engineering, synthetic-elastin-based materials, alternative methods of cross-linking tropoelastin, that utilize and modify the epsilon amino groups of resident lysines, have been explored including glutaraldehyde (GA) (Annabi et al. 2009a), 1-ethyl-3-(3-dimethylaminopropyl) carbodiimide (EDC) with N-hydroxysuccinimide (NHS) (Hafemann et al. 2001), genipin (GP) (Vieth et al. 2007), pyrroloquinoline quinone (PQQ) (Bellingham et al. 2003), bis(sulfosuccinimidyl) suberate (BS3) (Mithieux et al. 2004), ethylene glycol diglycidyl ether (EGDE) (Leach et al. 2005), pH-dependent cross-linker-free polymerization (Mithieux et al. 2009), and methacrylation-activated photo-cross-linking (Annabi et al. 2013).

GA has long been presented as a protein biomaterial cross-linking agent (Richards and Knowles 1968). For α-elastin, GA demonstrated that increasing cross-linker concentration increased pore size by approximately 50% (Annabi et al. 2009c). Additionally, the conjunctional use of high-pressure CO_2 facilitated coacervation of α-elastin, accelerated cross-linking, and substantially enhanced pore interconnectivity compared to scaffolds fabricated at atmospheric pressure (Annabi et al. 2009c).

One of the problems of cross-linking with a bifunctional agent, such as GA, is the release of toxic products on degradation of the oligomer bridges formed during cross-linking (Grimm et al. 1992, Speer et al. 1980). Alternative cross-linking strategies, such as a combination of water-soluble

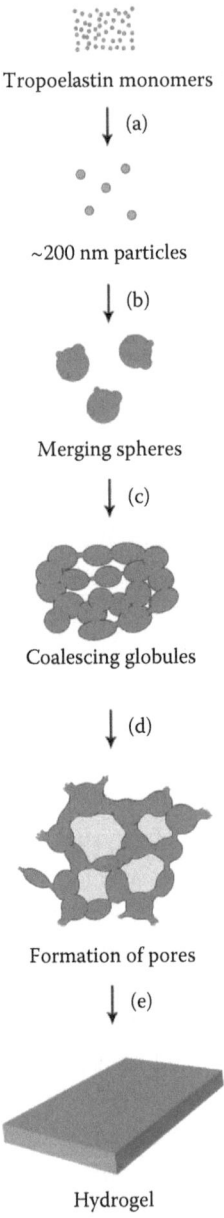

Tropoelastin monomers

(a)

~200 nm particles

(b)

Merging spheres

(c)

Coalescing globules

(d)

Formation of pores

(e)

Hydrogel

FIGURE 3.3 Schematic representation of the process of tropoelastin-based hydrogel formation. (a) The tropoelastin monomers form small spheres of approximately 200 nm in diameter. (b) The small spheres merge to form larger more stable micron-sized spheres. (c) The addition of chemical cross-linker facilitates coalescing globules that eventually (d) form networked pores, and (e) a hydrogel. (Adapted with permission from Tu, Y. et al., *Micron*, 41, 268, 2010.)

EDC mixed with NHS, may be employed instead. Compared to human split thickness grafts, xenogenic elastin/collagen membranes cross-linked in this way possessed a tensile strength that was significantly higher, approximately 12 MPa versus 5 MPa (Hafemann et al. 2001). The use of EDC additionally does not exhibit significant cytotoxicity (Park et al. 2002), highlighting a biocompatible alternative to bifunctional agents.

Similar to EDC, there are also other chemical cross-linkers that target the lysine residues in tropoelastin, emulating the *in vivo* cross-linking process. PQQ has been proposed as a cross-linker of lysine residues in elastin polypeptides in the presence of divalent copper (Shah et al. 1992). However, despite PQQ cross-linked scaffolds possessing similar mechanical properties to native elastin, it is also known to exhibit both beneficial and harmful effects on biological systems depending on the concentration of use (He et al. 2003). In light of this, GP has been proposed as an alternative cross-linking agent that demonstrates comparable cross-linking efficacy but reduced cytotoxicity (Nickerson et al. 2006). A study that compared PQQ and GP directly observed that GP cross-linked scaffolds possessed a Young's modulus closer to native elastin than PQQ cross-linked scaffolds (Vieth et al. 2007).

BS3 is another such chemical cross-linker that targets lysine residues of tropoelastin molecules (Snyder et al. 1987). Tropoelastin-based hydrogel fabrication using BS3 cross-linker demonstrated the ability to fabricate sponges, tubes, and sheets by employing a casting approach (Mithieux et al. 2004). These gels possessed Young's moduli ranging from 220 to 280 kPa compared to native elastin, typically 300–600 kPa (Mithieux and Weiss 2005). Furthermore, *in vivo* implantation of these scaffolds demonstrated fibroblast infiltration dependent on surface characteristics of the scaffolds; a smooth surface promoted monolayer growth, whereas an open-lattice surface allowed cellular infiltration followed by a slow breakdown of synthetic elastin (Mithieux et al. 2004). Ultimately, the elastin scaffolds were observed to be innocuous and well tolerated in an *in vivo* environment.

The need to scale up and commercialize elastin-based materials also brought relevance to using readily available materials such as α-elastin and diepoxy cross-linkers. For example, α-elastin hydrogels have been fabricated using EGDE cross-linker and alterations of pH conditions affected the degree of cross-linking; the inclusion of at least one alkaline step promoted higher extents of cross-linking and improved mechanical properties with elastic modulus reaching approximately 120 kPa (Leach et al. 2005). Ultimately, cross-linked α-elastin scaffolds were found to be mechanically fragile, compared to other elastin-based materials (Bellingham and Keeley 2004), and possessed an elastic modulus less than native elastin, hence limiting its biological application.

Other cross-linking strategies have also been explored, for example, targeting different cross-linking sites. Methacrylated human recombinant tropoelastin has been produced through the addition of methacrylate anhydride, which subsequently allowed the tropoelastin monomers to undergo cross-linking through UV radiation (Annabi et al. 2013). This MeTro gel (elastic modulus between 2.8 ± 0.6 kPa and 14.8 ± 1.9 kPa) was mechanically superior to other photo-cross-linked hydrogels, such as gelatin-based hydrogels, while supporting an average fibroblast and endothelial cell viability of over 92% measured across 7 days.

Alternative to chemical cross-linking, physical cross-linking avoids chemical cross-linker residues, resulting in a single-component biomaterial that shows comparable stability to that of chemically cross-linked tropoelastin in the presence of proteases. This presents distinct advantages such as uniformity of physical characteristics across the entire construct and simplification of *in vivo* interactions of the scaffold. Research into this area showed that under alkaline conditions, tropoelastin undergoes a sol–gel transition that leads to the formation of an irreversible hydrogel (Mithieux et al. 2009). Mechanically, the hydrogel formed under these conditions possessed a Young's modulus of 1.69 ± 0.04 MPa, which is comparable to native elastin.

3.4.1.3 Synthetic-Elastin-Based Hybrid Hydrogels

As the mechanical properties of hydrogels containing solely elastin or α-elastin are quite weak relative to the mechanical requirements of many *in vivo* tissues (Bellingham and Keeley 2004), their application in tissue regeneration or remodeling is limited. To address these shortcomings, there is increasing interest in hybrid or composite materials that combine the individual advantageous properties of different materials.

The addition of elastin imparts elasticity in composite with other materials in hybrid scaffolds, effectively decreasing energy loss and hysteresis (Annabi et al. 2011a) while also improving pore formation of relevant sizes to promote cellular growth and infiltration (Vasconcelos et al. 2012). The wide range of materials with which elastin may be combined offers much potential for tuning, both mechanically and structurally. Tropoelastin combined with α-elastin using high-pressure CO_2 during fabrication demonstrated that high-pressure gas enhanced compressive modulus and tensile strength by 2-fold and 2.5-fold, respectively, and promoted formation of larger pores in the hydrogel, supporting fibroblast infiltration, while tropoelastin/α-elastin ratios of 50/50 promoted structural preservation after swelling (Annabi et al. 2010). Additionally, the use of high-pressure CO_2 facilitated elastin penetration throughout poly(ε-caprolactone) (PCL) scaffolds, improving structural homogeneity (Annabi et al. 2011b). The physical cross-linking of tropoelastin to silk is another method for modification of mechanical properties, whereby increasing tropoelastin from 0% to 100% correlated to a Young's modulus ranging from 7.18 ± 2.61 to 2.11 ± 0.12 MPa, respectively (Hu et al. 2010).

In the context of structure and morphology, hybrid materials may be used to fabricate scaffolds that more closely resemble the complex architecture of natural tissues. A vascular graft constructed from multiple layers of type I collagen and elastic fibers purified from equine *ligamentum nuchae* demonstrated compatible suturability as well as ideal burst pressures of over 400 mmHg (Koens et al. 2010), which is above normal physiological blood pressures. Injectable hydrogels have also gained increasing attention for their potential of encapsulating cells, drugs, or growth factors while offering minimally invasive delivery methods. A study that incorporated α-elastin into a hybrid hydrogel with a copolymer, poly(N-isopropylacrylamide-*co*-polylactide-2-hydroxyethyl methacrylate-*co*-oligo(-ethylene glycol)monomethyl ether methacrylate) (PNIPAAm-*co*-PLA/HEMA) (synthesized inhouse), presented an interesting scaffold that was not only injectable through fine gauge needles but also cured *in situ* at 37°C in the absence of cross-linking reagents (Fathi et al. 2014). Most importantly, the physiochemical and gelation properties of this material can be finely tuned by altering the copolymer composition, while the ability to encapsulate cells provides potential clinical application such as dermal or cartilage regeneration.

Because of the emergence of different physical properties from elastin-based hybrid materials, the biological interface of these hydrogels is also affected and, in most cases, improved. The combination of silk and tropoelastin not only affects mechanical and morphological properties of scaffolds, but also electrical characteristics of the material. The combination of tropoelastin's net positive charge and silk's net negative charge in specific ratios enabled the attachment, proliferation, and formation of stable primary cortical neuronal networks, supporting optimal neuronal growth conditions (Hu et al. 2013). The surface topology and morphology of the constructs also exhibit dependence on the silk–tropoelastin ratio, significantly affecting human mesenchymal stem cell (hMSC) attachment and proliferation compared to pure silk or pure tropoelastin controls (Hu et al. 2010). Collectively, the effects of surface properties and mechanical elasticity also elicited different stem cell differentiation pathways; higher surface roughness was favored by hMSCs and facilitated osteogenic differentiation, whereas lower surface roughness promoted myoblast cell proliferation and myogenic differentiation (Hu et al. 2011). Synthetic-elastin-based hybrid constructs also favorably interface with other cell types, improving the range of potential clinical applications. The inclusion of α-elastin in PCL, for example, enabled primary articular cartilage chondrocyte attachment and proliferation, indicating potential utility in cartilage repair (Annabi et al. 2011a).

These studies have demonstrated that by combining synthetic elastomers with different copolymers in a hydrogel, the composite scaffold offers a high degree of tunability and customized properties ideal for a diverse range of tissue-specific regenerative applications.

3.4.2 Electrospun Materials

3.4.2.1 Principles

Electrospinning has proven to be a versatile tool in manufacturing fibrous scaffolds using synthetic and natural polymers to mimic the native ECM. In principle, a dissolved polymer solution is extruded through a syringe while a simultaneously applied voltage provides an impetus directing the ejected solution toward a target substrate (Figure 3.4). During the transit

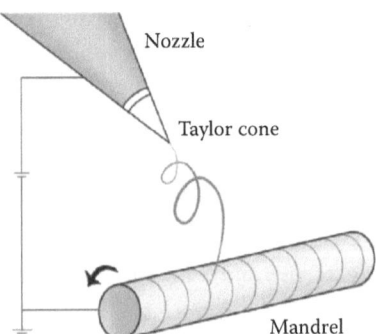

FIGURE 3.4 Schematic of how electrospinning is employed to fabricate elastin scaffolds. The voltage difference between the positively charged nozzle and the grounded substrate serves to guide the polymer stream across the gap. Different shaped collectors may be employed to generate different scaffold shapes; in this case, a rotating mandrel collector will generate tubular structures.

time of the polymer solution, the highly volatile solvent evaporates and the polymer is drawn to the substrate as a fiber.

Although electrospun constructs generally require some form of additional cross-linking to prevent dissolution post-electrospinning, the nature of electrospinning allows polymer coblending and, depending on the combination of polymers, avoids the need for additional cross-linking (Li et al. 2006). These coblends of polymer have the additional advantage of combining different properties of the created scaffolds by combining the appropriate base polymers.

3.4.2.2 Synthetic-Elastin-Based Electrospun Scaffolds

Soluble α-elastin and tropoelastin have been successfully utilized in electrospinning synthetic-elastin-based scaffolds. Electrospinning with synthetic elastin requires the protein to be dissolved in highly volatile organic solvents, such as 1,1,1,3,3,3-hexafluoro-2-propanol (HFP) (Boland et al. 2004), to allow extrusion through a nozzle while rapidly precipitating into a fiber as it travels to a collector.

Characterization of electrospun α-elastin highlighted a correlation between solution concentration and the resultant fiber morphology; 10% (w/v) resulted in beading and fragmented fibers, whereas 20% (w/v) resulted in continuous and uniform fibers that were also wider (Li et al. 2005). Tropoelastin-based electrospun scaffolds similarly demonstrated flat ribbon-like fibers at 20% (w/v) concentrations (Nivison-Smith et al. 2010). While electrospinning has been shown to denature collagen structure when electrospun from fluoroalcohols (Zeugolis et al. 2008), tropoelastin microfibers demonstrated preservation of secondary structures and biological function after electrospinning but prior to cross-linking (Nivison-Smith et al. 2010).

In terms of biological interfacing, human embryonic palatal mesenchymal (HEPM) cells displayed equal attachment, spreading, migration, and proliferation to confluence on α-elastin, tropoelastin- and collagen-based scaffolds, which were significantly higher than tissue-culture-treated polystyrene controls (Li et al. 2005). Other studies on tropoelastin scaffolds additionally indicated successful attachment and spreading of human fibroblasts, human umbilical vein endothelial cells (HUVECs), and human coronary artery smooth muscle cells (HCASMCs), with fibroblasts expressing collagen 1 and fibronectin by day 14 *in vitro* (Nivison-Smith et al. 2010, Rnjak-Kovacina et al. 2011). When the scaffolds were subcutaneously implanted into mice, the *in vivo* model also demonstrated a high level of fibroblast infiltration, native mouse collagen deposition, and no obvious immunological response (Rnjak-Kovacina et al. 2011).

3.4.2.3 Synthetic-Elastin-Based Hybrid Electrospun Scaffolds

While the previous studies demonstrate the potential for elastin-based electrospun materials, one of the major advantages of electrospinning is the ability to coblend various polymers together for hybrid materials and, thus, gain increasingly complex properties.

Initial studies explored the conditions for optimal hybrid fiber formation and postfabrication stability such as electrical field strength, use of different solvents, and viscosity of the spinning solution (Buttafoco et al. 2006). Tropoelastin and collagen coblends at different weight percentage ratios changed the solution viscosity and affected the efficiency of the electrospinning as well as the morphology of electrospun fibers, with increased collagen content resulting in wide fibers (Rnjak-Kovacina et al. 2012).

Depending on the composition of materials and their ratios, the resultant electrospun scaffolds can present very different mechanical properties. A study that incorporated polymer coblends of collagen type I, bovine neck ligament elastin, and PLGA demonstrated similar compliance to native vessels at 120 mmHg pressure (12%–14% diameter change of electrospun scaffolds vs. 9% of native vessels) while exhibiting a burst pressure of 1425 mmHg, which is nearly 12 times systolic pressure (Stitzel et al. 2006). More complex material combinations have also been explored through coblending collagen type I and bovine neck ligament elastin with a range of polymers including poly(L-lactide) (PLA), PCL, and poly(lactide-co-caprolactone) PLCL (Lee et al. 2007). Compared to the other polymers, PLA-blended scaffolds (45% collagen, 15% elastin, 40% polymer by weight) demonstrated superior tensile strength (0.83 MPa) as well as significantly higher elastic modulus (2.08 MPa) under comparable degrees of cross-linking and blend compositions. A scaffold of coblended PCL/tropoelastin layered with pure tropoelastin improved the ultimate tensile strength of hybrid constructs almost fourfold (approximately 50–200 kPa), while Young's modulus increased 12-fold (approximately 25–325 kPa) compared to tropoelastin-only constructs (Wise et al. 2011). Coblending bovine neck elastin and polydioxanone (PDO), which was selected to provide mechanical integrity (Sell et al. 2006), provided an elastic modulus of 9.64 ± 0.66 MPa, which closely matches that of native femoral artery (elastic modulus of 9–12 MPa; Hiroshi 1970, Fung 1984). The selection of appropriate materials for hybrid electrospinning has clear advantages for tunable mechanical properties and different clinical applications for these scaffolds.

While the mechanical properties of scaffolds are tuned by using different materials combined with elastin (*vide supra*), the biological activity is often significantly improved due to the elastin component. The necessity for elastin is exemplified in a study that showed that while 100% PDO scaffolds did not support dermal fibroblast infiltration, a 50/50 polymer–elastin mixture exhibited full-thickness cell infiltration within 7 days (Sell et al. 2006). As mentioned, the inclusion of tropoelastin can promote formation of porosity, improving cellular migration, and proliferation (Vasconcelos et al. 2012). When combined with collagen, the increased scaffold porosity demonstrated a level of cell infiltration and proliferation comparable to the standards of commercially available scaffolds when tested in subcutaneous implantation models (Rnjak-Kovacina et al. 2012). Blending of collagen type I, bovine neck ligament elastin, and PLGA enabled a 7-day average 80% survival for smooth muscle cells and endothelial cells, indicating a potential vascular for graft applications (Stitzel et al. 2006). In a different study, the addition of tropoelastin to PCL gave rise to a 3-fold increase in HUVEC attachment and proliferation (approximately $54.7 \pm 1.1\%$ by day 3) (Wise et al. 2011). When PCL was combined with elastin derived from bovine neck ligament, the electrospun scaffold enabled preferential attachment of chick dorsal root ganglia as well as neurite extension (Swindle-Reilly et al. 2014). A study that focused particularly on the immune response of tropoelastin/silk hybrids found significantly reduced levels of multiple inflammatory mediators including IL-1β, IL-6, MMP-2, and MMP-9 as well as reduced infiltration of inflammatory cells when tropoelastin was present compared to silk only electrospun scaffolds (Liu et al. 2014).

These discussed findings suggest that elastin imparts favorable biocompatibility features to hybrid electrospun scaffolds. Collectively, the combinations of elastin with mechanically strengthening hybrid materials implicate new outlooks and novel electrospun scaffolds for clinical applications.

3.4.3 Material Coatings

3.4.3.1 Principles

The ultimate goal in achieving biocompatibility is for a material to perform its function without eliciting an unfavorable host response or other forms of biologically related failure (Williams 2008). Following this argument, in certain contexts, it is feasible and practical to simply replace the pathological tissue with a synthetic polymer instead of regenerating the ECM. However, while there have been many polymers with ideal mechanical characteristics that have been clinically applied, the surface bioactivity of these polymeric materials may be inadequate for the facilitation of cellular activity or innocuous incorporation of the implant.

Surface modification techniques have been commonly used to enhance the biocompatibility of materials for purposes of implantation, for example, nanoscale patterning of metallic surfaces (Lu et al. 2008) or UV irradiation of polymer surfaces to enhance interactions with biological molecules (Nahar et al. 2004). However, these techniques generally result in passive cell adhesion, with little emphasis given to the biological signaling required for promoting cell survival or proliferation. Compared to passive surface modification strategies, surface coatings with relevant active biological motifs are much more effective in eliciting appropriate cellular activity. The observation that elastin, tropoelastin, and elastin derivatives readily adsorb onto a variety of polymer substrates (Woodhouse et al. 2004) serves as an impetus for exploring biologically derived coatings to improve the biocompatibility of a range of existing classes of materials. Namely, materials that are innately nonbiocompatible can be biologically activated through attachment of proteins such as tropoelastin. These modifications improve the range of applications for different materials that would otherwise be unacceptable for medical implants.

3.4.3.2 Tropoelastin-Based Coatings

Polymers, such as polyethylene, are typically too hydrophobic or negatively charged to facilitate direct cell adhesion (Walachova et al. 2002). For synthetic implants, many polymers can be surface modified for customized biocompatibility and bioactivity. Plasma immersion ion implantation (PIII) was originally a technique for surface engineering semiconductors, metals, and dielectrics (Conrad et al. 1987) by generating a plasma containing the ions of the species to be implanted while applying a net voltage to the substrate to attract the ions. In the context of binding biological molecules, nitrogen PIII treatment can be utilized to ionically modify a polymeric surface, subsequently modulating the cell binding activity of the substrate (Bax et al. 2011b, Gan et al. 2008, MacDonald et al. 2008) (Figure 3.5a).

PIII-based covalent attachment of proteins has been utilized with tropoelastin as a way to introduce active cell signaling properties to otherwise inert materials. Bound tropoelastin demonstrated increased human dermal fibroblast cell attachment and spreading compared to uncoated

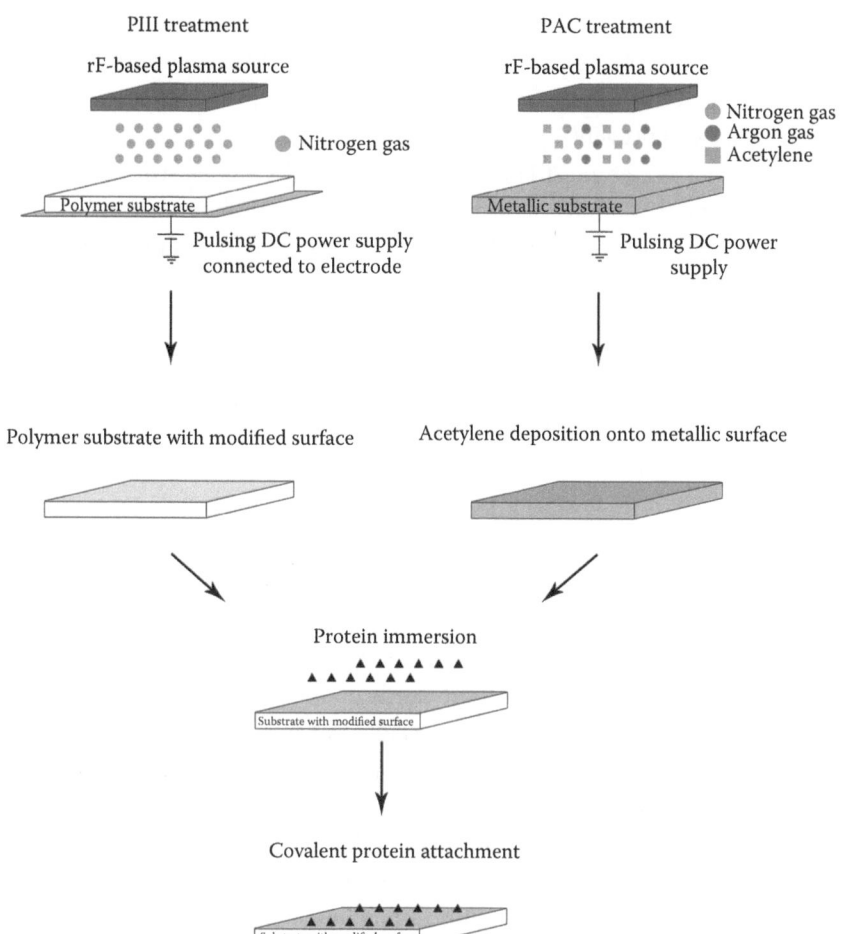

FIGURE 3.5 Process comparison between plasma immersion ion implantation (PIII) and plasma-activated coating (PAC). In PIII treatment, a polymeric substrate is placed on an electrode within a vacuum containing nitrogen gas that is ionized with radio frequency (rF) forming a plasma. A pulsing voltage supplied to the substrate allows implantation of highly energetic ions from the plasma onto the polymer surface, modifying the binding activity of the substrate. The substrate is then immersed in a solution containing the protein of interest that covalently attaches to the modified surface. In PAC treatment, a metallic substrate is placed within a vacuum containing nitrogen, argon, and acetylene that are ionized with rF forming a plasma. A pulsing voltage supplied to the substrate induces the acetylene to deposit onto the substrate, forming a polymer-like hydrocarbon coating containing free radicals on exposed surfaces. The substrate is then immersed in a solution containing the protein of interest that covalently attaches to the modified surface.

controls of both polystyrene and polytetrafluoroethylene (PTFE) surfaces (Bax et al. 2009, 2011b). Interestingly, the use of PIII treatment on PTFE also exhibited the ability to switch the state of bound tropoelastin between promoting and preventing fibroblast (Bax et al. 2011b) and endothelial cell attachment (Bax et al. 2011a). This dual role of tropoelastin modulating cell attachment can have significant implications on biomaterial behavior by providing context specific utility in different clinical applications, for example, cell attachment is preferred for dermal regeneration, however, may lead to lumen occlusion in vascular grafts.

Other polymers can also be functionalized using PIII-based deposition of tropoelastin. Polyurethanes and polyurethane blends have found extensive application in heart valves, vascular grafts, orthopedic, dental, and dermal contexts (Planck et al. 1984). PIII-based deposition of tropoelastin onto a polyurethane block copolymer Elast-Eon E2A allowed increased human dermal fibroblast and human umbilical vein endothelial cell adhesion, spreading and viability compared to untreated samples, while decreasing thrombogenicity (Bax et al. 2014).

While adhering biomolecules to polymers is possible through PIII, adhering biomolecules to metallic surfaces is much more difficult, a key limitation being that coatings are typically not robust enough to withstand *in vivo* exposure. Plasma-activated coating (PAC) is another surface modification technique based on plasma enhanced chemical vapor deposition that allows covalent immobilization of proteins onto metallic surfaces by first depositing a highly reactive polymer surface coating (Yin et al. 2009a,b) (Figure 3.5b). This method facilitates direct covalent immobilization of tropoelastin onto metallic implants (Bilek and McKenzie 2010, Bilek et al. 2011) that is of particular interest in modulating the blood–implant interface of cardiovascular devices. One study modified the surface of stainless steel with tropoelastin using PAC, which promoted endothelial cell attachment by $86.3\% \pm 10.5\%$ and proliferation by $76.9\% \pm 6.4\%$ at day 7 compared to uncoated controls (Yin et al. 2009b). In the context of coronary stents, where bare metal stents suffer not only from inherent thrombogenesis but also restenosis (Serruys et al. 1991), the use of PAC to covalently attach tropoelastin onto metallic stents gave rise to a $93\% \pm 1.2\%$ reduction in thrombogenicity (Waterhouse et al. 2010). Further exploration of PAC deposition with truncated specific functional domains of tropoelastin, as opposed to full-length tropoelastin, demonstrated preservation of low thrombogenicity while increasing resistance to blood protease degradation (Hiob et al. 2013), hence improving efficacy.

Functionalizing the surfaces of otherwise biologically inert materials with tropoelastin has proven to be a feasible strategy in directing cell activity and protein interfacing, significantly improving the variety of applications for already existing materials.

3.5 APPLICATIONS OF SYNTHETIC-ELASTIN MATERIALS

Despite the promise observed in synthetic-elastin biomaterials, there is yet to be widespread clinical application of these systems. The main contexts in which synthetic-elastin systems have been clinically applied include dermal substitutes and tubular constructs for vascular grafting; however, the utility of synthetic-elastic systems in repairing and regenerating other tissue types is also beginning to receive more interest. These studies are subsequently discussed.

3.5.1 Dermal Applications

The most common dermatological conditions that warrant skin substitute treatment include wounds, especially chronic wounds, and severe burns. Elastin is an essential component of the dermis that is often damaged in wounds and burns and, as previously discussed, is difficult to regenerate due to its inherently downregulated expression in adults. Additionally, elastin regeneration in skin substitutes is similarly inadequate (Casasco et al. 2004, Truong et al. 2005), for example, it can take 4–5 years for elastin expression to occur in burn wounds grafted with sheets of cultured epithelial autografts (Jones et al. 2002). Because of this, skin grafts that are sourced from biological sources (such as autografts, allografts, and xenografts) are favored due to their retention of elastic fibers. Although autologous skin grafting is the current gold standard for skin repair, there are alternative commercially available skin substitutes including decellularized porcine membranes (comprising 70% collagen, 30% insoluble elastin, and minor amounts of GAGs) (Bioplex Medical BV, Vaals, the Netherlands), decellularized human dermis (AlloDerm, LifeCell Corp., Bridgewater, NJ), and bovine type I collagen scaffold coated with 3% α-elastin (MatriDerm, Dr. Suwelack Skin & Health Care AG, Billerbeck, Germany).

Acellular dermal matrices of biological origin provide possibly the most direct alternative to using autologous skin grafts. Generally, these matrices are sourced from cadaver or porcine skin with the epidermal and dermal cells stripped without affecting the basement membrane or ECM, preserving many important biological proteins such as elastin (Wainwright 1995). Bioplex Medical's decellularized porcine membrane is one such example of a decellularized xenograft. When tested using a two-step procedure targeting both dermal and epidermal regeneration in a rat full-thickness excision model, the porcine membrane demonstrated successful basement membrane formation as well as histological organization of relevant dermal and epidermal cells (Hafemann et al. 1999). MatriDerm, constructed from porcine type I collagen scaffolds coated with 3% α-elastin, is another commercially available xenograft alternative. When tested in a human punch biopsy wound model, the MatriDerm scaffold demonstrated reduced wound contraction compared to native collagen sponges (De Vries et al. 1994). The inclusion of α-elastin additionally benefited dermal architecture by orchestrating collagen bundle organization (De Vries et al. 1995). MatriDerm has also demonstrated exceptional utility and efficacy in the treatment of hand burns; a 12-month follow-up study of MatriDerm grafted demonstrated no unstable scarring or blisters while retaining a full range of motion (Haslik et al. 2010).

As an alternative to decellularized xenografts, decellularized human dermis (AlloDerm) sourced from cadavers has also been tested on multiple animal models (Bannasch et al. 2008a,b) and has been applied to both full and partial thickness burn wounds. When tested in nude mouse models, AlloDerm demonstrated less wound contraction compared to other commercially available skin substitutes including Integra (bilayer artificial skin with bovine collagen gel dermis and polysiloxane polymer epidermis, Integra Life Sciences Corp., Plaisboro, NJ), Dermagraft-TC (woven bioabsorbable polymer membrane seeded with human dermal fibroblasts, Advanced Tissue Sciences, San Diego, CA), and Dermalogen (powdered human dermal collagen matrix, Collagenesis, Beverly, MA) (Truong et al. 2005). This may be correlated to the presence of elastic fibers within AlloDerm compared to other skin substitutes. In the context of human burns wounds, AlloDerm supports fibroblast infiltration, neovascularization as well as epithelial regeneration under a variety of application procedures (Callcut et al. 2006, Wainwright 1995). Although AlloDerm demonstrates successful clinical application, its high cost severely restricts its usage in reconstructive surgery and is usually limited to the most functionally crucial areas, such as joints (Jansen and Macadam 2011, Yim et al. 2010).

Despite the promising properties of synthetic-elastin systems as discussed in previous sections, there has been relatively limited research in further utilizing elastin-like materials or synthetic-elastin systems for skin substitutes. One of the more direct methods of employing this system is perhaps to supplement existing dermal substitute solutions with synthetic elastin.

The incorporation of tropoelastin into a dermal regeneration template, such as Integra, contributed to accelerated early stage angiogenesis in mouse and pig full-thickness repair models that significantly improves the efficacy of the dermal substitute in deep burn wounds (Wang et al. 2015). Hybrid peptides of elastin covalently linked to alginate dressings have been proposed as a possible enhancement to commercial wound dressings. Biological testing with normal human dermal fibroblasts demonstrated significantly increased cell attachment and proliferation on the hybrid peptide surface compared to noncoated controls. In an *in vivo* wound healing model, the hybrid peptide exhibited significantly higher epithelialization and a larger volume of tissue regeneration compared to controls (Hashimoto et al. 2004). Silk fibroin has been demonstrated to impart higher healing effects than silk only scaffolds when combined with alginate (Roh et al. 2006); however, when combined with elastin, the new hybrid material demonstrated increased utility in dermal burn and chronic wounds by supporting human skin fibroblast proliferation, accelerated re-epithelialization, and successful wound closure (Vasconcelos et al. 2012).

More recently, electrospun elastin–collagen composites have shown great potential as a new alternative for dermal substitutes. By controlling the flow rate of polymer extrusion during electrospinning of recombinant human tropoelastin, scaffolds of different porosity and tensile strength can be created that promoted migration and infiltration of dermal fibroblasts (Rnjak-Kovacina et al. 2011). Further optimization of the electrospun co-blend ratio of tropoelastin and collagen resulted in scaffolds of bioactivity that was comparable to commercially available dermal substitutes such as Integra (Rnjak-Kovacina et al. 2012).

There are many commercially available skin substitutes for dermal repair; however, it is increasingly apparent that elastin is also required for successful healing, most likely due to its inherent mechanical and signaling capacity. This was particularly exemplified by the significantly enhanced vascularization within commercially available Integra dermal scaffolds, after the addition of tropoelastin to the scaffold (Wang et al. 2015). With increasing understanding and application of synthetic-elastin composite scaffolds, the efficacy of dermal regeneration is also expected to improve.

3.5.2 Vascular Applications

There are many materials investigated for their potential use as synthetic vascular grafts; however, there are a number of reasons that can cause graft failure including the lack of endothelial cell lining or low-flow states in small diameter vessels. More commonly compliance mismatch between native vessels and synthetic grafts results in hemodynamic differences, such as turbulent flow and shear stresses, that can trigger neointimal hyperplasia at distal anastomoses (Abbott et al. 1987). The current gold standard used for clinical bypass grafting, as well as synthetic vascular graft design, are internal mammary arteries (elastic modulus: 268 ± 46 kPa, burst pressure: 2267 ± 215 mmHg) and saphenous veins (elastic modulus 683 ± 147 kPa, burst pressure 2295 ± 272 mmHg) (Wise et al. 2011).

In the space of vascular grafts, there is a growing demand for small-diameter vascular grafts (<6 mm diameter) that also exhibit long-term patency. The ideal properties for vascular graft solutions include off-the-shelf availability of various sizes, easy long-term storage, and manageable handling (Kakisis et al. 2005). Current clinically used synthetic graft materials include polyethylene terephthalate (Dacron) and expanded polytetrafluoroethylene (ePTFE). Despite success with large-diameter high-flow rate grafts (Prager et al. 2003), their performance in smaller diameter vessels is limited because of poor patency (Conte 1998) and unfavorable thrombogenic properties in the decreased flow rate conditions, increasing the likelihood of thrombus formation and intimal hyperplasia (Kannan et al. 2005). Additionally, their inelasticity leads to compliance mismatch resulting in complications as discussed previously.

One of the main missing components within tissue engineered vascular grafts is elastin, an important functional component of native vessel ECM both biologically, for modulating cell activity, and mechanically, for compliance and recoil properties (Mitchell and Niklason 2003). Through recent research, elastin has emerged as a potential new alternative material for vascular graft applications. The previous discussions have highlighted that in the context of biological interfacing, the nonthrombogenic interactions between elastin and blood are of especial significance in the interest of medical implants. In particular, this nonthrombogenic behavior is believed to stem from benign interactions with platelets (Baumgartner et al. 1976), which is significant because platelet-mediated mechanisms, rather than thrombin activation, are believed to be the main contributor to thrombosis of metallic prostheses (Schömig et al. 1996). Additionally, elastin signaling has been demonstrated to reduce the vascular proliferative response to arterial injury *in vivo* by modulating vascular smooth muscle cell activity and preventing fibrocellular pathology (Karnik et al. 2003). Ultimately, however, synthetic-elastic-based tissue engineered vascular grafts is still a lacking area (Patel et al. 2006) and has yet to find widespread commercial and/or clinical application.

The most commonly used materials for vascular grafts are of biological origin: autografts, allografts, or xenografts. This approach, similar to dermal grafting, is straightforward as the decellularized grafts possess the ideal size as well as mechanical and biological properties required for vascular applications. Two of the most widely used synthetic grafts include the ficin-digested, negatively charged glutaraldehyde-tanned (NCGT) bovine carotid graft and the GA-tanned human umbilical vein graft, both of which demonstrated high patency in clinical trials for treatment of peripheral vascular disease (Dardik et al. 2002, Sawyer et al. 1987). These grafts, however, have decreased in widespread usage due to tendencies for *in vivo* degeneration as well as aneurysm formation (Strobel et al. 1996). Counterintuitively, both of these grafts were intentionally depleted of both cells and elastin from the harvested vascular structures in the fabrication process, leaving behind a graft comprising of insoluble collagen (Sawyer et al. 1985). This lack of elastin may be ultimately correlated to their fundamental deficit. Alternative approaches have been subsequently explored in addressing the need to include elastin in vascular grafts. One such example proposed a potential small diameter vascular graft consisting of a purified elastin tubular conduit that has been strengthened with fibrin-bonded layers of acellular small intestinal submucosa, to address the low mechanical strength of elastin alone (Hinds et al. 2006). The graft was tested in a porcine acute thrombogenicity model and demonstrated occlusion; however, the thrombus appeared to be associated with the suture line rather than the material. Although the strength of such hybrid grafts appears to be promising, xenogenic grafts need to undergo extensive decellularization as foreign cell debris has been reported to initiate calcification (Schmidt and Baier 2000). Alternative to elastin materials, another strategy for attaining elastin in implanted vascular grafts is inducing *in vivo* elastin deposition. A study that developed arterial constructs using poly(glycerol sebacate) (PGS), of different pore sizes and cultured with smooth muscle cells, achieved mature elastin deposition within 3 weeks without the use of exogenous factors (Lee et al. 2011).

One of the main reasons for the lack of synthetic-elastin-based graft systems is the difficulty in isolating adequate amounts of elastin for manufacture. However, with the improvements in purifying recombinant tropoelastin as previously discussed, more recent strategies of synthetically fabricating vascular grafts have become possible. There are multiple methods of creating tubular constructs, such as wrapping a synthetic-elastin sheet into a tube (Mithieux et al. 2004); however, electrospinning has gained popularity due to its versatility of using hybrid materials as well as its conceptual simplicity. A review of the progress in electrospun synthetic-elastin-based vascular systems can be found in the previous discussion. With increasing understanding in this new approach, there is an expected increase in clinical and commercial application of synthetic-elastin vascular grafts in the future.

3.5.3 Other Tissue Applications

Although synthetic-elastin systems have mostly been clinically utilized in dermal and vascular regeneration, their application in regenerative medicine certainly expands to other tissue types conceptually. Complex hybrid hydrogels consisting of elastin, collagen, and GAGs have enabled adipose derived stem cell differentiation into nucleus pulposus cell phenotypes (Mercuri et al. 2014), while the scaffold's biomimetic and mechanical customizability can find potential application in cartilage repair (Daamen et al. 2003). The previous discussions have also described a range of other potential strategies for supporting alternative tissue repairs; the electrical charge tuning ability of tropoelastin combined with silk supported formation of stable primary cortical neuronal networks and neuronal growth (Hu et al. 2013), elastin combined with PCL showed dorsal root ganglia attachment as well as neurite extension (Swindle-Reilly et al. 2014), and the attachment of elastin to PCL in conjunction with gas foaming created scaffolds with relevant structural and biological properties to support chondrocyte attachment and potential cartilage repair (Annabi et al. 2011a,b).

3.6 CONCLUSIONS AND FUTURE DIRECTIONS

As a native protein in mammalian ECM, elastin exhibits paramount importance to normal physiology both mechanically and biologically. Consequently, there has been increasing interest in utilizing elastin-based materials for regenerative medicine and tissue repair. This was largely made feasible through such use as recombinant human tropoelastin in developing synthetic-elastin-based systems. Although synthetic-elastin-based biomaterials have demonstrated strong biological interfacing characteristics, it is their incorporation into hybrid systems with other synthetic or natural materials that has enhanced both the mechanical and biological potential of these constructs. Employing different fabrication techniques in conjunction with different material combinations translates to great customizability of material properties tuned specifically for a range of clinical applications. With increasing understanding of elastin fabrication and usage, there is great potential for the expansion of this new class of biomaterial with exciting implications for regenerative medicine and tissue engineering.

ACKNOWLEDGMENTS

ASW acknowledges funding from the Australian Research Council, National Health & Medical Research Council, National Institutes of Health (EB014283), and Wellcome Trust (103328). RW and JO acknowledge funding from the Australian Postgraduate Awards and University of Sydney Postgraduate Awards, respectively.

REFERENCES

Abbott, W.M., J. Megerman, J.E. Hasson, G. L'Italien, and D.F. Warnock. 1987. Effect of compliance mismatch on vascular graft patency. *Journal of Vascular Surgery*. 5(2): 376–382.

Annabi, N., A. Fathi, S.M. Mithieux, P. Martens, A.S. Weiss, and F. Dehghani. 2011a. The effect of elastin on chondrocyte adhesion and proliferation on poly (ε-caprolactone)/elastin composites. *Biomaterials*. 32(6): 1517–1525.

Annabi, N., A. Fathi, S.M. Mithieux, A.S. Weiss, and F. Dehghani. 2011b. Fabrication of porous PCL/elastin composite scaffolds for tissue engineering applications. *The Journal of Supercritical Fluids*. 59: 157–167.

Annabi, N., S.M. Mithieux, E.A. Boughton, A.J. Ruys, A.S. Weiss, and F. Dehghani. 2009a. Synthesis of highly porous crosslinked elastin hydrogels and their interaction with fibroblasts in vitro. *Biomaterials*. 30(27): 4550–4557.

Annabi, N., S.M. Mithieux, A.S. Weiss, and F. Dehghani. 2009b. Development and characterisation of a novel elastin hydrogel. *Proceedings of Material Research Society Fall Meeting Symposium*, Boston, MA.

Annabi, N., S.M. Mithieux, A.S. Weiss, and F. Dehghani. 2009c. The fabrication of elastin-based hydrogels using high pressure CO_2. *Biomaterials*. 30(1): 1–7.

Annabi, N., S.M. Mithieux, A.S. Weiss, and F. Dehghani. 2010. Cross-linked open-pore elastic hydrogels based on tropoelastin, elastin and high pressure CO2. *Biomaterials*. 31(7): 1655–1665.

Annabi, N., S.M. Mithieux, P. Zorlutuna, G. Camci-Unal, A.S. Weiss, and A. Khademhosseini. 2013. Engineered cell-laden human protein-based elastomer. *Biomaterials*. 34(22): 5496–5505.

Baldock, C., A.F. Oberhauser, L. Ma, D. Lammie, V. Siegler, S.M. Mithieux, Y. Tu, J.Y.H. Chow, F. Suleman, and M. Malfois. 2011. Shape of tropoelastin, the highly extensible protein that controls human tissue elasticity. *Proceedings of the National Academy of Sciences*. 108(11): 4322–4327.

Bannasch, H., G. Stark, F. Knam, R. Horch, and M. Föhn. 2008a. Decellularized dermis in combination with cultivated keratinocytes in a short-and long-term animal experimental investigation. *Journal of the European Academy of Dermatology and Venereology*. 22(1): 41–49.

Bannasch, H., T. Unterberg, M. Föhn, B. Weyand, R.E. Horch, and G.B. Stark. 2008b. Cultured keratinocytes in fibrin with decellularised dermis close porcine full-thickness wounds in a single step. *Burns.* 34(7): 1015–1021.

Baumgartner, H.R., R. Muggli, T.B. Tschopp, and V.T. Turitto. 1976. Platelet adhesion, release and aggregation in flowing blood: Effects of surface properties and platelet function. *Thrombosis and Haemostasis.* 35(1): 124–138.

Bax, D.V., A. Kondyurin, A. Waterhouse, D.R. McKenzie, A.S. Weiss, and M.M. Bilek. 2014. Surface plasma modification and tropoelastin coating of a polyurethane copolymer for enhanced cell attachment and reduced thrombogenicity. *Biomaterials.* 35(25): 6797–6809.

Bax, D.V., S.J. Liu, D.R. McKenzie, M.M. Bilek, and A.S. Weiss. 2011a. Tropoelastin switch and modulated endothelial cell binding to PTFE. *BioNanoScience.* 1(4): 123–127.

Bax, D.V., D.R. McKenzie, A.S. Weiss, and M.M. Bilek. 2009. Linker-free covalent attachment of the extracellular matrix protein tropoelastin to a polymer surface for directed cell spreading. *Acta Biomaterialia.* 5(9): 3371–3381.

Bax, D.V., Y. Wang, Z. Li, P.K. Maitz, D.R. McKenzie, M.M. Bilek, and A.S. Weiss. 2011b. Binding of the cell adhesive protein tropoelastin to PTFE through plasma immersion ion implantation treatment. *Biomaterials.* 32(22): 5100–5111.

Bellingham, C. and F. Keeley. 2004. Self-ordered polymerization of elastin-based biomaterials. *Current Opinion in Solid State and Materials Science.* 8(2): 135–139.

Bellingham, C.M., M.A. Lillie, J.M. Gosline, G.M. Wright, B.C. Starcher, A.J. Bailey, K.A. Woodhouse, and F.W. Keeley. 2003. Recombinant human elastin polypeptides self-assemble into biomaterials with elastin-like properties. *Biopolymers.* 70(4): 445–455.

Bilek, M.M., D.V. Bax, A. Kondyurin, Y. Yin, N.J. Nosworthy, K. Fisher, A. Waterhouse, A.S. Weiss, C.G. dos Remedios, and D.R. McKenzie. 2011. Free radical functionalization of surfaces to prevent adverse responses to biomedical devices. *Proceedings of the National Academy of Sciences.* 108(35): 14405–14410.

Bilek, M.M. and D.R. McKenzie. 2010. Plasma modified surfaces for covalent immobilization of functional biomolecules in the absence of chemical linkers: Towards better biosensors and a new generation of medical implants. *Biophysical Reviews.* 2(2): 55–65.

Boland, E.D., J.A. Matthews, K.J. Pawlowski, D.G. Simpson, G.E. Wnek, and G.L. Bowlin. 2004. Electrospinning collagen and elastin: Preliminary vascular tissue engineering. *Frontiers in Bioscience.*(9): 1422–1432.

Brown, P.L., L. Mecham, C. Tisdale, and R.P. Mecham. 1992. The cysteine residues in the carboxy terminal domain of tropoelastin form an intrachain disulfide bond that stabilizes a loop structure and positively charged pocket. *Biochemical and Biophysical Research Communications.* 186(1): 549–555.

Buttafoco, L., N. Kolkman, P. Engbers-Buijtenhuijs, A. Poot, P. Dijkstra, I. Vermes, and J. Feijen. 2006. Electrospinning of collagen and elastin for tissue engineering applications. *Biomaterials.* 27(5): 724–734.

Callcut, R., M. Schurr, M. Sloan, and L. Faucher. 2006. Clinical experience with Alloderm: A one-staged composite dermal/epidermal replacement utilizing processed cadaver dermis and thin autografts. *Burns*. 32(5): 583–588.

Casasco, M., A. Casasco, A.I. Cornaglia, A. Farina, and A. Calligaro. 2004. Differential distribution of elastic tissue in human natural skin and tissue-engineered skin. *Journal of Molecular Histology*. 35(4): 421–428.

Chung, M.I., M. Miao, R.J. Stahl, E. Chan, J. Parkinson, and F.W. Keeley. 2006. Sequences and domain structures of mammalian, avian, amphibian and teleost tropoelastins: Clues to the evolutionary history of elastins. *Matrix Biology*. 25(8): 492–504.

Clarke, A.W., E.C. Arnspang, S.M. Mithieux, E. Korkmaz, F. Braet, and A.S. Weiss. 2006. Tropoelastin massively associates during coacervation to form quantized protein spheres. *Biochemistry*. 45(33): 9989–9996.

Conrad, J.R., J. Radtke, R. Dodd, F.J. Worzala, and N.C. Tran. 1987. Plasma source ion-implantation technique for surface modification of materials. *Journal of Applied Physics*. 62(11): 4591–4596.

Conte, M.S. 1998. The ideal small arterial substitute: A search for the Holy Grail? *FASEB Journal*. 12(1): 43–45.

Cox, B., B. Starcher, and D. Urry. 1973. Coacervation of α-elastin results in fiber formation. *Biochimica et Biophysica Acta (BBA)-protein structure*. 317(1): 209–213.

Daamen, W., H.T.B. Van Moerkerk, T. Hafmans, L. Buttafoco, A. Poot, J. Veerkamp, and T. Van Kuppevelt. 2003. Preparation and evaluation of molecularly-defined collagen–elastin–glycosaminoglycan scaffolds for tissue engineering. *Biomaterials*. 24(22): 4001–4009.

Dardik, H., K. Wengerter, F. Qin, A. Pangilinan, F. Silvestri, F. Wolodiger, M. Kahn, B. Sussman, and I.M. Ibrahim. 2002. Comparative decades of experience with glutaraldehyde-tanned human umbilical cord vein graft for lower limb revascularization: an analysis of 1275 cases. *Journal of Vascular Surgery*. 35(1): 64–71.

Davidson, J., S. Shibahara, C. Boyd, M. Mason, P. Tolstoshev, and R. Crystal. 1984. Elastin mRNA levels during foetal development of sheep nuchal ligament and lung. Hybridization to complementary and cloned DNA. *The Biochemical Journal*. 220: 653–663.

De Vries, H.J., E. Middelkoop, J.R. Mekkes, R.P. Dutrieux, C.H. Wildevuur, and W. Westerhof. 1994. Dermal regeneration in native non-cross-linked collagen sponges with different extracellular matrix molecules. *Wound Repair and Regeneration*. 2(1): 37–47.

De Vries, H.J., J. Zeegelaar, E. Middelkoop, G. Gijsbers, J. Marle, C. Wildevuur, and W. Westerhof. 1995. Reduced wound contraction and scar formation in punch biopsy wounds. Native collagen dermal substitutes. A clinical study. *British Journal of Dermatology*. 132(5): 690–697.

Debelle, L., A.J. Alix, M.P. Jacob, J.P. Huvenne, M. Berjot, B. Sombret, and P. Legrand. 1995. Bovine elastin and kappa-elastin secondary structure determination by optical spectroscopies. *Journal of Biological Chemistry*. 270(44): 26099–26103.

Debelle, L., A.J. Alix, S.M. Wei, M.P. Jacob, J.P. Huvenne, M. Berjot, and P. Legrand. 1998. The secondary structure and architecture of human elastin. *European Journal of Biochemistry.* 258(2): 533–539.

Debelle, L. and A. Tamburro. 1999. Elastin: Molecular description and function. *The International Journal of Biochemistry & Cell Biology.* 31(2): 261–272.

Duca, L., N. Floquet, A.J. Alix, B. Haye, and L. Debelle. 2004. Elastin as a matrikine. *Critical Reviews in Oncology/Hematology.* 49(3): 235–244.

Fathi, A., S.M. Mithieux, H. Wei, W. Chrzanowski, P. Valtchev, A.S. Weiss, and F. Dehghani. 2014. Elastin based cell-laden injectable hydrogels with tunable gelation, mechanical and biodegradation properties. *Biomaterials.* 35(21): 5425–5435.

Foster, J.A., C.B. Rich, S. Fletcher, S.R. Karr, M.D. DeSa, T. Oliver, and A. Przybyla. 1981. Elastin biosynthesis in chick embryonic lung tissue: Comparison to chick aortic elastin. *Biochemistry.* 20(12): 3528–3535.

Fung, Y. 1984. Blood flow in arteries: Pressure and velocity waves in large arteries and the effects of geometric nonuniformity. In *Biodynamics—Circulation.* New York: Springer. pp. 133–136.

Gan, B., N. Nosworthy, D. McKenzie, C. Dos Remedios, and M. Bilek. 2008. Plasma immersion ion implantation treatment of polyethylene for enhanced binding of active horseradish peroxidase. *Journal of Biomedical Materials Research Part A.* 85(3): 605–610.

Gauvin, R., R. Parenteau-Bareil, M.R. Dokmeci, W.D. Merryman, and A. Khademhosseini. 2012. Hydrogels and microtechnologies for engineering the cellular microenvironment. *Wiley Interdisciplinary Reviews: Nanomedicine and Nanobiotechnology.* 4(3): 235–246.

Giro, M., A. Oikarinen, H. Oikarinen, G. Sephel, J. Uitto, and J. Davidson. 1985. Demonstration of elastin gene expression in human skin fibroblast cultures and reduced tropoelastin production by cells from a patient with atrophoderma. *Journal of Clinical Investigation.* 75(2): 672.

Grimm, M., E. Eybl, M. Grabenwöger, H. Spreitzer, W. Jäger, G. Grimm, P. Böck, M. Müller, and E. Wolner. 1992. Glutaraldehyde affects biocompatibility of bioprosthetic heart valves. *Surgery.* 111(1): 74–78.

Hafemann, B., S. Ensslen, C. Erdmann, R. Niedballa, A. Zühlke, K. Ghofrani, and C. Kirkpatrick. 1999. Use of a collagen/elastin-membrane for the tissue engineering of dermis. *Burns.* 25(5): 373–384.

Hafemann, B., K. Ghofrani, H.-G. Gattner, H. Stieve, and N. Pallua. 2001. Crosslinking by 1-ethyl-3-(3-dimethylaminopropyl)-carbodiimide (EDC) of a collagen/elastin membrane meant to be used as a dermal substitute: Effects on physical, biochemical and biological features in vitro. *Journal of Materials Science: Materials in Medicine.* 12(5): 437–446.

Hashimoto, T., Y. Suzuki, M. Tanihara, Y. Kakimaru, and K. Suzuki. 2004. Development of alginate wound dressings linked with hybrid peptides derived from laminin and elastin. *Biomaterials.* 25(7): 1407–1414.

Haslik, W., L.-P. Kamolz, F. Manna, M. Hladik, T. Rath, and M. Frey. 2010. Management of full-thickness skin defects in the hand and wrist region: First long-term experiences with the dermal matrix Matriderm®. *Journal of Plastic, Reconstructive & Aesthetic Surgery.* 63(2): 360–364.

He, K., H. Nukada, T. Urakami, and M.P. Murphy. 2003. Antioxidant and pro-oxidant properties of pyrroloquinoline quinone (PQQ): Implications for its function in biological systems. *Biochemical Pharmacology.* 65(1): 67–74.

Hinds, M.T., R.C. Rowe, Z. Ren, J. Teach, P.C. Wu, S.J. Kirkpatrick, K.D. Breneman, K.W. Gregory, and D.W. Courtman. 2006. Development of a reinforced porcine elastin composite vascular scaffold. *Journal of Biomedical Materials Research Part A.* 77(3): 458–469.

Hiob, M.A., S.G. Wise, A. Kondyurin, A. Waterhouse, M.M. Bilek, M.K. Ng, and A.S. Weiss. 2013. The use of plasma-activated covalent attachment of early domains of tropoelastin to enhance vascular compatibility of surfaces. *Biomaterials.* 34(31): 7584–7591.

Hiroshi, Y. 1970. *Strength of Biological Materials.* Baltimore, MD: Williams & Wilkins.

Holst, J., S. Watson, M.S. Lord, S.S. Eamegdool, D.V. Bax, L.B. Nivison-Smith, A. Kondyurin, L. Ma, A.F. Oberhauser, and A.S. Weiss. 2010. Substrate elasticity provides mechanical signals for the expansion of hemopoietic stem and progenitor cells. *Nature Biotechnology.* 28(10): 1123–1128.

Hu, X., S.-H. Park, E.S. Gil, X.-X. Xia, A.S. Weiss, and D.L. Kaplan. 2011. The influence of elasticity and surface roughness on myogenic and osteogenic-differentiation of cells on silk-elastin biomaterials. *Biomaterials.* 32(34): 8979–8989.

Hu, X., M.D. Tang-Schomer, W. Huang, X.X. Xia, A.S. Weiss, and D.L. Kaplan. 2013. Charge-tunable autoclaved silk-tropoelastin protein alloys that control neuron cell responses. *Advanced Functional Materials.* 23(31): 3875–3884.

Hu, X., X. Wang, J. Rnjak, A.S. Weiss, and D.L. Kaplan. 2010. Biomaterials derived from silk–tropoelastin protein systems. *Biomaterials.* 31(32): 8121–8131.

Indik, Z., W.R. Abrams, U. Kucich, C.W. Gibson, R.P. Mecham, and J. Rosenbloom. 1990. Production of recombinant human tropoelastin: Characterization and demonstration of immunologic and chemotactic activity. *Archives of Biochemistry and Biophysics.* 280(1): 80–86.

Indik, Z., H. Yeh, N. Ornstein-Goldstein, P. Sheppard, N. Anderson, J.C. Rosenbloom, L. Peltonen, and J. Rosenbloom. 1987. Alternative splicing of human elastin mRNA indicated by sequence analysis of cloned genomic and complementary DNA. *Proceedings of the National Academy of Sciences.* 84(16): 5680–5684.

Jansen, L.A. and S.A. Macadam. 2011. The use of AlloDerm in postmastectomy alloplastic breast reconstruction: Part II. A cost analysis. *Plastic and Reconstructive Surgery.* 127(6): 2245–2254.

Jones, I., L. Currie, and R. Martin. 2002. A guide to biological skin substitutes. *British Journal of Plastic Surgery.* 55(3): 185–193.

Kakisis, J.D., C.D. Liapis, C. Breuer, and B.E. Sumpio. 2005. Artificial blood vessel: The Holy Grail of peripheral vascular surgery. *Journal of Vascular Surgery*. 41(2): 349–354.

Kannan, R.Y., H.J. Salacinski, P.E. Butler, G. Hamilton, and A.M. Seifalian. 2005. Current status of prosthetic bypass grafts: A review. *Journal of Biomedical Materials Research Part B: Applied Biomaterials*. 74(1): 570–581.

Karnik, S.K., B.S. Brooke, A. Bayes-Genis, L. Sorensen, J.D. Wythe, R.S. Schwartz, M.T. Keating, and D.Y. Li. 2003. A critical role for elastin signaling in vascular morphogenesis and disease. *Development*. 130(2): 411–423.

Koens, M., K. Faraj, R. Wismans, J. Van der Vliet, A. Krasznai, V. Cuijpers, J. Jansen, W. Daamen, and T. Van Kuppevelt. 2010. Controlled fabrication of triple layered and molecularly defined collagen/elastin vascular grafts resembling the native blood vessel. *Acta Biomaterialia*. 6(12): 4666–4674.

Kozel, B.A., H. Wachi, E.C. Davis, and R.P. Mecham. 2003. Domains in tropoelastin that mediate elastin deposition in vitro and in vivo. *Journal of Biological Chemistry*. 278(20): 18491–18498.

Leach, J.B., J.B. Wolinsky, P.J. Stone, and J.Y. Wong. 2005. Crosslinked α-elastin biomaterials: Towards a processable elastin mimetic scaffold. *Acta Biomaterialia*. 1(2): 155–164.

Lee, K.-W., D.B. Stolz, and Y. Wang. 2011. Substantial expression of mature elastin in arterial constructs. *Proceedings of the National Academy of Sciences*. 108(7): 2705–2710.

Lee, S.J., J.J. Yoo, G.J. Lim, A. Atala, and J. Stitzel. 2007. In vitro evaluation of electrospun nanofiber scaffolds for vascular graft application. *Journal of Biomedical Materials Research Part A*. 83(4): 999–1008.

Li, M., M.J. Mondrinos, X. Chen, M.R. Gandhi, F.K. Ko, and P.I. Lelkes. 2006. Co-electrospun poly (lactide-co-glycolide), gelatin, and elastin blends for tissue engineering scaffolds. *Journal of Biomedical Materials Research Part A*. 79(4): 963–973.

Li, M., M.J. Mondrinos, M.R. Gandhi, F.K. Ko, A.S. Weiss, and P.I. Lelkes. 2005. Electrospun protein fibers as matrices for tissue engineering. *Biomaterials*. 26(30): 5999–6008.

Liu, H., S.G. Wise, J. Rnjak-Kovacina, D.L. Kaplan, M.M. Bilek, A.S. Weiss, J. Fei, and S. Bao. 2014. Biocompatibility of silk-tropoelastin protein polymers. *Biomaterials*. 35(19): 5138–5147.

Livingstone, C.D. and G.J. Barton. 1993. Protein sequence alignments: A strategy for the hierarchical analysis of residue conservation. *Computer Applications in the Biosciences: CABIOS*. 9(6): 745–756.

Lu, J., M.P. Rao, N.C. MacDonald, D. Khang, and T.J. Webster. 2008. Improved endothelial cell adhesion and proliferation on patterned titanium surfaces with rationally designed, micrometer to nanometer features. *Acta Biomaterialia*. 4(1): 192–201.

Lucero, H. and H. Kagan. 2006. Lysyl oxidase: An oxidative enzyme and effector of cell function. *Cellular and Molecular Life Sciences CMLS*. 63(19–20): 2304–2316.

MacDonald, C., R. Morrow, A.S. Weiss, and M.M. Bilek. 2008. Covalent attachment of functional protein to polymer surfaces: A novel one-step dry process. *Journal of The Royal Society Interface.* 5(23): 663–669.

McGowan, S.E., S.K. Jackson, P.J. Olson, T. Parekh, and L.I. Gold. 1997. Exogenous and endogenous transforming growth factors-β influence elastin gene expression in cultured lung fibroblasts. *American Journal of Respiratory Cell and Molecular Biology.* 17(1): 25–35.

Martin, S.L., B. Vrhovski, and A.S. Weiss. 1995. Total synthesis and expression in Escherichia coli of a gene encoding human tropoelastin. *Gene.* 154(2): 159–166.

Mecham, R.P. and J.A. Foster. 1979. Characterization of insoluble elastin from copper-deficient pigs: Its usefulness in elastin sequence studies. *Biochimica et Biophysica Acta (BBA)-Protein Structure.* 577(1): 147–158.

Mercuri, J., C. Addington, R. Pascal, S. Gill, and D. Simionescu. 2014. Development and initial characterization of a chemically stabilized elastin-glycosaminoglycan-collagen composite shape-memory hydrogel for nucleus pulposus regeneration. *Journal of Biomedical Materials Research Part A.* 102(12): 4380–4393.

Mitchell, S.L. and L.E. Niklason. 2003. Requirements for growing tissue-engineered vascular grafts. *Cardiovascular Pathology.* 12(2): 59–64.

Mithieux, S.M., J.E. Rasko, and A.S. Weiss. 2004. Synthetic elastin hydrogels derived from massive elastic assemblies of self-organized human protein monomers. *Biomaterials.* 25(20): 4921–4927.

Mithieux, S.M., Y. Tu, E. Korkmaz, F. Braet, and A.S. Weiss. 2009. In situ polymerization of tropoelastin in the absence of chemical cross-linking. *Biomaterials.* 30(4): 431–435.

Mithieux, S.M. and A.S. Weiss. 2005. Elastin. *Advances in Protein Chemistry.* 70: 437–461.

Mithieux, S.M., S.G. Wise, M.J. Raftery, B. Starcher, and A.S. Weiss. 2005. A model two-component system for studying the architecture of elastin assembly in vitro. *Journal of Structural Biology.* 149(3): 282–289.

Muiznieks, L.D., S.A. Jensen, and A.S. Weiss. 2003. Structural changes and facilitated association of tropoelastin. *Archives of Biochemistry and Biophysics.* 410(2): 317–323.

Nahar, P., A. Naqvi, and S.F. Basir. 2004. Sunlight-mediated activation of an inert polymer surface for covalent immobilization of a protein. *Analytical Biochemistry.* 327(2): 162–164.

Nickerson, M., R. Farnworth, E. Wagar, S. Hodge, D. Rousseau, and A. Paulson. 2006. Some physical and microstructural properties of genipin-cross-linked gelatin–maltodextrin hydrogels. *International Journal of Biological Macromolecules.* 38(1): 40–44.

Nivison-Smith, L., J. Rnjak, and A.S. Weiss. 2010. Synthetic human elastin microfibers: Stable cross-linked tropoelastin and cell interactive constructs for tissue engineering applications. *Acta Biomaterialia.* 6(2): 354–359.

Park, S.-N., J.-C. Park, H.O. Kim, M.J. Song, and H. Suh. 2002. Characterization of porous collagen/hyaluronic acid scaffold modified by 1-ethyl-3-(3-dimethylaminopropyl) carbodiimide cross-linking. *Biomaterials.* 23(4): 1205–1212.

Parks, W.C., H. Secrist, L.C. Wu, and R. Mecham. 1988. Developmental regulation of tropoelastin isoforms. *Journal of Biological Chemistry.* 263(9): 4416–4423.

Pasquali-Ronchetti, I., M. Baccarani-Contri, C. Fornieri, G. Mori, and D. Quaglino Jr. 1993. Structure and composition of the elastin fibre in normal and pathological conditions. *Micron.* 24(1): 75–89.

Patel, A., B. Fine, M. Sandig, and K. Mequanint. 2006. Elastin biosynthesis: The missing link in tissue-engineered blood vessels. *Cardiovascular Research.* 71(1): 40–49.

Piontkivska, H., Y. Zhang, E.D. Green, and L. Elnitski. 2004. Multi-species sequence comparison reveals dynamic evolution of the elastin gene that has involved purifying selection and lineage-specific insertions/deletions. *BMC Genomics.* 5(1): 31–44.

Planck, H., G. Egbers, and I. Syre. 1984. Polyurethanes in Biomedical Engineering: Proceedings of the International Colloquium "Polyurethane in Medical Technics," Organized by the *Biomedical Branch of the Institute for Textile Technology and Chemical Engineering,* Denkdorf, West Germany, January 27–29, 1983, Stuttgart, Germany: Elsevier.

Prager, M.R., T. Hoblaj, J. Nanobashvili, E. Sporn, P. Polterauer, O. Wagner, H.-J. Böhmig, H. Teufelsbauer, M. Ploner, and I. Huk. 2003. Collagen-versus gelatine-coated Dacron versus stretch PTFE bifurcation grafts for aortoiliac occlusive disease: Long-term results of a prospective, randomized multicenter trial. *Surgery.* 134(1): 80–85.

Richards, F. and J. Knowles. 1968. Glutaraldehyde as a protein cross-linking reagent. *Journal of Molecular Biology.* 37(1): 231–233.

Rnjak-Kovacina, J., S.G. Wise, Z. Li, P.K. Maitz, C.J. Young, Y. Wang, and A.S. Weiss. 2011. Tailoring the porosity and pore size of electrospun synthetic human elastin scaffolds for dermal tissue engineering. *Biomaterials.* 32(28): 6729–6736.

Rnjak-Kovacina, J., S.G. Wise, Z. Li, P.K. Maitz, C.J. Young, Y. Wang, and A.S. Weiss. 2012. Electrospun synthetic human elastin: Collagen composite scaffolds for dermal tissue engineering. *Acta Biomaterialia.* 8(10): 3714–3722.

Rodríguez-Cabello, J., M. Alonso, M. Díez, M. Caballero, and M. Herguedas. 1999. Structural investigation of the poly (pentapeptide) of elastin, poly (GVGVP), in the solid state. *Macromolecular Chemistry and Physics.* 200: 1831–1838.

Roh, D.-H., S.-Y. Kang, J.-Y. Kim, Y.-B. Kwon, H.Y. Kweon, K.-G. Lee, Y.-H. Park, R.-M. Baek, C.-Y. Heo, and J. Choe. 2006. Wound healing effect of silk fibroin/alginate-blended sponge in full thickness skin defect of rat. *Journal of Materials Science: Materials in Medicine.* 17(6): 547–552.

Sawyer, P.N., J. Fitzgerald, M.J. Kaplitt, R.J. Sanders, G.M. Williams, R.P. Leather, A. Karmody, R.W. Hallin, R. Taylor, and C.C. Fries. 1987. Ten year experience with the negatively charged glutaraldehyde-tanned vascular graft in peripheral vascular surgery: Initial multicenter trail. *The American Journal of Surgery.* 154(5): 533–537.

Sawyer, P.N., A.M. O'Shaughnessy, and Z. Sophie. 1985. Development and performance characteristics of a new vascular graft. *Journal of Biomedical Materials Research.* 19(9): 991–1010.

Schmidt, C.E. and J.M. Baier. 2000. Acellular vascular tissues: natural biomaterials for tissue repair and tissue engineering. *Biomaterials.* 21(22): 2215–2231.

Schömig, A., F.-J. Neumann, A. Kastrati, H. Schühlen, R. Blasini, M. Hadamitzky, H. Walter, E.-M. Zitzmann-Roth, G. Richardt, and E. Alt. 1996. A randomized comparison of antiplatelet and anticoagulant therapy after the placement of coronary-artery stents. *New England Journal of Medicine.* 334(17): 1084–1089.

Sell, S., M.J. McClure, C.P. Barnes, D.C. Knapp, B.H. Walpoth, D.G. Simpson, and G.L. Bowlin. 2006. Electrospun polydioxanone–elastin blends: Potential for bioresorbable vascular grafts. *Biomedical Materials.* 1(2): 72–80.

Serruys, P.W., B.H. Strauss, K.J. Beatt, M.E. Bertrand, J. Puel, A.F. Rickards, B. Meier, J.-J. Goy, P. Vogt, and L. Kappenberger. 1991. Angiographic follow-up after placement of a self-expanding coronary-artery stent. *New England Journal of Medicine.* 324(1): 13–17.

Shah, M.A., P.R. Bergethon, A.M. Boak, P.M. Gallop, and H.M. Kagan. 1992. Oxidation of peptidyl lysine by copper complexes of pyrroloquinoline quinone and other quinones: A model for oxidative pathochemistry. *Biochimica et Biophysica Acta (BBA)-Protein Structure and Molecular Enzymology.* 1159(3): 311–318.

Snyder, S.R., E.V. Welty, R.Y. Walder, L.A. Williams, and J.A. Walder. 1987. HbXL99 alpha: A hemoglobin derivative that is cross-linked between the alpha subunits is useful as a blood substitute. *Proceedings of the National Academy of Sciences.* 84(20): 7280–7284.

Speer, D.P., M. Chvapil, C. Eskelson, and J. Ulreich. 1980. Biological effects of residual glutaraldehyde in glutaraldehyde-tanned collagen biomaterials. *Journal of Biomedical Materials Research.* 14(6): 753–764.

Stitzel, J., J. Liu, S.J. Lee, M. Komura, J. Berry, S. Soker, G. Lim, M. Van Dyke, R. Czerw, and J.J. Yoo. 2006. Controlled fabrication of a biological vascular substitute. *Biomaterials.* 27(7): 1088–1094.

Stone, P.J., S.M. Morris, S. Griffin, S. Mithieux, and A.S. Weiss. 2001. Building elastin: Incorporation of recombinant human tropoelastin into extracellular matrices using nonelastogenic rat-1 fibroblasts as a source for lysyl oxidase. *American Journal of Respiratory Cell and Molecular Biology.* 24(6): 733–739.

Strobel, R., A. Boontje, and J. Van Den Dungen. 1996. Aneurysm formation in modified human umbilical vein grafts. *European Journal of Vascular and Endovascular Surgery.* 11(4): 417–420.

Swee, M.H., W.C. Parks, and R.A. Pierce. 1995. Developmental regulation of elastin production. Expression of tropoelastin pre-mRNA persists after down-regulation of steady-state mRNA levels. *Journal of Biological Chemistry.* 270(25): 14899–14906.

Swindle-Reilly, K.E., C.S. Paranjape, and C.A. Miller. 2014. Electrospun poly (caprolactone)-elastin scaffolds for peripheral nerve regeneration. *Progress in Biomaterials.* 3(1): 1–8.

Truong, A.-T.N., A. Kowal-Vern, B.A. Latenser, D.E. Wiley, and R.J. Walter. 2005. Comparison of dermal substitutes in wound healing utilizing a nude mouse model. *Journal of Burns and Wounds.* 4(e4): 72–82.

Tu, Y., S.G. Wise, and A.S. Weiss. 2010. Stages in tropoelastin coalescence during synthetic elastin hydrogel formation. *Micron.* 41(3): 268–272.

Uitto, J., H.-P. Hoffmann, and D.J. Prockop. 1976. Synthesis of elastin and procollagen by cells from embryonic aorta: Differences in the role of hydroxyproline and the effects of proline analogs on the secretion of the two proteins. *Archives of Biochemistry and Biophysics.* 173(1): 187–200.

Vasconcelos, A., A.C. Gomes, and A. Cavaco-Paulo. 2012. Novel silk fibroin/elastin wound dressings. *Acta biomaterialia.* 8(8): 3049–3060.

Vieth, S., C. Bellingham, F. Keeley, S. Hodge, and D. Rousseau. 2007. Microstructural and tensile properties of elastin-based polypeptides cross-linked with Genipin and pyrroloquinoline quinone. *Biopolymers.* 85(3): 199–206.

Vrhovski, B. and A.S. Weiss. 1998. Biochemistry of tropoelastin. *European Journal of Biochemistry.* 258(1): 1–18.

Wainwright, D. 1995. Use of an acellular allograft dermal matrix (AlloDerm) in the management of full-thickness burns. *Burns.* 21(4): 243–248.

Walachova, K., V. Švorčík, L. Bačáková, and V. Hnatowicz. 2002. Colonization of ion-modified polyethylene with vascular smooth muscle cells in vitro. *Biomaterials.* 23(14): 2989–2996.

Wang, Y., S.M. Mithieux, Y. Kong, X.Q. Wang, C. Chong, A. Fathi, F. Dehghani, E. Panas, J. Kemnitzer, and R. Daniels. 2015. Tropoelastin incorporation into a dermal regeneration template promotes wound angiogenesis. *Advanced Healthcare Materials.* 4(4): 577–584.

Waterhouse, A., Y. Yin, S.G. Wise, D.V. Bax, D.R. McKenzie, M.M. Bilek, A.S. Weiss, and M.K. Ng. 2010. The immobilization of recombinant human tropoelastin on metals using a plasma-activated coating to improve the biocompatibility of coronary stents. *Biomaterials.* 31(32): 8332–8340.

Williams, D.F. 2008. On the mechanisms of biocompatibility. *Biomaterials.* 29(20): 2941–2953.

Wise, S.G., M.J. Byrom, A. Waterhouse, P.G. Bannon, M.K. Ng, and A.S. Weiss. 2011. A multilayered synthetic human elastin/polycaprolactone hybrid vascular graft with tailored mechanical properties. *Acta Biomaterialia.* 7(1): 295–303.

Wise, S.G., S.M. Mithieux, M.J. Raftery, and A.S. Weiss. 2005. Specificity in the coacervation of tropoelastin: solvent exposed lysines. *Journal of Structural Biology.* 149(3): 273–281.

Wise, S.G., G.C. Yeo, M.A. Hiob, J. Rnjak-Kovacina, D.L. Kaplan, M.K. Ng, and A.S. Weiss. 2014. Tropoelastin: A versatile, bioactive assembly module. *Acta Biomaterialia.* 10(4): 1532–1541.

Woodhouse, K.A., P. Klement, V. Chen, M.B. Gorbet, F.W. Keeley, R. Stahl, J.D. Fromstein, and C.M. Bellingham. 2004. Investigation of recombinant human elastin polypeptides as non-thrombogenic coatings. *Biomaterials.* 25(19): 4543–4553.

Wrenn, D., W.C. Parks, L.A. Whitehouse, E.C. Crouch, U. Kucich, J. Rosenbloom, and R. Mecham. 1987. Identification of multiple tropoelastins secreted by bovine cells. *Journal of Biological Chemistry.* 262(5): 2244–2249.

Yim, H., Y.S. Cho, C.H. Seo, B.C. Lee, J.H. Ko, D. Kim, J. Hur, W. Chun, and J.H. Kim. 2010. The use of AlloDerm on major burn patients: AlloDerm prevents post-burn joint contracture. *Burns.* 36(3): 322–328.

Yin, Y., M.M. Bilek, D.R. McKenzie, N.J. Nosworthy, A. Kondyurin, H. Youssef, M.J. Byrom, and W. Yang. 2009a. Acetylene plasma polymerized surfaces for covalent immobilization of dense bioactive protein monolayers. *Surface and Coatings Technology.* 203(10): 1310–1316.

Yin, Y., S.G. Wise, N.J. Nosworthy, A. Waterhouse, D.V. Bax, H. Youssef, M.J. Byrom, M.M. Bilek, D.R. McKenzie, and A.S. Weiss. 2009b. Covalent immobilisation of tropoelastin on a plasma deposited interface for enhancement of endothelialisation on metal surfaces. *Biomaterials.* 30(9): 1675–1681.

Zeugolis, D.I., S.T. Khew, E.S. Yew, A.K. Ekaputra, Y.W. Tong, L.-Y.L. Yung, D.W. Hutmacher, C. Sheppard, and M. Raghunath. 2008. Electro-spinning of pure collagen nano-fibres—just an expensive way to make gelatin? *Biomaterials.* 29(15): 2293–2305.

CHAPTER 4

Biomolecular Regulation of Elastic Matrix Regeneration and Repair

Ganesh Swaminathan, Balakrishnan Sivaraman, and Anand Ramamurthi

CONTENTS

4.1 INTRODUCTION

The extracellular matrix (ECM) of tissues is the structural framework that provides cell support and sustenance. In soft connective tissues, the ECM is composed of structural proteins (e.g., elastin and collagen), and proteoglycans (PGs) and glycosaminoglycans (GAGs). Besides contributing to tissue mechanical properties, the ECM is a reservoir for growth factors (GFs) and other cell signaling biomolecules, and exerts dynamic spatiotemporal control on GF bioavailability, toward intimately guiding cell signaling, tissue homeostasis, and tissue regenerative processes (Lutolf and Hubbell 2005, Lee et al. 2011). While matrix generation or regeneration involves *de novo* cellular matrix synthesis and organization, matrix repair involves positive cellular remodeling of existing, matrix-compromised structures *in vivo* toward restoring tissue homeostasis. ECM components are synthesized, secreted, and remodeled by cells in most tissues, in response to perceived biochemical and biomechanical transductive cues. However, this response is highly specific to the ECM component, tissue type, and state of health.

Tissue engineering technologies proffer significant promise and potential to generate ECM structures using autologous patient-derived cells toward custom-fabricating tissue and organ replacements on demand. Differently, principles of regenerative medicine employ autologous or allogeneic cell types or their secretions, *in situ* repair or regeneration of the ECM of tissues that are structurally compromised by disease, trauma, or aging, to restore their form and function (Greenwood et al. 2006, Mason and Dunnill 2008). Despite nearly three decades of progressive innovation and refinements in pertinent tools and methodologies, the promise of tissue engineering and regenerative medicine remains unfulfilled due to significant challenges to replicating the complex matrix composition and architecture of various soft tissues, particularly those containing cell types that may be classified as permanent or stable cell (e.g., cardiac and vascular cells). One yet unsurmounted roadblock is the poor capacity of postneonatal cells, barring exceptions such as smooth muscle cells (SMCs) of the bladder (Wognum et al. 2009) and vaginal wall (Rahn et al. 2008), to synthesize elastin precursors (tropoelastin) and to recruit and organize these precursors into mature elastic fibers and tissue-specific higher order architectures (e.g., sheets, lamellae) in a manner that recapitulates developmental elastogenesis (Parks et al. 1993, Swee et al. 1995). These intrinsic deficiencies are exacerbated in cells within a disease milieu (Huffman et al. 2000), and can have serious ramifications to our ability to restore healthy tissue function because elastic fibers critically maintain native tissue structure, enable their stretch and recoil following release of stretching forces, and also regulate behavior of contacting cells via biomechanical transductive contacting cues (Robert et al. 1995, Faury et al. 1998, Li et al. 1998a,b).

The mechanical and biological properties of elastic fibers are critically mediated by their complex compositional profile comprising elastin protein, glycoprotein microfibrils (fibrillin), and nearly 30 other components (Kielty et al. 2002). In light of the poor synthesis/assembly of elastic matrix by adult cell types, biomaterials assembled from recombinant elastin and synthetic elastin-like peptides (ELPs) (Daamen et al. 2003, 2007, Berglund et al. 2004, Buijtenhuijs et al. 2004, Leach et al. 2005) have been developed to provide mechanical/structural properties similar to elastic matrix, and mediate cell adhesion and signaling through interaction with elastin receptors on cell surfaces (Mithieux et al. 2004, Almine et al. 2010). However, a major perceived limitation of these materials is that they do not replicate the compositional biocomplexity of native elastic fibers and are thus unlikely to mimic healthy-cell–elastic-fiber interactions, thus contributing to aberrant matrix homeostasis (Bashur et al. 2012). This highlights the need for cell involvement in elastic matrix assembly. Considering poor elastogenicity of most elastin-generating adult cell types (e.g., SMCs and fibroblasts) (Sephel and Davidson 1986) there is a critical need for approaches to augment elastin synthesis and fiber assembly, and to provide the impetus and guidance necessary for cells to organize these fibers into tissue-type-specific three-dimensional architectures.

This chapter is intended to provide an overview of technologies in development aimed at mimicking robust developmental elastic matrix assembly. Because Chapters 1 through 3 in this book will focus on aspects of elastin biology and biomaterials-based approaches to elastic tissue engineering, this chapter will emphasize biomolecule (e.g., GFs, cytokines)-based proelastogenic and antiproteolytic approaches to facilitate biomimetic elastic matrix assembly and matrix repair. The chapter will provide a succinct overview of the steps involved in cellular elastic fiber assembly and highlight critical aberrations that must be overcome or circumvented via GF therapy and the advances that have been made in this regard. Biomaterial scaffolds and nanovehicles will be discussed in the context of their role as structural frameworks for targeted and sustained delivery of proelastogenic and antiproteolytic agents for tissue-localized regenerative elastic matrix repair. Attenuating chronic matrilysis at the intended site of tissue repair through these delivery modalities, concurrent with providing a regenerative stimulus, is critical to facilitate significant accumulation of new elastic matrix structures for lasting improvements to tissue structure and function. Intrinsic to use of these approaches is the need to spatiotemporally control bioavailability of proelastogenic/antiproteolytic biomolecules and also the patterns of induced cellular elastic matrix assembly at the *in vivo* tissue site, which is also discussed. In light of evidence of (a) the tissue reparative potential of stem cells (SCs) and their derivatives, (b) their active role in developmental elastogenesis, which suggests high elastogenic potential versus terminally differentiated, adult cells, and evidence that (c) their tissue regenerative/reparative effects are mediated through their secretions that can include GFs known to stimulate elastogenesis or inhibit proteolysis, this chapter also reviews prospects, challenges, and recent advances toward clinical use of SC-based or stem-cell-inspired approaches for elastic matrix engineering and regenerative repair.

4.2 HIERARCHICAL ASSEMBLY OF ELASTIC FIBERS

A thorough understanding of the highly complex process of elastin precursor synthesis and elastic fiber formation is a requisite to identifying inherent deficiencies in the process when affected by stable, adult cell types, toward developing strategies to overcome the same. The process of elastic matrix assembly occurs primarily during development and is virtually complete by adolescence. It is a complex, hierarchical process as illustrated in Figure 1.2 (Chapter 1). The process of elastin synthesis and elastic matrix assembly is regulated at multiple levels, which are described in detail in other review articles (Swee et al. 1995, Davidson 2002). Elastin is first secreted as precursor molecules called tropoelastin into the extracellular space. Tropoelastin, a 72 kDa protein, is encoded by a single copy gene *ELN* in humans and synthesized by many cell types, but primarily SMCs (Jones et al. 1979) and fibroblasts (Sephel and Davidson 1986). Three different isoforms of tropoelastin exist, which correspond to alternative splicing patterns of the transcripts that are affected by posttranscription (Davidson 2002). Approximately 75% of the amino acid content of the tropoelastin molecules is made up of hydrophobic amino acids; the remainder is composed of hydrophilic amino acids containing lysine and alanine residues, with the former involved in intermolecular crosslinking (Suyama and Nakamura 1990, Brown-Augsburger et al. 1995).

In the extracellular space, through their hydrophobic VGVAPG domain (Hinek et al. 1991), tropoelastin molecules engage with and bind a chaperone protein, elastin-binding protein (EBP). EBP protects the precursors from degradation (Hinek et al. 1991, Hinek and Rabinovitch 1994). The EBP binds both the cell membrane, and at its galactolectin-binding site, galactosugars. Galactosugars present on microfibrillar glycoprotein (e.g., fibrillin) prescaffolds that form extracellular linear arrays engage the galactolectin-binding site. This serves to reduce strength of EBP binding to tropoelastin as well as the cell membrane to cause disassociation of bound precursor molecules from the EBP and the EBP itself from the cell membrane (Figure 4.1a). The disassociated tropoelastin molecules coalesce on the microfibril prescaffold (Clarke et al. 2005), and their lysine side chains undergo oxidative cross-linking by lysyl oxidase (LOX), a Cu^{2+}-dependent enzyme (Kagan and Li 2003), to form desmosine and isodesmosine linkages. The microfibrillar prescaffold serves to (a) provide spatial coordination and alignment to coalescing tropoelastin nuclei toward their extension and cross-linking to form mature elastic fibers, (b) maintain fiber integrity, and (c) facilitate biomechanical transduction of contacting cells by the elastic fibers. In cross section, mature elastic fibers exhibit a diameter of 300 nm^{-2} μm and contain a central core of electron-dense alkali-insoluble cross-linked elastin surrounded by microfibrils in the periphery. Desmosine cross-linking of adjacent elastin molecules within these fibers allow them to stretch and recoil as a single unit. In addition, in the presence of cross-links, forces and stress levels that are transduced by cells are dramatically increased (Armentano et al. 1991). The mature elastic fibers that form a fundamental structural unit of tissue elastic matrix then interconnect via a process mediated by cells to organize into higher order structures such as discrete fiber networks, and denser, fibrous membranes or sheets (Kielty et al. 2002). The unique structural organization of elastic fibers contribute to their unique mechanics, particularly high elasticity (i.e., long-range deformability, passive recoil, low hysteresis) compared to other structural ECM components (e.g., collagen) within connective tissues. In contrast, collagen fibers exhibit a more viscoelastic response that can cause interfibrillar slippage (Freeman et al. 2007).

Repair of proteolytically disrupted elastic matrix structures in diseased tissues occurs through a similar process. Newly synthesized elastin precursors are deposited and cross-linked with pre-existing microfibril scaffolds at the site of tissue repair, which emphasizes the importance of existing fiber framework to the repair process. Differently, Berk et al. (2005)

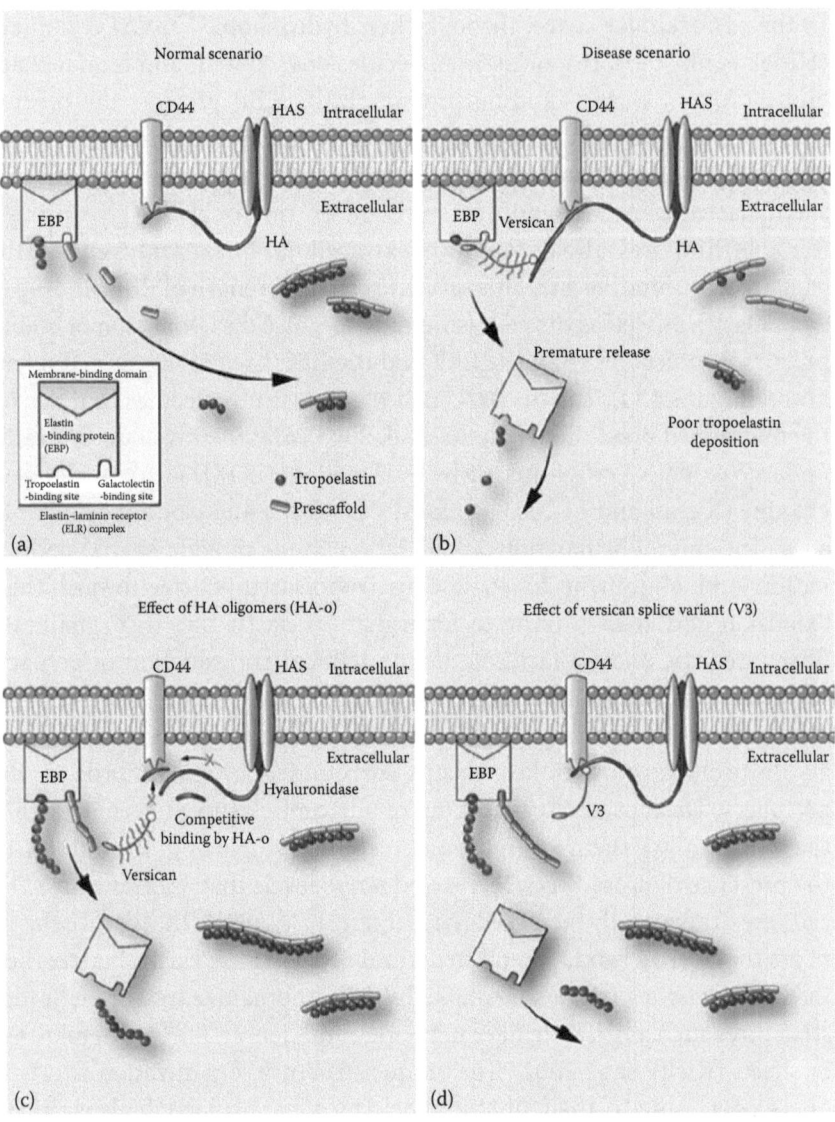

FIGURE 4.1 Regulation of elastic fiber assembly by hyaluronan and versican. (a) In a healthy tissue microenvironment, galacotosugar moieties of extracellular microfibrils engage the galactolectin-binding site on the elastin–laminin receptor (ELR) complex to result in the release of tropoelastin nuclei bound to the tropoelastin-binding site on the ELR. These nuclei deposit and are cross-linked on the fibrillin-prescaffold, and further coalesce and extend to form mature elastic fibers.   (Continued)

have shown that degraded desmosine and isodesmosine cross-links can be reformed or salvaged, though little is known of its mechanistic basis. In addition, the extent of remodeling that occurs has been shown to depend on the degree of elastic matrix disruption (Gacchina and Ramamurthi 2011). Because the ECM serves as a reservoir for matrix regenerative GFs, the role of these biomolecules in augmenting and modulating aspects of elastic matrix repair in a proteolytic tissue milieu is unique and differentiates it from *de novo* elastic matrix assembly.

4.3 CHALLENGES IN ENABLING *DE NOVO* ELASTIC MATRIX ASSEMBLY

The foremost roadblock to growing elastic tissue constructs in controlled culture microenvironments *in vitro* pertains to poor stability of tropoelastin mRNA (Johnson et al. 1995) and its rather limited translation to protein synthesis by most postneonatal, stable cell types, with SMCs of the bladder (Wognum et al. 2009) and vaginal wall (Rahn et al. 2008) representing significant exemptions. Other key impediments lie in the poor (<1%–10%) recruitment of tropoelastin precursors by cells and their nucleation, and poor precursor engagement of fibrillin glycoproteins and cross-linking into an elastic matrix (Fornieri et al. 1992). To emphasize the importance of the cross-linking aspect, we evoke the disorganized, amyloid pseudoelastic fibers generated within neointimal vascular plaques (Deb and

FIGURE 4.1 (Continued) (b) In cell cultures and within diseased tissues, the chondroitin sulfate (CS)-bearing proteoglycan, versican, accumulates. In the extracellular space, versican binds to long-chain hyaluronan (HA), whose production is also increased, and which in turn is bound to its cell surface receptor CD44, and its component CS side chains containing galactosugars, engages the galactolectin-binding site on the elastin-binding protein of the ELR in preference to microfibrillar glycoproteins (e.g., fibrillin). This prompts the premature release of the EBP from the cell membrane and of tropoelastin precursors for the EBP, the latter preventing tropoelastin from depositing on the microfibrillar scaffold and undergoing cross-linking by LOX to form mature fibers. (c) Although hyaluronan oligomers (HA-o) are not synthesized by cells, their delivery to cell cultures/tissues can competitively inhibit binding of long-chain HA to their CD44 receptors and further binding of versican to HA. The net outcome of improved elastic matrix assembly in such a scenario is similar to that which results on supplementation of splice variants of versican (V3). (d) V3 that lacks the chondroitin sulfate chain-bearing domain fails to engage the EBP thus improving engagement of the EBP galactolectin-binding site by fibrillin microfibrils toward facilitating tropoelastin nucleation and timely release for improved elastic fiber assembly.

Ramamurthi 2014), where their limited cross-linking renders them susceptible to proteolysis. To date, no convincing solution to these issues has been found in terms of cellular substrates (e.g., biomaterial scaffolds) and culture conditions (e.g., biomolecular cues, biomechanical conditioning) that augment mature elastic fiber assembly and further facilitate the organization of these fibers into higher order elastic matrix structures specific to tissue type. The latter outcome is particularly important because elastic matrix content and more so architecture differ significantly based on tissue location and role, and critically determine the biomechanics essential to fulfill their intended function. For example, in blood vessels, the elastic matrix is organized into concentric, circumferentially organized sheets, in the dermis of the skin, in pulmonary tissues, and in the vaginal wall as meshes of loosely intertwined elastic fibers, and in aortic heart valve leaflets as dense fibrous sheets (Kielty et al. 2002). Thus, poor ability to generate or regenerate mature elastic fibers, or replicate their size, density, and relative orientation and alignment can adversely impact mechanics of engineered elastic tissue replacements or of tissues subject to regenerative repair *in vivo*. As an illustrative example, vascular tissue constructs generated using tissue engineering principles lack sufficient elastin, mature and complete elastic fibers, and poor lamellar organization of elastic fibers, despite application of biaxial stretch conditioning regimens during culture to coax circumferential cellular orientation and elastic matrix deposition. These aberrations of the elastic matrix contribute to wall weakening and dilatation to form an aneurysm when implanted *in vivo*. Evoking developmental patterns of elastogenesis in adult tissues can also present unique challenges due to nonexpression of key developmental elastic matrix assembly proteins in adulthood. For example, while fibrillin-2 is primarily expressed in the fetus where robust elastogenesis occurs, fibrillin-1 is primarily expressed in adult tissues (Kielty et al. 2002). There are also significant challenges to controlling spatial patterns and alignments of the microfibrillar components *in vitro*, and much more so *in vivo*. Interaction of cultured cells with unnatural scaffolding materials *in vitro*, or inflammatory responses to the scaffold when implanted *in vivo*, can also prompt cellular overexpression of matrix degradative enzymes, which in turn prevents accumulation of *de novo* synthesized elastic matrix. Modalities to suppress elastolysis concurrent with providing a proelastogenic stimulus to cells within tissue-engineered constructs is thus important to augment elastic matrix content toward improving tissue elasticity and restoring healthy mechanical and biological function.

Enabling regenerative repair (i.e., new fiber formation and restoring disrupted cross-links) of elastic matrix *in situ* within proteolytically ECM-disrupted tissues, in absence of in-born defects of elastic matrix assembly proteins, represents its unique set of challenges. In the diseased tissue *milieu*, a subset of parenchymal cells (e.g., SMCs, fibroblasts) may switch to an activated phenotype characterized by (a) poor elastogenicity compared to even cells of a healthy phenotype (Beamish et al. 2010), and (b) poor production and impaired activity of LOX, the elastin and collagen-cross-linking enzyme. In addition, the extracellular microenvironment in diseased tissues may show drastic changes relative to healthy tissues that can adversely impact elastic matrix assembly. For example, a first response to tissue injury includes in-tissue buildup of GAGs and PGs (Hinek et al. 1991), which can interfere with the precursor nucleation, coalescing, and fiber formation steps of the elastic matrix assembly process (Figure 4.1a,b). The chronic overexpression of elastin targeting matrix metalloproteinases (MMPs; specifically MMPs 2, 9, and 12) enzymes by parenchymal and inflammatory cells at the site of tissue injury can reduce net accumulation of new elastin deposits and disrupt new and pre-existing elastic matrix structures. Because intact elastic fibers have been found to serve as nucleation sites for guiding growth of new elastic fibers (Kielty et al. 2002), this aspect of elastogenesis can be impaired by chronically upregulated MMP activity at the site of tissue repair. Chronic elastolysis also generates soluble elastin peptides that unlike intact elastic fibers, promote cell proliferation, cytokine, chemokine, and MMP release, and intracellular Ca^{2+} intake resulting in cell/matrix calcification (Aikawa et al. 2009); the elastin peptides, through a positive feedback loop involving MMP increases, serve to further elastic matrix degradation (Senior et al. 1980). In this light, restoring elastin homeostasis in injured/diseased tissues is contingent on attenuating elastolysis concurrent with providing a regenerative impetus to shift the balance between these two contradictory processes to favor net accumulation of intact new elastic matrix.

4.4 BIOMOLECULAR STIMULATION OF ELASTIC MATRIX REGENERATION

Controlled delivery of GFs in tandem with other approaches (e.g., novel biomaterial scaffolds, topographic cues, and biomechanical stimuli) is emerging as a useful strategy to improve elastic matrix content and structure within tissue-engineered constructs and to restore elastic matrix homeostasis at tissue injury sites. Engagement of extracellular GFs with cell surface receptors trigger intracellular changes wherein signaling proteins and pathways are either activated or inhibited to augment or attenuate aspects of elastic matrix assembly. Several biological moieties have been documented to influence elastic matrix assembly across tissue types. A noncomprehensive list of biomolecular agents that promote and/ or inhibit different aspects of elastic matrix assembly as a function of dose or depending on the regenerative microenvironment is given in Table 4.1. The list includes a variety of nucleotides, GFs, cytokines, cell-derived or exogenously provided enzymes, vitamins, steroids, and matrix GAGs and PGs. For example, there is evidence that galactosugar-bearing GAGs such as chondroitin sulfate (CS), and PGs (e.g., versican) presenting CS serve to inhibit mature elastic fiber formation by adult vascular SMCs (Hinek et al. 1991). To the contrary, neonatal vascular SMCs that produce very limited amounts of versican, robustly synthesize elastic matrix (Wight and Merrilees 2004). This can be well explained on the basis of the schematic shown in Figure 4.1. In healthy tissues (Figure 4.1a), tropoelastin precursors engage and bind to the EBP where they undergo nucleation till a point when the prescaffold of fibrillin glycoproteins bearing galactosugar moieties engages the galactolectin-binding site on the EBP to release the tropoelastin nuclei for coacervation on to the adjacent prescaffold to be cross-linked and extended to form a fiber. In disease and/or injury response scenarios, GAGs (e.g., long-chain hyaluronan or HA with molecular weights >2 million daltons; CS) and PGs (e.g., versican) are abundantly synthesized in the extracellular space. The HA secreted by the cells forms a pericellular sheath and binds to the HA receptor (CD44) on the cell surface. The long-chain HA has been shown to have no stimulatory effect on tropoelastin synthesis itself, though it provides some benefit to recruitment and cross-linking of these precursor molecules (Joddar and Ramamurthi 2006a,b) via opposite charge interaction that physically coacervate them (Fornieri et al. 1987). Even though long-chain HA may provide an impetus to elastin protein cross-linking, fiber formation is impeded. Briefly, versican chains bind to HA via their HA-binding domain and the attached CS chains engage the galactolectin-binding site on the EBP to reduce affinity of bound tropoelastin to the EBP and affinity of the EBP for the cell membrane. This results in their premature release before nucleation of tropoelastin molecules has sufficiently occurred, so that these nuclei do not engage the microfibrillar prescaffolding to initiate fiber assembly (Figure 4.1b). Differently, in the presence of short HA oligomers (HA-o),

TABLE 4.1 Listing of Biological Factors That Regulate Elastin Homeostasis

Biological Factor	Target Cells	Effects	References
		Antielastogenic Factors	
Ascorbic acid	Aortic SMCs, dermal fibroblasts, pulmonary arterial SMCs	↓ LOX activity, ↓ cross-linking of tropoelastin, ↓ tropoelastin synthesis and matrix assembly	Barone et al. (1985), Bergethon et al. (1989), Davidson et al. (1997), Dunn and Franzblau (1982), Faris et al. (1984), Keire et al. (2010)
bFGF	Lung fibroblasts	→ tropoelastin synthesis, ↓ elastin mRNA	Brettell and McGowan (1994)
cAMP	Ligament fibroblasts	→ tropoelastin synthesis, cGMP antagonist	Mecham et al. (1985)
Chondroitin sulfate	Vascular SMCs	→ elastin synthesis	Hinek et al. (1991)
Theophylline	Ligament fibroblasts	→ tropoelastin synthesis, dexamethasone antagonist	Mecham et al. (1981)
Monensin	Ligament fibroblasts, chondrocytes, aortic SMCs	→ tropoelastin synthesis	Davis and Mecham (1998), Frisch et al. (1985)
Bafilomycin A1	Ligament fibroblasts, chondrocytes	→ tropoelastin synthesis	Davis and Mecham (1998)
Cycloheximide	Ligament fibroblasts	→ elastin synthesis	Mecham et al. (1981)
Chloroquine	Ligament fibroblasts, chondrocytes	→ tropoelastin synthesis	Davis and Mecham (1998)
EGF	Lung fibroblasts	→ tropoelastin synthesis and → elastin deposition	DiCamillo et al. (2006)
NH_4Cl	Ligament fibroblasts, chondrocytes	→ tropoelastin synthesis	Davis and Mecham (1998)

(Continued)

TABLE 4.1 (*Continued*)   Listing of Biological Factors That Regulate Elastin Homeostasis

Biological Factor	Target Cells	Effects	References
Versican	Aortic SMCs	Release of EBP from cell surface leading to ↓ elastin fiber assembly	Hinek et al. (1991)
Elastogenesis-Stimulatory Factors			
IGF-1	Aortic SMCs	↑ tropoelastin and matrix assembly	Kothapalli and Ramamurthi (2008), Rich et al. (1993), Wolfe et al. (1993)
HA oligomers	Aortic SMCs	↑ tropoelastin synthesis and matrix assembly	Joddar and Ramamurthi (2006a,b), Joddar et al. (2007), Kothapalli et al. (2009a,b), Kothapalli and Ramamurthi (2008)
LOX	Aortic SMCs	↑ tropoelastin synthesis and matrix assembly	Kothapalli and Ramamurthi (2009b)
Retinoic acid	Vascular SMCs, dermal fibroblasts	↑ tropoelastin synthesis, ↑ fibrillin	Hayashi et al. (1995), Tajima et al. (1997)
Insulin	Vascular SMCs	↑ elastin synthesis	Shi et al. (2012)
Aldosterone	Dermal fibroblasts	↑ tropoelastin synthesis and fiber formation	Mitts et al. (2010)
HGF	Vocal fold fibroblasts	↑ tropoelastin synthesis	Hirano et al. (2003a,b,c), Luo et al. (2006)
cGMP	Ligament fibroblasts	↑ elastin synthesis in presence of intracellular Ca^{2+}	Mecham et al. (1985)
Cdk4 inhibitor	Dermal fibroblasts	↑ elastin synthesis	Sen et al. (2011)
Coenzyme Q	Dermal fibroblasts	↑ tropoelastin mRNA	Zhang et al. (2012)
FCS	Ligament fibroblasts	≥5% w/v ↑ elastin synthesis	Mecham et al. (1981)
Dexamethasone	Ligament fibroblasts	↑ tropoelastin synthesis	Mecham et al. (1981)

(*Continued*)

TABLE 4.1 (*Continued*) Listing of Biological Factors That Regulate Elastin Homeostasis

Biological Factor	Target Cells	Effects	References
Heparin sulfate	Dermal fibroblasts	Elastin synthesis	Annovi et al. (2012)
Bleomycin	Ligament fibroblasts	↑ tropoelastin synthesis	Mecham et al. (1981)
		Factors with Contradictory Effects	
HA-long chain	Aortic SMCs	↑ tropoelastin, ↑ tropoelastin cross-linking; ↑ versican binding, ↓ elastin fiber assembly	Joddar and Ramamurthi (2006a,b)
TGF-β1	Aortic SMCs	↑ LOX expression and activity; ↓ MMP-2, -9;	Dai et al. (2005), Kothapalli et al. (2009a,b),
	Fibroblasts, SMCs	↑ TIMP-1, -2, -3; ↑ elastin synthesis	Losy et al. (2003), Sales et al. (2006)
		Matrix mineralization at high doses	Brown et al. (2002), Simionescu et al. (2005)
Cu2+ ion	Aortic SMCs	↑ cross-linking; toxic at high doses	Cortizo et al. (2004), Kothapalli and Ramamurthi (2009a,c)
IL-1β	Dermal fibroblasts	↑ tropoelastin	Mauviel et al. (1993), Berk et al. (1991)
	Lung fibroblasts	↓ tropoelastin expression	

IGF-1, insulin-like growth factor-1; HA, hyaluronan; HGF, hepatocyte growth factor; FCS, fetal calf serum; bFGF, basic fibroblast growth factor; EGF, epidermal growth factor; IL-1β, interleukin; SMC, smooth muscle cells; LOX, lysyl oxidase; EBP, elastin-binding protein, cGMP, cyclic GMP; TGF, transforming growth factor; MMP, matrix metalloprotease; TIMP, tissue inhibitors of MMP.

which are not synthesized as such but rather generated by depolymerization of long-chain HA, often by hyaluronidase, or when exogenously delivered, the oligomers compete with long-chain HA for binding to cell surface CD44 receptors and through the process, reduce prospects for versican binding and engagement of EBP. Thus, premature release of EBP and tropoelastin is avoided and mature elastic fiber assembly is improved (Figure 4.1c). The same outcomes have been evoked by treating cells with a splice variant of versican (V3), which lacks the HA-binding domain. Here too, with impedance of versican binding and consequent engagement of the EBP, elastic fiber assembly is improved (Figure 4.1d).

The effects of many of these proelastogenic biomolecules have been shown to be dose dependent. For example, transforming growth factor-beta (TGF-β) has been shown to have biphasic effects with procollagen-regenerative and promitotic properties, besides adverse procalcific effects at doses lower than 1 ng/ml and greater than 15 ng/ml (Brown et al. 2002, Simionescu et al. 2005) and to augment tropoelastin synthesis and cross-linking via augmentation of LOX mRNA expression and enzyme activity at intermediate doses (Shanley et al. 1997). Similarly, the demonstrated antielastogenic effects of ascorbic acid and ascorbates on SMCs and fibroblasts from various tissues have been shown to be closely dose dependent, and withdrawal of ascorbate increased elastic matrix deposition by cultured cells (Dunn and Franzblau 1982, Faris et al. 1984, Barone et al. 1985, Bergethon et al. 1989). These outcomes have served as a basis for designing a novel culture regimen for tissue-engineered vascular constructs, wherein the initial period of ascorbate dosing promotes high cellularity of the scaffolding material and its stiffening via new collagen deposition, and a subsequent switch to culture under ascorbate-free conditions augments elastic matrix synthesis and tissue elasticity (Keire et al. 2010). Insulin growth factor-1 (IGF-1) has also been demonstrated to provide significant proelastogenic stimuli to vascular SMCs, by augmenting elastin mRNA expression, protein translation, and matrix deposition (Wolfe et al. 1993). Other agents, such as the steroid aldosterone, have been shown to provide proelastogenic stimuli through an IGF-1 receptor-mediated signaling pathway (Mitts et al. 2010). Further research by Ramamurthi and his co-workers has also demonstrated significant synergy of action of biomolecules with proelastogenic properties. For example, both IGF-1 and TGF-β effects on improving (a) tropoelastin synthesis, (b) proportion of tropoelastin cross-linked into matrix structures, and (c) elastic fiber assembly were shown to be synergistically enhanced when these factors were co-delivered with HA-o *in vitro*; likely, these effects occur through several combinatory mechanisms. In light of the dose-dependent possible adverse effect of TGF-β and IGF-1 and potentially inflammatory effects of HA-o at higher doses (Noble 2002), controlled presentation of these agents to cells at safe per cell doses is necessary. Retinoic acid delivery to fibroblasts and vascular SMCs has also been shown to augment elastin gene expression, protein synthesis, and improve fiber formation by enhancing fibrillin-1 prescaffold assembly (Hayashi et al. 1995, Tajima et al. 1997).

Despite progress toward identifying biomolecular agents that stimulate elastin precursor synthesis, recruitment and cross-linking of these molecules by cells into matrix structures remains a challenge. Typical yields of elastic matrix (i.e., percentage ratio of matrix elastin deposited per unit amount of tropoelastin precursor synthesized) generated by healthy vascular cells lie in the range of 10%–15% (Joddar and Ramamurthi 2006b), while that by cells of a diseased phenotype can be much lower (e.g., 1%–2% for human aneurysmal SMCs) (Gacchina et al. 2011a). In this situation, our ability to generate finite-sized elastic tissue constructs on demand for human use, or repair large defects in elastic tissues *in situ,* is contingent on augmenting yield of elastic matrix. One manner of accomplishing this is through augmenting production, activity, or spatial bioavailability of LOX and its homologues (see Section 4.2) in the vicinity of the cell toward improving elastin precursor capture and cross-linking and promoting elastic fiber renewal (Kagan and Li 2003). Building on early findings as to feasibility of cross-linking recombinant tropoelastin with exogenous, purified LOX, Ramamurthi's research group has previously demonstrated that purified exogenous LOX protein when supplemented to cultured rat vascular SMCs significantly improves yield of elastic matrix beyond that achievable in control cultures wherein tropoelastin cross-linking is mediated by endogenous LOX/LOX homologues alone (Kothapalli and Ramamurthi 2009b). As mentioned in Section 4.2, the LOX enzyme requires copper ions (Cu^{2+}) for its extracellular transport. In addition, Cu^{2+} is essential to activity of LOX (endogenous and exogenous) in its role in facilitating oxidative deamination of lysine residues on the tropoelastin molecules, a necessary step in cross-link formation (Kagan and Li 2003). Capitalizing on this information, Kothapalli and Ramamurthi (2009a) delivered soluble copper salts to vascular SMC cultures and demonstrated significant increases in tropoelastin cross-linking, which was attributed to increased LOX production and activity in the presence of exogenous Cu^{2+}. However, at the useful doses (0.1 M) of the delivered copper salts, cell death was noted

(Cortizo and Fernandez Lorenzo de Mele 2004). This problem was circumvented by delivering the equivalent cumulative exposure dose of Cu^{2+} through extended steady-state release from copper nanoparticles (CuNP), which was shown to not only prevent cytotoxicity but also dramatically improve the percentage fraction of tropoelastin precursors that were cross-linked from ~10% to nearly 45% (Kothapalli and Ramamurthi 2009a). Co-delivery of HA-o and CuNP was shown to further improve elastic matrix deposition, likely due to a combination of (a) benefits provided by HA-o to elastic fiber formation, described earlier in this section, and (b) enhancement of LOX activity by CuNP-released Cu^{2+} ions in the vicinity of cells on electrostatic interactions between the cationic CuNP and negatively charged pericellular GAGs and HA-o (Kothapalli and Ramamurthi 2009a).

While much of the literature reported above pertains to delivery of pro-elastogenic factors to enhance elastic fiber assembly by healthy cells, of direct relevance to improving elastic matrix content and structure within tissue-engineered constructs, these factors may also be useful to affect *in situ* regenerative repair of elastic matrix at sites of chronic proteolytic disruption. Even compared to their healthy counterparts, elastogenesis by cells of a diseased phenotype tends to be orders of magnitude lower with significant limitations to both tropoelastin synthesis and efficiency of cross-linking of these precursor molecules (Gacchina et al. 2011a,b). In addition, significant compromises in the content and structural integrity of the pre-existing ECM framework within these diseased tissues not only adversely impact new fiber formation based on nucleation sites presented by pre-existing elastic fibers (Bressan et al. 1986), but have been shown to further diminish response of the parenchymal cells to proelasto-genic stimuli (Gacchina and Ramamurthi 2011). This is directly related to aberrations in elastic fiber regulation of cell phenotype and GF/cytokine bioavailability (Eble and Niland 2009). For example, the microfibril components of intact elastic fibers (e.g., fibulin-5) bind latent TGF-β-binding protein (LTBP), which bind and serve as a reservoir of TGF-β (Ono et al. 2009). The interaction between LTBP and fibrillin-1 glycoproteins is essential to TGF-β sequestration (Ono et al. 2009). When the fibrillin-1 component is lost as in disrupted or aberrant elastic fibers, TGF-β storage in the ECM is reduced and its bioavailability in an active form is increased with adverse implications to cellular health and viability (e.g., apoptosis), and ECM quality (e.g., matrix mineralization). As a result of proteolytic injury, other elastic fiber components essential to regulating cell phenotype and function and elastic fiber assembly are also compromised. For example, with disruption of the microfibrillar component of elastic fibers composed primarily of RGD-motif-presenting fibrillin-1, interactions with cell surface integrins are interrupted (Halper and Kjaer 2014). Other microfibrillar components, MAGP-1 and fibulins, are known to bind both tropoelastin and LOX to facilitate cross-linking while interacting with components of the ECM (e.g., collagen VI, PGs) (Wagenseil and Mecham 2007). In a proteolytic *milieu*, etching of elastic fibers by MMPs can compromise these vital elastic matrix assembly functions associated with intact elastic fibers. Still further, concomitant signaling by endogenous GFs, cytokines and other chemokines within the diseased tissue *milieu* can interfere with elastogenic factor–receptor interaction-induced intracellular signaling pathways leading to improved elastic matrix assembly outcomes.

Despite these many constraints, augmenting bioavailability of proelastogenic factors such as TGF-β1, either by supplementing exogenous GFs or by increasing endogenous factor production, has been shown to significantly augment tropoelastin synthesis, and cross-linked elastic fiber assembly by cells of a diseased phenotype, both *in vitro* (Kothapalli et al. 2009b, Gacchina et al. 2011a,b) and *in vivo* (Dai et al. 2011). For example, healthy SMCs seeded within aortic xenografts in rats that developed abdominal aortic aneurysms (AAAs) transiently produced TGF-β1 that stimulated matrix production and LOX-mediated cross-linking by host fibroblasts and SMCs within (Losy et al. 2003). Similarly, via gene therapy strategies, TGF-β1 has been overexpressed with formed AAAs, again in rats, toward achieving some degree of elastic matrix regenerative repair in the vessel wall (Dai et al. 2005). While these outcomes clearly demonstrate the responsiveness of activated or diseased cells to elastogenic stimulation, Ramamurthi's group has shown that significantly higher per cell doses of proelastogenic factors are required for tangible regenerative effect with these cells relative to their healthy counterparts, and that their responsiveness is inversely related to the degree of injury to their ECM (Gacchina and Ramamurthi 2011), for the reasons outlined in the previous paragraph.

A unique requirement to ensuring successful *in situ* regenerative elastic tissue repair in a proteolytic *milieu* lies in providing a deterrent to MMPs concurrent with a proelastogenic stimulus. Chronic MMP overexpression can also occur as a response to seeding cells on unnatural tissue engineering scaffolding materials *in vitro* and through the auspices of inflammatory cell recruitment to these materials when implanted *in vivo*. If not attenuated, proteolytic disruption and loss of the elastic matrix can overwhelm stimulated elastogenesis to prevent accumulation of new or repaired elastic matrix structures. In this context, many GFs with known proelastogenic properties have also been shown to influence MMP production and activity as listed in Table 4.1. The key factor to be considered in using a singular biological agent to fulfill these dual requirements for effective regenerative elastic matrix repair—providing both proelastogenic and anti-MMP stimuli—lies in selecting and ensuring tight control over the delivery dose, because the overlapping dose range for the respective effects may be slim. At the very least, if a given proelastogenic factor is also found to upregulate MMPs, dosing must be tightly controlled to limit its effect to enhancing elastic matrix assembly. At this time, several other options are available for inhibiting chronic proteolysis. *In vivo*, MMP balance is effected naturally through tissue inhibitors of MMPs (TIMPs). Although delivery of purified TIMP proteins could be a theoretically useful anti-MMP strategy, there are issues with their ability to be reliably manufactured (Coussens et al. 2002), and possible adverse effects including upregulation of MMP2 (Butler et al. 1998) and induction of apoptosis (Baker et al. 1998). Several cationic amphiphile compounds that mimic the anti-MMP effects of TIMPs have also been identified, which could find useful application in the regenerative space. The catalytically active site of MMPs contains anionic glutamic acid and histidine residues important for substrate binding and enzyme activity. TIMPs are compounds with a strong net positive charge that act in part by electrostatically engaging these anionic residues to inactivate MMPs (Murphy and Nagase 2008). Cationic amphiphile compounds such as quaternary glucosamine derivatives (Kagan et al. 1981a), and other synthetic compounds such as didodecyldimethyl ammonium bromide (DMAB) (Kagan et al. 1981b), have been shown to significantly inhibit activity of elastolytic MMPs (MMPs 2, 9), likely by mimicking the anti-MMP mechanisms of action of TIMPs. Recently, Sivaraman and Ramamurthi (2013) showed that in addition to its anti-MMP effects, DMAB, when functionalized on a substrate, also provides an impetus to cellular elastic matrix deposition by cultured aneurysmal vascular SMCs by attracting negatively charged LOX and augmenting LOX-mediated cross-linking (Kagan et al. 1981a,b), and by electrostatic repulsion of elastases (Kagan et al. 1979). As described by Kagan et al. (1981a), binding of hydrocarbon chains of these amphiphiles to the hydrophobic residues on the tropoelastin molecules also causes a conformational twist that exposes their lysine side chains for efficient cross-linking by LOX. MMPs can also be inhibited by the action of exogenous MMP antibodies and small molecule/drug-based inhibitors.

While MMP antibodies provide high specificity of targeting, they are cost-prohibitive (Clutterbuck et al. 2009) and not as yet validated by clinical trials. Nonsteroid anti-inflammatory drugs, statins, and other drug classes have been shown to inhibit upstream signaling pathways leading to MMP synthesis (Clutterbuck et al. 2009). Tetracycline derivatives such as doxycycline (DOX) have been widely studied in recent years in the context of inhibiting MMPs for treatment growth stabilization of AAAs (Curci et al. 1998, Manning et al. 2003, Bartoli et al. 2006) and treatment of chronic obstructive pulmonary disease (Dalvi et al. 2011), another condition that involves chronic breakdown of elastic matrix structures. DOX and similar compounds (e.g., minocycline; Wojtowicz-Praga et al. 1997) at least partly act by directly engaging the catalytic Zn^{2+} ion within the active site of the MMP enzyme (Wojtowicz-Praga et al. 1997). Despite its benefits, there are issues relating to its broad inhibition of all MMPs, not only those associated with elastolytic activity, and uncertainties as to its modes of action, of which there are several (Baxter et al. 2002). Another concern is that at the systemic doses deemed useful for inhibiting MMPs (Bartoli et al. 2006), DOX appears to inhibit cellular deposition of new elastic matrix (Franco et al. 2006). To circumvent this problem, Sivaraman and Ramamurthi (2013) developed nanoparticles for sustained, predictable, low-level (<5 μM) dosing of DOX. At this dosing level, DOX both maintained its MMP inhibitory activity and surprisingly also provided a proelastogenic stimulus. DOX delivery via this modality thus proffers attractive prospects for augmenting elastic matrix regenerative repair. Targeting microRNAs (miRNAs) is emerging now as a useful modality for regulating multiple downstream ECM homeostatic events. For example, overexpression of microRNA 29-b has recently been shown to result in overexpression of MMPs 2 and 9, and increased elastin mRNA expression and matrix synthesis, which likely accounts for its ability to stabilize murine AAAs against growth. Gene therapy approaches such as this are discussed in greater detail in Chapter 9.

4.5 MODALITIES FOR DELIVERY OF PROELASTOGENIC AND ANTIPROTEOLYTIC AGENTS

In seeking to achieve regenerative repair of elastic matrix *in vivo*, it is critical that proelastogenic and antiproteolytic agents be delivered to cells at the correct stage and precise location to elicit the desired reparative outcomes. This is especially important considering that cell responses, which are intimate functions of the extracellular microenvironment, are influenced by spatial heterogeneity and spatiotemporal changes in GF/cytokine bioavailability and autocrine/paracrine signaling, ECM composition and quality, and tissue cellularity. In addition, achieving sustained, predictable release of regenerative factors over the necessary duration over which the matrix/tissue is expected to regenerate, while minimizing their inactivation and ready clearance by the body, is essential, which cannot be achieved by delivery of exogenous factors. Developing modalities for protecting and exerting spatiotemporal control over the bioavailability of proregenerative agents is thus essential for functional tissue regeneration. In this context, biomaterials, both synthetic and natural, have been investigated extensively as scaffolds and nanovehicles for delivery of physically encapsulated, chemically tethered, or surface-adsorbed matrix regenerative biomolecules. Although in addition to serving as a delivery vehicle for biomolecules, scaffolding materials provide a mechanical framework within an injured tissue to allow cell binding, spreading, and *de novo* matrix deposition, and serve to provide biomechanical transductive cues to modulate cell phenotype, fate, and regenerative responses; these aspects are discussed in detail in Chapter 5. The present discussion of biomaterial scaffold and nanocarrier properties will thus be limited to the context of their providing spatiotemporal control over delivery of biomolecules for matrix regeneration.

4.5.1 Properties of Biomaterial Vehicles for Delivery of Matrix Regenerative Factors

The principal properties of nanoparticle vehicles and biomaterial scaffolds that must be considered in their selection tend to be interdependent and include chemistry, surface charge and topography, wetting properties, degradability, and mechanics (compliance and failure characteristics). While surface charge of biomaterial scaffolds is a more important factor for determining attachment of cells presenting hydrophilic surfaces than those that are hydrophobic (Panyam et al. 2002), in general, most cell types show affinity for attachment to hydrophilic surfaces (Healy et al. 1994). Cell attachment only shows differences in response to changes in charge and wettability for hydrophilic surfaces (Dowling et al. 2011). The chemistry, topography, and compliance of a scaffold also impact cell adherence, spreading, and integrin-mediated cellular mechanotransduction (Flemming et al. 1999, Safran et al. 2005). Inflammatory responses to scaffolding materials is a major factor determining their selection, which in turn is a critical function of their (a) degradation characteristics and by-products, and compliance match and integration with native tissue, both of which can determine stability or failure of the tissue site of regeneration, and (b) surface characteristics including roughness, surface charge, pore size/porosity, and wettability properties (Mikos et al. 1998). These factors are important in choosing whether to use synthetic (e.g., polyurethanes or PUs, polyesters, polyglycerol sebacate, synthetic elastomers) or natural (e.g., collagen, elastin, fibrin, chitosan) materials as drug delivery vehicles for regenerative applications. In addition, of direct import to the degradation characteristics of these materials is the issue of cross-linking, which is particularly important to ensure long-term stability of implantation of ECM-based biomaterials. For example, while cross-linked small intestinal submucosa (SIS) scaffolds elicit a proinflammatory response mediated by M1 macrophages, lack of cross-linking instead evokes a pro-tissue remodeling response by M2 macrophages (Badylak et al. 2008).

4.5.2 Scaffolds for Delivery of Proelastogenic and Antiproteolytic Agents

Scaffolds are intended to serve four major functions from a matrix/tissue regenerative perspective. The first role is to provide mechanical support to the tissue to be repaired until a time the tissue regenerates and takes over load bearing function, and provide a framework for cell adherence and infiltration by presenting cell-binding sites (Langer and Tirrell 2004). The second role is to ensure sustained and predictable release of biological agents in a spatiotemporally appropriate manner to influence cell fate processes and phenotype and augment aspects of new matrix assembly and pre-existing matrix repair (Lutolf and Hubbell 2005). The third role is to provide contacting cells necessary topographical cues and biomechanical transductive cues to influence their phenotype and orientation, and alignment and hence that of the matrix fibers they assemble (Cannizzaro et al. 1998). Finally, on their breakdown, the scaffolds are expected to, in a favorable scenario, generate degradation by-products (e.g., of structural components such as collagen or incorporated proregenerative biomolecules) that can themselves serve as cues to beneficially modulate cell behavior and/or matrix regeneration (Ahmann et al. 2010). At the very least, scaffold degradation by-products would be expected to not induce any adverse tissue remodeling, inflammatory responses, or toxicological effects and be rapidly cleared from the body (Martinon 2010). The simplest mode of incorporating biomolecular agents into scaffolds is physical surface adsorption (Ji et al. 2011). For example, the components of the elastic matrix such as tropoelastin, fibrillin-1, and fibulin-5 have been physically adsorbed on to PU-polycaprolactone (PCL) scaffolds to regulate SMC adherence and phenotype (Stephan et al. 2006). Adsorbed microfibrils on PLGA scaffolds are influenced by the scaffold surface chemistry in assuming structural conformations similar to their native hydrated form (Sherratt et al. 2005). Likewise, short elastin peptides organize into fibrillar structures on hydrophobic scaffolding surfaces due to hydrophobic interactions (Yang et al. 2002). In a variant approach, fibronectin has been adsorbed on to scaffolding surfaces to encourage binding of endogenous cell-generated proelastogenic factors such as IGF-1; in cases such as this, care must be exercised in ensuring that conformational changes to the fibronectin on adsorption do not occur, which can potentially expose binding sites for other endogenous factors such as epidermal growth factor-1 (EGF-1) with known antielastogenic effects (Mitsi et al. 2006). Other disadvantages of surface adsorption include challenges to creating and maintaining homogeneity of the adsorbed layer, possible removal from the surface, deactivation of exposed biological factors *in vivo*, or their masking through nonspecific protein adsorption *in vivo*, and limitations to sustained delivery to cells. An alternate approach is to covalently bind factors to the scaffold, which can serve to prolong their bioavailability to cells prior to scaffold degradation toward improving cell responses, as also shown by studies in Ramamurthi's lab that have sought to present proelastogenic HA-o through surface tethering, in preference to delivery of exogenous oligomers (Joddar and Ramamurthi 2006b, Joddar et al. 2007). In this case, the tethered HA-o not only maintained their proelastogenic signaling effects but also improved elastic matrix cross-linking due to (a) intimate, nontransient interactions between HA-o and cells (Joddar et al. 2007), and (b) colocalization of both LOX and tropoelastin molecules on the anionic HA-o tethered surface due to opposite charge interactions. Other GFs such as TGF-β and ECM components with proelastogenic properties such as fibronectin have also been tethered to scaffolds toward augmenting elastic matrix synthesis (Mann et al. 2001, Michael et al. 2003, Ma et al. 2007). Despite the advantages that covalent tethering provides, here too there are concerns, which include compromised or lost biological activity of tethered biomolecules due to (a) need to chemically modify or derive the biological factors to render them amenable to covalent tethering and cross-linking, which can result in conformational changes, and (b) cross-linking of amino acid sequences vital to cell adhesion (Lee et al. 2011). A third approach to deliver biomolecules from scaffolds is to encapsulate biomolecules in the bulk of the scaffolding material leading to the surface, which can be very advantageous because the biological effects of these factors can be extended to cells penetrating the interior of the scaffolds even after degradation of the scaffolding surface. For example, proelastogenic basic fibroblast growth factor (bFGF) and IGF-1 have been encapsulated within hydrogels for controlled release (Nuttelman et al. 2006). While a number of research groups have successfully demonstrated ability of GFs encapsulated within the fibers of electrospun polymer scaffolds to be released in a sustained and steady manner to provide functional benefit to scaffold-adherent cells, to date, no proelastogenic factors have been delivered in this manner toward stimulating elastic matrix synthesis. Ibrahim et al. (2011) showed significant increases in elastic fiber formation by vascular SMCs within hydrogels of methacrylated high molecular weight HA with increases in content of encapsulated proelastogenic HA-o. In another study, solubilized elastin was introduced into the bulk of collagen scaffold and was shown to augment new elastic matrix formation within compared to control collagen constructs when implanted in rats, and to promote matrix calcification, a response elicited by elastin peptides (Aikawa et al. 2009), unlike intact elastin. In creating scaffolds encapsulating proelastogenic factors, however, extreme care must be taken to maintain their structural integrity and biological activity due to use of solvents and temperatures during formulation that cause protein denaturation. As an illustrative example, fabricating electrospun collagen fiber scaffolds requires dissolution of collagen in hexafluoro-2-propanol (HFIP), which however breaks the cross-links within and denatures the protein. Such problems can be circumvented or reduced by innovative formulation strategies using alternative solvents and conditions such as encapsulation of the GF in an aqueous buffer and the polymer in the requisite HFIP solvent, as done in incorporating bFGF within PLGA scaffolds (Sahoo et al. 2010).

4.5.3 Nanoparticles for Induced Regenerative Elastic Matrix Repair

Nanoparticles (also called nanocarriers; typically <100 nm) and their slightly larger counterparts, submicroparticles (100 nm to <1 μm) are emerging as efficient vehicles to enable localized and targeted delivery of biological factors to cells *in vivo*. As polymer nanoparticles or liposomes, they are ideally suited for targeting cells in diseased tissues due to their increased permeability owing to enhanced vascularity or disrupted ECM. Nano- and submicron particles provide several advantages in the context of drug delivery that include (a) large surface area per unit volume for high rate of drug release that can be sustained over several months, (b) predictable polymer degradation profiles and drug out-diffusion characteristics, (c) amenability to be surface-modified to target specific cell or extracellular targets, and (d) small size that minimizes generation of potentially cytotoxic polymer degradation by-products (Grottkau et al. 2013). As with drug delivery scaffolds, covalent tethering of biomolecules to the nanoparticle surface is possible. For the purpose of targeting regenerative repair of elastic matrix, nanoparticles for release of proelastogenic and/or antiproteolytic agents can be surface-modified to incorporate functional groups that bind to specific amino acid sequences or hydrophobic domains in the exposed elastin core of proteolytically disrupted elastic fibers. Elastin protein is made up of interlinked, highly hydrophobic polypeptide chains (Jordan et al. 1974). On this basis, long-chain hydrophobic compounds (e.g., sodium dodecyl sulfate or SDS) (Kagan et al. 1972, Jordan et al. 1974) and compounds bearing hydrocarbon chains show strong affinity for binding to elastin (Jordan et al. 1974). A disadvantage of using SDS for targeted elastin binding however is that such binding imparts a net anionic charge to the complex, imparted by anionic groups on the SDS molecules, and subsequently attracts cationic elastases that can serve to further elastic fiber disruption (Gertler 1971). In the 1970s, Kagan et al. (1981a) showed that long-chain hydrocarbons (fatty acids) present on cationic amphiphiles (e.g., DMAB, dodecyltrimethylammonium bromide or DTAB, dodecylamine hydrochloride or DAH) similarly bind to elastin. However, on account of the cationic charge presented by these molecules, they tend to cause electrostatic repulsion of positively charged elastases and MMPs, while the long-chain hydrocarbon chains can also interfere with the conformation of MMPs to cause their inactivation. In addition, LOX-mediated cross-linking was shown to be augmented by these molecules due to (a) electrostatic attraction of the elastin cross-linking enzyme, LOX (Kagan et al. 1979, Kagan and Li 2003) that bears a net negative charge at physiologic pH, and (b) conformational twist of elastin molecules on binding of hydrophobic moieties on the cationic amphiphiles that exposes lysine side groups for cross-linking through LOX-mediated oxidative deamination (Kagan and Li 2003). Seeking to capitalize on these phenomena, Sivaraman and Ramamurthi (2013) functionalized PLGA nanoparticle surfaces with cationic amphiphiles (DMA, DTAB, or DAH) and demonstrated *in vitro* cultures of rat aneurysmal SMCs as to their functional benefit, independent of the effects of the delivered drug (in this case, DOX, an MMP inhibitor) in terms of (a) enabling targeted binding to the hydrophobic elastic matrix, (b) inhibiting elastolytic MMP (MMPs 2, 9) protein synthesis and enzyme activity, and (c) augmenting LOX activity toward significantly enhancing cellular assembly of cross-linked elastic matrix structures (Figure 4.2). In the context of discussing the elastic matrix regenerative benefits of imparting a positive surface charge to the nanoparticles, care must be taken that the surface zeta potential does not exceed 45–50 mV, because this can increase interactions between such nanoparticles and the generally anionic cell membrane that can cause

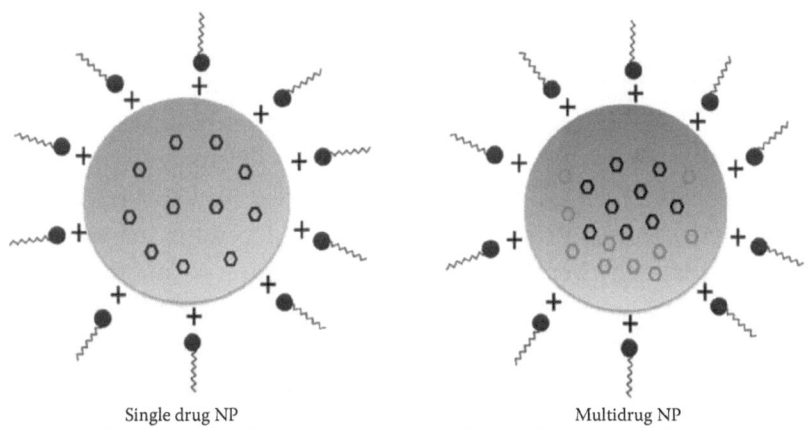

Component	Description	Function
⟨chain⟩	Hydrocarbon chain	Binds to elastic matrix and facilitates elastin cross-linking
+	Cationic group	Enhances NP uptake in select tissue (vascular), inhibits elastase and MMPs, and increases LOX activity
○	Anti-MMP drug	Inhibits MMP synthesis and activity
○	Proelastogenic factor	Stimulates elastic matrix deposition and assembly

FIGURE 4.2 Design of nanoparticles (NPs) for elastin regenerative therapy. The NPs are surface modified with cationic amphiphiles. While the positive surface charge enhances vessel wall uptake from circulation, contributes to repulsion of positively charged elastases, and engages anionic groups on the active site of matrix metalloproteinases (MMPs) to reduce their activity, and attracts lysyl oxidase (LOX) enzyme for improved tropoelastin cross-linking, the hydrocarbon chains of the amphiphiles bind to hydrophobic domains in the exposed elastin core of disrupted elastic fibers at the site of tissue repair, and conformationally change elastin molecules to expose their lysine side chains for more efficient cross-linking by LOX. The NPs can be loaded with active drugs to stimulate elastic matrix regenerative repair via sustained release of encapsulated proelastogenic and/or anti-MMP molecules.

depolarization, disruption, and cell death (De Jong and Borm 2008, Arvizo et al. 2010, Mura et al. 2011). In addition, in some cases, the magnitude of the positive charge may need to be significantly lowered to a near neutral value, to allow the proregenerative nanoparticles to penetrate through tissues rich in anionic GAGs and PGs.

EBP (Hinek and Rabinovitch 1994) or peptides with specific amino acid sequences that recognize SMC or fibroblast surface receptors (Buck and Horwitz 1987, Hersel et al. 2003) can also be used a nanoparticle targeting modality. In seeking to achieve regenerative elastic matrix repair concurrent with treating the underlying disease etiology (e.g., tissue inflammation), it is important to keep in mind the deleterious effects of certain anti-inflammatory agents (e.g., imidazoles, Ohta et al. 1996; rofecoxib, Oitate et al. 2007) on elastic matrix fate. These drugs have been reported to engage allysine residues on elastin to interrupt existing intermolecular cross-links and new cross-link formation (Oitate et al. 2007), resulting in disruption of elastic matrix structures in a dose-dependent manner.

Despite the many benefits that covalent tethering of biomolecules to the nanoparticle surface provides, there are several disadvantages including the possible need to chemically derivatize the biomolecules, which could alter or compromise their biological function, and their reduced half-life *in vivo* (Sivaraman et al. 2012). For these reasons, encapsulation of biomolecules within the nanocarrier matrix is preferred. Among the parameters that influence the rate of release of encapsulated matrix regenerative biologics and the fraction of their theoretically loaded amounts that is cumulatively released at any point in time, are biomolecule loading density, nanocarrier dose, and their properties such as molecular weight, monomer mixture composition, and porosity and pore size. Nanoparticle size in particular critically decides site of nanoparticle localization in tissue (inside or outside cells), their amenability to phagocytosis, and consequent immune response. For example, for nanoparticles targeting stimulation of regenerative elastic matrix assembly, which occurs in the extracellular space, nanoparticles of 300–500 nm have been deemed appropriate (Sivaraman and Ramamurthi 2013), while nanoparticles larger than 500 nm are typically phagocytosed (Nguyen et al. 2009); those smaller than 100 nm in size tend to be immunogenic (Fahmy et al. 2008). On the other hand, release of encapsulated proelastogenic or antiproteolytic agents is augmented at higher nanoparticle bolus concentrations and when loading levels of the encapsulated biologics are reduced, so that in-penetration of water from the tissue microenvironment and subsequent out-diffusion of dissolved drugs from the nanoparticle interior are both enhanced (Sivaraman and Ramamurthi 2013).

Although delivery of encapsulated GFs from nanoparticles has been widely described in the literature, very few of these have targeted improved elastic matrix/fiber assembly. TGF-β1 has been delivered from liposomes and PEG-PLGA microparticles, to generate TGF-β1 concentrations in the range of 1 ng/ml, which Ramamurthi and his co-workers has previously shown to be proelastogenic (Lu et al. 2000, Tanaka et al. 2005). Similarly, predictable release of IGF-1, a proelastogenic GF (Silva et al. 2009), from PLGA nanoparticles (Eley and Mathew 2007) and microspheres (Meinel et al. 2003) has been successfully demonstrated, though these nanoparticles were not investigated for providing matrix regenerative benefit. In yet other work, *trans*-retinoic acid (*trans*-RA), which is known to improve fibrillin-1 deposition, was delivered from liposomes (Mehta et al. 1994, Parthasarathy and Mehta 1998), though the resultant benefits to elastic fiber assembly have not yet been studied. In a series of publications, the previously described cationic amphiphile—surface-modified PLGA nanoparticles developed by the Ramamurthi's group were shown to provide an additional impetus to *de novo* elastic matrix assembly through release of encapsulated proelastogenic biomolecules (TGF-β (Dai et al. 2005) and HA oligomers (Zimmermann et al. 1994)) or MMP inhibitors (e.g., DOX) (Ding et al. 2005).

As discussed earlier in this chapter, MMP inhibition concurrent with provision of a GF stimulus to elastogenesis is useful to shift the balance between elastolysis and elastic matrix regeneration within a proteolytic tissue *milieu* to favor net accumulation of new elastic matrix structures. Although controlled release of MMP inhibitors such as DOX from PLGA (Patel et al. 2008, 2012), PLGA-hydroxyapatite (Wang et al. 2012) and PLGA-PCL microparticles (Mundargi et al. 2007), and liposomes (Sangare et al. 2001) has been amply demonstrated both *in vitro* and *in vivo* (Mundargi et al. 2007) microenvironments, DOX release from nanoparticles was first described by Sivaraman and Ramamurthi (2013). This group demonstrated that unlike its elastin (Bendeck et al. 2002) and ECM synthesis-inhibitory effects (Davies et al. 1996, TeKoppele et al. 1998) at tissue equivalents (16–54 µg/ml) of systemic circulating doses, DOX released from nanoparticles at levels <5 µg/ml maintains its MMP inhibitory activity but additionally has a stimulatory effect on *de novo* cellular elastic matrix deposition by cultured rat aneurysmal SMCs. Although effective, DOX is a broad-spectrum MMP inhibitor that inhibits several MMPs not relevant to elastic matrix homeostasis, and which may be involved in healthy tissue remodeling. Thus, for elastic matrix regenerative repair applications, localized, nanoparticle-based delivery of MMP inhibitors that selectively target elastolytic MMPs alone is likely to be useful. For example, Ro 28-2653, a drug that inhibits elastolytic MMPs 2 and 9, has been released from liposomes (Piette et al. 2007). Recently, microRNAs such as miRNA-29b have been identified as targets for downstream inhibition of MMPs with implied benefit to elastic matrix regeneration (Maegdefessel et al. 2012). With evidence that microRNA release from nanoliposomes is useful to provide therapeutic benefit in cancer, there are definite future opportunities to utilize this model of miRNA delivery to augment elastic matrix regenerative repair (Anand et al. 2010).

4.6 ELASTIC MATRIX REGENERATION DRIVEN BY CELLULAR SECRETIONS

The use of terminally differentiated cells derived from most adult tissues for the purpose of populating scaffolds for growing tissue constructs *in vitro*, or for the purpose of delivery to proteolytically compromised tissue sites to facilitate regenerative repair, particularly of the elastic matrix, is limited by our inability to sufficiently stimulate them to generate sufficient functional elastic fibers in a limited time period. Deploying alternative cell types that retain their high elastogenic potential throughout life as surrogates may be an option, if they can be noninvasively biopsied and expanded in culture. For example, bladder SMCs (Wognum et al. 2009) and SMCs within the vaginal wall retain their elastogenicity in adults; vaginal SMCs facilitate remodeling and repair of the vaginal wall during parturition (Rahn et al. 2008). These cells could be used to affect regenerative repair, say within aortic aneurysms, if they can be reconditioned, perhaps *in situ*, to assume a more vascular SMC phenotype, though this could also potentially have negative implications to their innate high elastogenic potential. Macrophage-type cells derived from the peritoneal fluid have also been shown to be recruited to intraperitoneally implanted scaffolds to assume a myofibroblastic/SMC-like phenotype capable of generating some elastic matrix, though this was observed only following autologous intra-aortal transplantation of the semimatured tissue construct. Bashur and Ramamurthi (2014) showed that functionalization of intraperitoneal scaffolds with proelastogenic biomolecules such as TGF-β, served to not only increase elastic matrix production by recruited peritoneal cells but also drive them to assume a more myofibroblastic/SMC-like phenotype.

Despite the positive nature of these outcomes, an uncertainty with this approach is the lack of knowledge as to the origin and phenotype of recruited cells, the conditions (e.g., scaffold type, structure) that drive their recruitment and phenotypic switch, and most of all the inherent intrapatient and patient-to-patient variability of these necessary processes.

Evidence of the involvement of SCs in tissue repair processes involving generation of greater than normal amounts of elastic matrix (Shanahan et al. 1993), though highly disorganized, and not necessarily in the form of mature elastic fibers, and in robust developmental elastogenesis (Owens et al. 2004) prompts their investigation as a novel source of autologous cells for *in vitro* elastic tissue engineering or *in vivo* regenerative elastic matrix repair. In light of the above pieces of evidence, it is certainly possible that SCs and possibly their derivatives retain the high capacity for tropoelastin mRNA expression, protein synthesis, and fiber assembly that terminally differentiated cell types (e.g., vascular SMCs) lose with the aging process. The high elastogenicity of neonatal SMCs relative to adult SMCs rationalizes this hypothesis (Johnson et al. 1995). Although there is ample published literature describing successful derivation of SMC-like cells from a variety of SC types including those from the bone marrow, peripheral blood, and adipose tissues (Kane et al. 2011), very little study has gone into investigating the abilities of these cells to generate elastic matrix, beyond demonstrating their ability to express elastin mRNA. Recent work by Swaminathan et al. (2014) has shown that conditions employed for directed differentiation of these SCs into SMC-like cells can influence the phenotypic coordinates of the derived cells on a synthetic to contractile phenotype scale that in turn influences their elastogenic potential. In recent years, induced pluripotent stem cell (iPSC) techniques have enabled generation of individualized cell lines of specific lineages (e.g., SMCs) by reprogramming somatic cells from patients including fibroblasts, adipose SCs from human and murine sources (Xie et al. 2009, Lee et al. 2010, Sugii et al. 2011). Pluripotent iPSCs can potentially circumvent some disadvantages of multipotent adult SC such as their low incidence in source tissues, low yields during isolation, and difficulties in scaling up their production pre- or postdifferentiation for application to tissue engineering or cell therapy applications (Kane et al. 2011). While there are several requirements for autologous SCs to be used for regenerative tissue repair, these will be discussed elsewhere in a dedicated chapter in this book. Rather, this chapter will provide a broad overview of what is known regarding the GF secretions from the different SC types discussed above that could provide an impetus to one or more aspects of elastic matrix neoassembly or, alternately, regenerative elastic matrix repair.

Pluripotent SC used to stimulate elastic matrix regenerative repair in the dynamic proteolytic space would be expected to fulfill key functions in a sustained fashion, as shown in Figure 4.3. While sorted and purified populations of undifferentiated SCs could be directly introduced *in vivo*, their differentiation toward an SMC-progenitor lineage, or into functional SMCs exhibiting defined phenotypic coordinates may alternately be pursued, if the derived cells prove to be elastogenically superior to the undifferentiated SCs and have more impressive proelastogenic characteristics, as demonstrated in a recent study by Swaminathan et al. (2014), or in the case of iPSCs, as a safety measure to avoid potential tumorigenesis *in vivo*. To protect the cells from inflammatory cytokines and other biomolecules peculiar to a diseased tissue microenvironment, it is advisable that the cells be encapsulated (e.g., alginate microcapsules) prior to *in vivo* delivery. Once in the diseased tissue space, the cells will be expected to serve both as a source of new elastin and elastic fibers, and also provide the necessary impetus for elastin producing parenchymal cells (e.g., SMCs, fibroblasts) within the tissue to upregulate elastin synthesis and formation of mature, cross-linked elastic fibers. This may occur either through a combination of juxtacrine and paracrine signaling between the delivered SC/derivatives and the parenchymal cells within the tissues, although signaling by encapsulated SCs/derivatives will primarily be through the paracrine mode. Juxtacrine signaling would occur later as the microcapsules degrade to allow contact between the delivered and resident cell types. As examples, we evoke recent studies that have shown that mesenchymal stem cells (MSCs) encapsulated within alginate microcapsules release proelastogenic molecules such as TGF-β and others, which contrarily inhibit elastogenesis such as fibroblast growth factor (FGF-1 and FGF-2) (Yu et al. 2010). While TGF-β stimulation of tropoelastin synthesis occurs through increased activity of phosphatidylinositol 3-kinase/Akt (Kuang et al. 2007), anti-elastogenic effects of FGF-2 have been attributed to increased Fra-1/c-Jun repressor complex binding to the tropoelastin promoter sequence (Rich et al. 1999). Because cell phenotype is dictated by its microenvironment, the compositional and temporal GF release profile of encapsulated SCs/derivatives can be modulated by appropriate choice of encapsulating agent and through inclusion of other biomolecules or cell adherence factors (Yu et al. 2010). In another *in vitro* study, MSCs were shown to release IGF-1 (Chen et al. 2008), which is known to upregulate tropoelastin mRNA

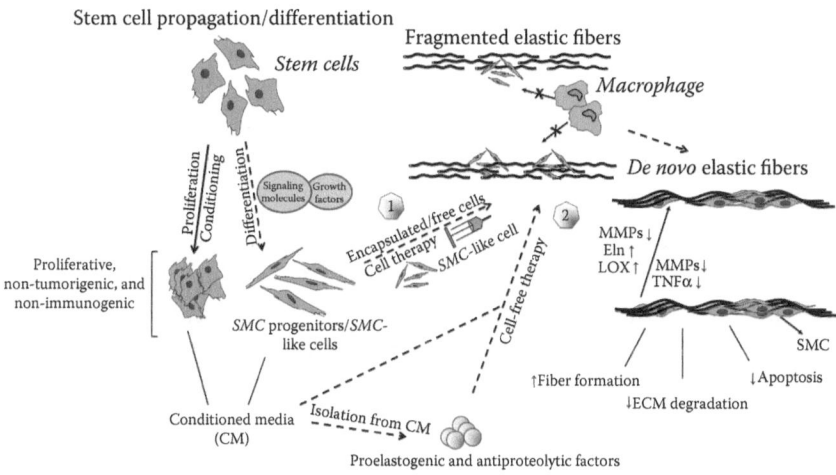

FIGURE 4.3 Stem-cell-based approaches for *in situ* elastin regenerative repair. The schematic shows the expected roles of stem cells or their differentiated smooth muscle cells (SMC)-like derivatives for the purpose. While physical delivery of purified, undifferentiated stem cells might be possible, their predifferentiation into SMC progenitors or SMC-like cells may be warranted should they exhibit superior elastogenic and proelastin synthesis-inductive characteristics, or in the case of pluripotent stem cells that may be tumorigenic, for safety reasons. The stem cells or their SMC-like derivatives could also be encapsulated within a protective microenvironment (e.g., microbeads) to initially shield them the adverse effects of cytokines in the proteolytic tissue repair microenvironment. Within the tissue, the delivered cells are expected to both serve as a source of new elastin precursors and elastic fibers, and upregulate elastic fiber neoassembly and repair, and attenuate proteolytic enzyme activity by SMCs and macrophages already present in the tissue. The overall goal is that elastic fiber formation occurs faster than degradation of the existing elastic matrix. A second possible regenerative approach is based on identifying the key biomolecular factors in stem cell/derivative secretome responsible for their paracrine proelastogenic and antiproteolytic effects on tissue parenchymal cells and delivering these factors in a predictable and sustained delivery from micro- or nanoparticles and polymer scaffolds. This latter approach could have fewer risks and complications than stem cell therapies and would eliminate the associated demand for significant innovation in methods and quality control for stem cell sourcing, processing, delivery, and tracking.

expression by decreasing binding of a transcription factor, Sp3, that in turn suppresses elastin gene expression (Conn et al. 1996).

Recent evidence with bone marrow MSCs (BM-MSCs) has demonstrated that their tissue reparative benefits in animal models and in humans (Salazar et al. 2009), and proelastin regenerative effects of these cells (Wada et al. 2011), the latter demonstrated in our own studies (Swaminathan et al. 2014), can be at least partially accounted for by the action of their secreted trophic factors and that the physical presence of the SCs may not be required for tissue regenerative repair (Maguire 2013). This motivates development of cell-free approaches (e.g., controlled release from scaffolds or using micro/nanoparticles) to augment elastin regenerative repair based on delivery of key GF components of the SC/derivative secretome (Figure 4.3). Such an approach would (a) circumvent need for extensive innovation in methods for cell processing, scale-up, purification, and quality control, and for targeted, and efficient *in vivo* cell delivery and tracking, and (b) alleviate concerns of the adverse effects of the proteolytic/inflammatory *milieu* at the repair site on fate and performance of delivered cells. The stumbling block in pursuing this regenerative strategy lies in identifying beyond doubt, the key secretome components necessary and sufficient for such effects, and replicating the spatiotemporal pattern of release of one or more of these factors sequentially or in combination in a manner that replicates their release from SCs/derivatives.

Table 4.2 provides a summary of the very limited body of the available literature that has focused on the study of SCs and their derivatives in the context of their application toward generating or repairing elastic matrix structures. In general, most literature has been biased toward the study of BM-MSCs. There is evidence that (a) SCs can be successfully differentiated toward an SMC-progenitor lineage or to assume SMC-like phenotypic and functional characteristics (Galmiche et al. 1993, Kurpinski et al. 2006, Kurpinski et al. 2010, Gong and Niklason 2011), (b) both SCs and their SMC-like derivatives are capable of positive elastin gene expression (Xie et al. 2008), (c) elastin mRNA expression by SCs increases as they differentiate progressively toward an SMC lineage (unpublished data from the Ramamurthi's lab), (d) SCs and SC-derived SMCs produce elastin protein precursors (Ross et al. 2006, Popova et al. 2010), and (e) secrete trophic factors that may have proelastogenic effects or which may have antiproteolytic and anti-inflammatory properties. For example, murine BM-MSCs were reported to attenuate overexpression of elastolytic MMPs-2 and -9 and production of inflammatory cytokine tumor necrosis factor-alpha by macrophages both *in vitro* culture models and *in vivo* within induced mouse AAAs and to stimulate *de novo* elastic matrix assembly by aortic SMCs in culture toward slowing AAA growth (Hashizume et al. 2011). At this time, there is little, if any, information on elastic matrix synthesis potential of pluripotent SC types (iPSCs and embryonic stem cells or ESCs

TABLE 4.2 Selected Studies Investigating Elastic Matrix Assembly by Undifferentiated and Differentiated Stem Cells

Source	Species	Study	Outcomes	References
Neonatal stem cells from bone marrow	Mouse	Delivered at AAA site	Increased *Eln* and decreased *Mmp2* and *Mmp9*, while quantity of elastic matrix was preserved	Kuang et al. (2007)
Neonatal SMC-like cells derived from bone marrow	Rat	Treated with TGF-β and PDGF-BB	Increased *Eln* but elastic fibers were undetected with histological stain	Kielty (2006)
		5% circumferential strain for 3 weeks	No difference in elastin levels compared to static conditions	Kielty (2006)
	Sheep	Implant lamb jugular vein for 6 weeks	Highly organized, fibrillar elastin similar to normal veins (histology)	Bashur et al. (2012)
Autologous cells from bone marrow	Pig	Delivered to AAA	Fragmentation of elastic fibers with AAA, outcomes due to MSC treatment was not analyzed	Boucher et al. (2012)
	Human	After 8 days at a cutaneous wound	Elastic fibers (histology) increased with MSCs but not without	Salazar et al. (2009)
SMC-like cells derived from bone marrow MSCs	Rat	Treated with TGF-β and PDGF-BB	Increased elastic matrix synthesis and assembly and also stimulated elastogenesis by AAA SMCs	Swaminathan et al. (2014)
Adipose-derived stem cells	Rat	Delivered at AAA site	Increased elastic matrix deposition and preserved elastic fibers	Tian et al. (2014)
	Rat	Delivered to urethra	Increased elastic matrix with cell therapy, but not without (histology)	Hashizume et al. (2011)
	Human	Injected into mice skin	Increased tropoelastin and fibrillin-1 synthesis	Jeong et al. (2014)
SMC-like cells derived from peripheral blood	Rat	Treated with PDGF-BB	Increased *Eln* mRNA, but no quantification was done	Wada et al. (2011)

(Continued)

TABLE 4.2 (*Continued*) Selected Studies Investigating Elastic Matrix Assembly by Undifferentiated and Differentiated Stem Cells

Source	Species	Study	Outcomes	References
Bone marrow MSCs	Rat	Delivered as concentrated conditioned medium intraperitoneally	Promoted urethral elastogenesis	Deng et al. (2015)
	Mouse	Delivered intravenously toward AAA site	Increased elastin content and preserved elastic fibers within aorta	Fu et al. (2013)
Umbilical cord MSCs	Human	Treated with connective tissue growth factor	Increased *Eln* mRNA	Caballero et al. (2013)
Placental MSCs	Human	Delivered to mouse AAA	Prevented lymphocyte activation and attenuated AAA formation	Turnbull et al. (2011)
iPSC-derived MSCs	Human	Subcutaneously injected exosomes from MSCs at rat wound sites	Increased *Eln* and tropoelastin content	Zhang et al. (2015)
Neonatal MSCs from lung	Human	Treated with TGF-β	Increased *Eln*	Ross et al. (2006)

AAA, abdominal aortic aneurysm; SMC, smooth muscle cell; TGF, transforming growth factor; MSC, mesenchymal stem cell; iPSC, induced pluripotent stem cell.

and their SMC-like derivatives). Future investigation in this direction may open up new avenues for successful regenerative repair or tissue engineering of elastic matrix-rich tissues.

4.7 CONCLUSIONS

The last several decades have seen significant advances in our understanding of the biomolecular factor-mediated regulation of the highly complex process of elastic fiber assembly and fiber repair, which we have summarized in Table 4.1. However, there may be several other biomolecules than those we have listed, which likely also play a role in elastin synthesis and fiber assembly. The key to moving forward without doubt is developing an intimate understanding of how elastic fiber assembly proceeds during fetal and neonatal development, and in systematically profiling biomolecular signaling agents in the developing tissue microenvironment and correlating elastic matrix assembly outcomes to spatiotemporal changes in GF signaling. Developing modalities for modulating gene and protein level expression of upstream signaling molecules leading to downstream effects of stimulating elastogenesis and attenuating MMP-mediated proteolysis represent new, emerging strategies for elastic matrix regenerative repair. Strategies in development based on the use of biomaterial scaffolds and drug delivery carriers allow spatiotemporal control of GF bioavailability and also enable sustained and predictable release of one or more GFs in combination or sequence. However, for these approaches to work, further innovation is required to conjugate or incorporate biomolecules within these controlled-release polymer vehicles without change in their bioactivity and functional effects.

REFERENCES

Ahmann, K. A., Weinbaum, J. S., Johnson, S. L., and Tranquillo, R. T. 2010. Fibrin degradation enhances vascular smooth muscle cell proliferation and matrix deposition in fibrin-based tissue constructs fabricated in vitro. *Tissue Eng Part A* 16(10): 3261–3270.

Aikawa, E., Aikawa, M., Libby, P. et al. 2009. Arterial and aortic valve calcification abolished by elastolytic cathepsin S deficiency in chronic renal disease. *Circulation* 119(13): 1785–1794.

Almine, J. F., Bax, D. V., Mithieux, S. M. et al. 2010. Elastin-based materials. *Chem Soc Rev* 39(9): 3371–3379.

Anand, S., Majeti, B. K., Acevedo, L. M. et al. 2010. MicroRNA-132-mediated loss of p120RasGAP activates the endothelium to facilitate pathological angiogenesis. *Nat Med* 16(8): 909–914.

Annovi, G., Boraldi, F., Moscarelli, P. et al. 2012. Heparan sulfate affects elastin deposition in fibroblasts cultured from donors of different ages. *Rejuvenation Res* 15(1): 22–31.

Armentano, R. L., Levenson, J., Barra, J. G. et al. 1991. Assessment of elastin and collagen contribution to aortic elasticity in conscious dogs. *Am J Physiol* 260(6 Pt 2): H1870–H1877.

Arvizo, R. R., Miranda, O. R., Thompson, M. A. et al. 2010. Effect of nanoparticle surface charge at the plasma membrane and beyond. *Nano Lett* 10(7): 2543–2548.

Badylak, S. F., Valentin, J. E., Ravindra, A. K., McCabe, G. P., and Stewart-Akers, A. M. 2008. Macrophage phenotype as a determinant of biologic scaffold remodeling. *Tissue Eng Part A* 14(11): 1835–1842.

Baker, A. H., Zaltsman, A. B., George, S. J., and Newby, A. C. 1998. Divergent effects of tissue inhibitor of metalloproteinase-1, -2, or -3 overexpression on rat vascular smooth muscle cell invasion, proliferation, and death in vitro. TIMP-3 promotes apoptosis. *J Clin Invest* 101(6): 1478–1487.

Barone, L. M., Faris, B., Chipman, S. D. et al. 1985. Alteration of the extracellular matrix of smooth muscle cells by ascorbate treatment. *Biochim Biophys Acta* 840(2): 245–254.

Bartoli, M. A., Parodi, F. E., Chu, J. et al. 2006. Localized administration of doxycycline suppresses aortic dilatation in an experimental mouse model of abdominal aortic aneurysm. *Ann Vasc Surg* 20(2): 228–236.

Bashur, C. A. and Ramamurthi, A. 2014. Composition of intraperitoneally implanted electrospun conduits modulates cellular elastic matrix generation. *Acta Biomater* 10(1): 163–172.

Bashur, C. A., Venkataraman, L., and Ramamurthi, A. 2012. Tissue engineering and regenerative strategies to replicate biocomplexity of vascular elastic matrix assembly. *Tissue Eng Part B Rev* 18(3): 203–217.

Baxter, B. T., Pearce, W. H., Waltke, E. A. et al. 2002. Prolonged administration of doxycycline in patients with small asymptomatic abdominal aortic aneurysms: Report of a prospective (Phase II) multicenter study. *J Vasc Surg* 36(1): 1–12.

Beamish, J. A., He, P., Kottke-Marchant, K., and Marchant, R. E. 2010. Molecular regulation of contractile smooth muscle cell phenotype: Implications for vascular tissue engineering. *Tissue Eng Part B Rev* 16(5): 467–491.

Bendeck, M. P., Conte, M., Zhang, M. et al. 2002. Doxycycline modulates smooth muscle cell growth, migration, and matrix remodeling after arterial injury. *Am J Pathol* 160(3): 1089–1095.

Bergethon, P. R., Mogayzel, P. J., Jr., and Franzblau, C. 1989. Effect of the reducing environment on the accumulation of elastin and collagen in cultured smooth-muscle cells. *Biochem J* 258(1): 279–284.

Berglund, J. D., Nerem, R. M., and Sambanis, A. 2004. Incorporation of intact elastin scaffolds in tissue-engineered collagen-based vascular grafts. *Tissue Eng* 10(9–10): 1526–1535.

Berk, J. L., Franzblau, C., and Goldstein, R. H. 1991. Recombinant interleukin-1 beta inhibits elastin formation by a neonatal rat lung fibroblast subtype. *J Biol Chem* 266(5): 3192–3197.

Berk, J. L., Hatch, C. A., Morris, S. M., Stone, P. J., and Goldstein, R. H. 2005. Hypoxia suppresses elastin repair by rat lung fibroblasts. *Am J Physiol Lung Cell Mol Physiol* 289(6): L931–L936.

Boucher, J., Gridley, T., and Liaw, L. 2012. Molecular pathways of notch signaling in vascular smooth muscle cells. *Front Physiol* 3: 81.

Bressan, G. M., Pasqualironchetti, I., Fornieri, C. et al. 1986. Relevance of aggregation properties of tropoelastin to the assembly and structure of elastic fibers. *J Ultrastruct Mol Struct Res* 94(3): 209–216.

Brettell, L. M. and McGowan, S. E. 1994. Basic fibroblast growth factor decreases elastin production by neonatal rat lung fibroblasts. *Am J Respir Cell Mol Biol* 10(3): 306–315.

Brown-Augsburger, P., Tisdale, C., Broekelmann, T., Sloan, C., and Mecham, R. P. 1995. Identification of an elastin cross-linking domain that joins three peptide chains. Possible role in nucleated assembly. *J Biol Chem* 270(30): 17778–1783.

Brown, R. A., Sethi, K. K., Gwanmesia, I. et al. 2002. Enhanced fibroblast contraction of 3D collagen lattices and integrin expression by TGF-beta1 and -beta3: Mechanoregulatory growth factors? *Exp Cell Res* 274(2): 310–322.

Buck, C. A. and Horwitz, A. F. 1987. Cell surface receptors for extracellular matrix molecules. *Annu Rev Cell Biol* 3: 179–205.

Buijtenhuijs, P., Buttafoco, L., Poot, A. A. et al. 2004. Tissue engineering of blood vessels: Characterization of smooth-muscle cells for culturing on collagen-and-elastin-based scaffolds. *Biotechnol Appl Biochem* 39: 141–149.

Butler, G. S., Butler, M. J., Atkinson, S. J. et al. 1998. The TIMP2 membrane type 1 metalloproteinase "receptor" regulates the concentration and efficient activation of progelatinase A. A kinetic study. *J Biol Chem* 273(2): 871–880.

Caballero, M., Skancke, M. D., Halevi, A. E. et al. 2013. Effects of connective tissue growth factor on the regulation of elastogenesis in human umbilical cord-derived mesenchymal stem cells. *Ann Plast Surg* 70(5): 568–573.

Cannizzaro, S. M., Padera, R. F., Langer, R. et al. 1998. A novel biotinylated degradable polymer for cell-interactive applications. *Biotechnol Bioeng* 58(5): 529–535.

Chen, L., Tredget, E. E., Wu, P. Y., and Wu, Y. 2008. Paracrine factors of mesenchymal stem cells recruit macrophages and endothelial lineage cells and enhance wound healing. *PLoS One* 3(4): e1886.

Clarke, A. W., Wise, S. G., Cain, S. A., Kielty, C. M., and Weiss, A. S. 2005. Coacervation is promoted by molecular interactions between the PF2 segment of fibrillin-1 and the domain 4 region of tropoelastin. *Biochemistry* 44(30): 10271–10281.

Clutterbuck, A. L., Asplin, K. E., Harris, P., Allaway, D., and Mobasheri, A. 2009. Targeting matrix metalloproteinases in inflammatory conditions. *Curr Drug Targets* 10(12): 1245–1254.

Conn, K. J., Rich, C. B., Jensen, D. E. et al. 1996. Insulin-like growth factor-I regulates transcription of the elastin gene through a putative retinoblastoma control element. A role for Sp3 acting as a repressor of elastin gene transcription. *J Biol Chem* 271(46): 28853–28860.

Cortizo, M. C. and Fernandez Lorenzo de Mele, M. 2004. Cytotoxicity of copper ions released from metal: Variation with the exposure period and concentration gradients. *Biol Trace Elem Res* 102(1–3): 129–141.

Coussens, L. M., Fingleton, B., and Matrisian, L. M. 2002. Matrix metalloproteinase inhibitors and cancer: Trials and tribulations. *Science* 295(5564): 2387–2392.

Curci, J. A., Petrinec, D., Liao, S. X., Golub, L. M., and Thompson, R. W. 1998. Pharmacologic suppression of experimental abdominal aortic aneurysms: A comparison of doxycycline and four chemically modified tetracyclines. *J Vasc Surg* 28(6): 1082–1093.

Daamen, W. F., van Moerkerk, H. T. B., Hafmans, T. et al. 2003. Preparation and evaluation of molecularly-defined collagen-elastin-glycosaminoglycan scaffolds for tissue engineering. *Biomaterials* 24(22): 4001–4009.

Daamen, W. F., Veerkamp, J. H., van Hest, J. C. M., and van Kuppevelt, T. H. 2007. Elastin as a biomaterial for tissue engineering. *Biomaterials* 28(30): 4378–4398.

Dai, J., Losy, F., Guinault, A. M. et al. 2005. Overexpression of transforming growth factor-beta1 stabilizes already-formed aortic aneurysms: A first approach to induction of functional healing by endovascular gene therapy. *Circulation* 112(7): 1008–1015.

Dai, J., Michineau, S., Franck, G. et al. 2011. Long term stabilization of expanding aortic aneurysms by a short course of cyclosporine A through transforming growth factor-beta induction. *PLoS One* 6(12): e28903.

Dalvi, P. S., Singh, A., Trivedi, H. R. et al. 2011. Effect of doxycycline in patients of moderate to severe chronic obstructive pulmonary disease with stable symptoms. *Ann Thorac Med* 6(4): 221–226.

Davidson, J. M. 2002. Smad about elastin regulation. *Am J Respir Cell Mol Biol* 26(2): 164–166.

Davidson, J. M., LuValle, P. A., Zoia, O., Quaglino, D., and Giro, M. G. 1997. Ascorbate differentially regulates elastin and collagen biosynthesis in vascular smooth muscle cells and skin fibroblasts by pretranslational mechanisms. *J Biol Chem* 272(1): 345–352.

Davies, S. R., Cole, A. A., and Schmid, T. M. 1996. Doxycycline inhibits type X collagen synthesis in avian hypertrophic chondrocyte cultures. *J Biol Chem* 271(42): 25966–25970.

Davis, E. C. and Mecham, R. P. 1998. Intracellular trafficking of tropoelastin. *Matrix Biol* 17(4): 245–254.

De Jong, W. H. and Borm, P. J. 2008. Drug delivery and nanoparticles: Applications and hazards. *Int J Nanomedicine* 3(2): 133–149.

Deb, P. P. and Ramamurthi, A. 2014. Spatiotemporal mapping of matrix remodelling and evidence of in situ elastogenesis in experimental abdominal aortic aneurysms. *J Tissue Eng Regen Med*, 2014 / 05 / 07.

Deng, K., Lin, D. L., Hanzlicek, B. et al. 2015. Mesenchymal stem cells and their secretome partially restore nerve and urethral function in a dual muscle and nerve injury stress urinary incontinence model. *Am J Physiol Renal Physiol* 308(2): F92-F100.

DiCamillo, S. J., Yang, S., Panchenko, M. V. et al. 2006. Neutrophil elastase-initiated EGFR/MEK/ERK signaling counteracts stabilizing effect of autocrine TGF-beta on tropoelastin mRNA in lung fibroblasts. *Am J Physiol Lung Cell Mol Physiol* 291(2): L232–L243.

Ding, R., McGuinness, C. L., Burnand, K. G., Sullivan, E., and Smith, A. 2005. Matrix metalloproteinases in the aneurysm wall of patients treated with low-dose doxycycline. *Vascular* 13(5): 290–297.

Dowling, D. P., Miller, I. S., Ardhaoui, M., and Gallagher, W. M. 2011. Effect of surface wettability and topography on the adhesion of osteosarcoma cells on plasma-modified polystyrene. *J Biomater Appl* 26(3): 327–347.

Dunn, D. M. and Franzblau, C. 1982. Effects of ascorbate on insoluble elastin accumulation and cross-link formation in rabbit pulmonary artery smooth muscle cultures. *Biochemistry* 21(18): 4195–4202.

Eble, J. A. and Niland, S. 2009. The extracellular matrix of blood vessels. *Curr Pharm Des* 15(12): 1385–1400.

Eley, J. G. and Mathew, P. 2007. Preparation and release characteristics of insulin and insulin-like growth factor-one from polymer nanoparticles. *J Microencapsul* 24(3): 225–234.

Fahmy, T. M., Demento, S. L., Caplan, M. J., Mellman, I., and Saltzman, W. M. 2008. Design opportunities for actively targeted nanoparticle vaccines. *Nanomedicine (Lond)* 3(3): 343–355.

Faris, B., Ferrera, R., Toselli, P. et al. 1984. Effect of varying amounts of ascorbate on collagen, elastin and lysyl oxidase synthesis in aortic smooth muscle cell cultures. *Biochim Biophys Acta* 797(1): 71–75.

Faury, G., Garnier, S., Weiss, A. S. et al. 1998. Action of tropoelastin and synthetic elastin sequences on vascular tone and on free Ca^{2+} level in human vascular endothelial cells. *Circ Res* 82(3): 328–336.

Flemming, R. G., Murphy, C. J., Abrams, G. A., Goodman, S. L., and Nealey, P. F. 1999. Effects of synthetic micro- and nano-structured surfaces on cell behavior. *Biomaterials* 20(6): 573–588.

Fornieri, C., Baccarani-Contri, M., Quaglino, D., Jr., and Pasquali-Ronchetti, I. 1987. Lysyl oxidase activity and elastin/glycosaminoglycan interactions in growing chick and rat aortas. *J Cell Biol* 105(3): 1463–1469.

Fornieri, C., Quaglino, D., Jr., and Mori, G. 1992. Role of the extracellular matrix in age-related modifications of the rat aorta. Ultrastructural, morphometric, and enzymatic evaluations. *Arterioscler Thromb* 12(9): 1008–1016.

Franco, C., Ho, B., Mulholland, D. et al. 2006. Doxycycline alters vascular smooth muscle cell adhesion, migration, and reorganization of fibrillar collagen matrices. *Am J Pathol* 168(5): 1697–1709.

Freeman, J. W., Woods, M. D., and Laurencin, C. T. 2007. Tissue engineering of the anterior cruciate ligament using a braid-twist scaffold design. *J Biomech* 40(9): 2029–2036.

Frisch, S. M., Davidson, J. M., and Werb, Z. 1985. Blockage of tropoelastin secretion by monensin represses tropoelastin synthesis at a pretranslational level in rat smooth muscle cells. *Mol Cell Biol* 5(1): 253–258.

Fu, X. M., Yamawaki-Ogata, A., Oshima, H. et al. 2013. Intravenous administration of mesenchymal stem cells prevents angiotensin II-induced aortic aneurysm formation in apolipoprotein E-deficient mouse. *J Transl Med* 11: 175.

Gacchina, C., Brothers, T., and Ramamurthi, A. 2011a. Evaluating smooth muscle cells from CaCl2-induced rat aortal expansions as a surrogate culture model for study of elastogenic induction of human aneurysmal cells. *Tissue Eng Part A* 17(15–16): 1945–1958.

Gacchina, C. E., Deb, P., Barth, J. L., and Ramamurthi, A. 2011b. Elastogenic inductability of smooth muscle cells from a rat model of late stage abdominal aortic aneurysms. *Tissue Eng Part A* 17(13–14): 1699–1711.

Gacchina, C. E. and Ramamurthi, A. 2011. Impact of pre-existing elastic matrix on TGFbeta1 and HA oligomer-induced regenerative elastin repair by rat aortic smooth muscle cells. *J Tissue Eng Regen Med* 5(2): 85–96.

Galmiche, M. C., Koteliansky, V. E., Briere, J., Herve, P., and Charbord, P. 1993. Stromal cells from human long-term marrow cultures are mesenchymal cells that differentiate following a vascular smooth muscle differentiation pathway. *Blood* 82(1): 66–76.

Gertler, A. 1971. The non-specific electrostatic nature of the adsorption of elastase and other basic proteins on elastin. *Eur J Biochem* 20(4): 541–546.

Gong, Z. and Niklason, L. E. 2011. Use of human mesenchymal stem cells as alternative source of smooth muscle cells in vessel engineering. *Methods Mol Biol* 698: 279–294.

Greenwood, H. L., Singer, P. A., Downey, G. P. et al. 2006. Regenerative medicine and the developing world. *PLoS Med* 3(9): e381.

Grottkau, B. E., Cai, X., Wang, J., Yang, X., and Lin, Y. 2013. Polymeric nanoparticles for a drug delivery system. *Curr Drug Metab* 14(8): 840–846.

Halper, J. and Kjaer, M. 2014. Basic components of connective tissues and extracellular matrix: Elastin, fibrillin, fibulins, fibrinogen, fibronectin, laminin, tenascins and thrombospondins. *Adv Exp Med Biol* 802: 31–47.

Hashizume, R., Yamawaki-Ogata, A., Ueda, Y., Wagner, W. R., and Narita, Y. 2011. Mesenchymal stem cells attenuate angiotensin II-induced aortic aneurysm growth in apolipoprotein E-deficient mice. *J Vasc Surg* 54(6): 1743–1752.

Hayashi, A., Suzuki, T., and Tajima, S. 1995. Modulations of elastin expression and cell proliferation by retinoids in cultured vascular smooth muscle cells. *J Biochem* 117(1): 132–136.

Healy, K. E., Lom, B., and Hockberger, P. E. 1994. Spatial distribution of mammalian cells dictated by material surface chemistry. *Biotechnol Bioeng* 43(8): 792–800.

Hersel, U., Dahmen, C., and Kessler, H. 2003. RGD modified polymers: Biomaterials for stimulated cell adhesion and beyond. *Biomaterials* 24(24): 4385–4415.

Hinek, A., Mecham, R. P., Keeley, F., and Rabinovitch, M. 1991. Impaired elastin fiber assembly related to reduced 67-kD elastin-binding protein in fetal lamb ductus arteriosus and in cultured aortic smooth muscle cells treated with chondroitin sulfate. *J Clin Invest* 88(6): 2083–2094.

Hinek, A. and Rabinovitch, M. 1994. 67-kD elastin-binding protein is a protective "companion" of extracellular insoluble elastin and intracellular tropoelastin. *J Cell Biol* 126(2): 563–574.

Hirano, S., Bless, D., Heisey, D., and Ford, C. 2003a. Roles of hepatocyte growth factor and transforming growth factor beta 1 in production of extracellular matrix by canine vocal fold fibroblasts. *Laryngoscope* 113(1): 144–148.

Hirano, S., Bless, D. M., Heisey, D., and Ford, C. N. 2003b. Effect of growth factors on hyaluronan production by canine vocal fold fibroblasts. *Ann Otol Rhinol Laryngol* 112(7): 617–624.

Hirano, S., Bless, D. M., Massey, R. J., Hartig, G. K., and Ford, C. N. 2003c. Morphological and functional changes of human vocal fold fibroblasts with hepatocyte growth factor. *Ann Otol Rhinol Laryngol* 112(12): 1026–1033.

Huffman, M. D., Curci, J. A., Moore, G. et al. 2000. Functional importance of connective tissue repair during the development of experimental abdominal aortic aneurysms. *Surgery* 128(3): 429–438.

Ibrahim, S., Kothapalli, C. R., Kang, Q. K., and Ramamurthi, A. 2011. Characterization of glycidyl methacrylate—Crosslinked hyaluronan hydrogel scaffolds incorporating elastogenic hyaluronan oligomers. *Acta Biomater* 7(2): 653–665.

Jeong, J. H., Fan, Y., You, G. Y., Choi, T. H., and Kim, S. 2014. Improvement of photoaged skin wrinkles with cultured human fibroblasts and adipose-derived stem cells: A comparative study. *Journal of Plastic, Reconstructive & Aesthetic Surgery* 68(3): 372–381.

Ji, W., Sun, Y., Yang, F. et al. 2011. Bioactive electrospun scaffolds delivering growth factors and genes for tissue engineering applications. *Pharm Res* 28(6): 1259–1272.

Joddar, B., Ibrahim, S., and Ramamurthi, A. 2007. Impact of delivery mode of hyaluronan oligomers on elastogenic responses of adult vascular smooth muscle cells. *Biomaterials* 28(27): 3918–3927.

Joddar, B. and Ramamurthi, A. 2006a. Fragment size- and dose-specific effects of hyaluronan on matrix synthesis by vascular smooth muscle cells. *Biomaterials* 27(15): 2994–3004.

Joddar, B. and Ramamurthi, A. 2006b. Elastogenic effects of exogenous hyaluronan oligosaccharides on vascular smooth muscle cells. *Biomaterials* 27(33): 5698–5707.

Johnson, D. J., Robson, P., Hew, Y., and Keeley, F. W. 1995. Decreased elastin synthesis in normal development and in long-term aortic organ and cell cultures is related to rapid and selective destabilization of mRNA for elastin. *Circ Res* 77(6): 1107–1113.

Jones, P. A., Scott-Burden, T., and Gevers, W. 1979. Glycoprotein, elastin, and collagen secretion by rat smooth muscle cells. *Proc Natl Acad Sci U S A* 76(1): 353–357.

Jordan, R. E., Hewitt, N., Lewis, W., Kagan, H., and Franzblau, C. 1974. Regulation of elastase-catalyzed hydrolysis of insoluble elastin by synthetic and naturally occurring hydrophobic ligands. *Biochemistry* 13(17): 3497–3503.

Kagan, H. M., Crombie, G. D., Jordan, R. E., Lewis, W., and Franzblau, C. 1972. Proteolysis of elastin-ligand complexes. Stimulation of elastase digestion of insoluble elastin by sodium dodecyl sulfate. *Biochemistry* 11(18): 3412–3418.

Kagan, H. M. and Li, W. 2003. Lysyl oxidase: Properties, specificity, and biological roles inside and outside of the cell. *J Cell Biochem* 88(4): 660–672.

Kagan, H. M., Simpson, D. E., and Tseng, L. 1981a. Substrate-directed modulation of elastin oxidation by lysyl oxidase. *Connect Tissue Res* 8(3–4): 213–217.

Kagan, H. M., Sullivan, K. A., Olsson, T. A., 3rd, and Cronlund, A. L. 1979. Purification and properties of four species of lysyl oxidase from bovine aorta. *Biochem J* 177(1): 203–214.

Kagan, H. M., Tseng, L., and Simpson, D. E. 1981b. Control of elastin metabolism by elastin ligands. Reciprocal effects on lysyl oxidase activity. *J Biol Chem* 256(11): 5417–5421.

Kane, N. M., Xiao, Q., Baker, A. H. et al. 2011. Pluripotent stem cell differentiation into vascular cells: A novel technology with promises for vascular re(generation). *Pharmacol Ther* 129(1): 29–49.

Keire, P. A., L'Heureux, N., Vernon, R. B. et al. 2010. Expression of versican isoform V3 in the absence of ascorbate improves elastogenesis in engineered vascular constructs. *Tissue Eng Part A* 16(2): 501–512.

Kielty, C. M. 2006. Elastic fibres in health and disease. *Expert Rev Mol Med* 8(19): 1–23.

Kielty, C. M., Sherratt, M. J., and Shuttleworth, C. A. 2002. Elastic fibres. *J Cell Sci* 115(Pt 14): 2817–2828.

Kothapalli, C. R., Gacchina, C. E., and Ramamurthi, A. 2009a. Utility of hyaluronan oligomers and transforming growth factor-beta1 factors for elastic matrix regeneration by aneurysmal rat aortic smooth muscle cells. *Tissue Eng Part A* 15(11): 3247–3260.

Kothapalli, C. R. and Ramamurthi, A. 2008. Benefits of concurrent delivery of hyaluronan and IGF-1 cues to regeneration of crosslinked elastin matrices by adult rat vascular cells. *J Tissue Eng Regen Med* 2(2–3): 106–116.

Kothapalli, C. R. and Ramamurthi, A. 2009a. Copper nanoparticle cues for biomimetic cellular assembly of crosslinked elastin fibers. *Acta Biomater* 5(2): 541–553.

Kothapalli, C. R. and Ramamurthi, A. 2009b. Lysyl oxidase enhances elastin synthesis and matrix formation by vascular smooth muscle cells. *J Tissue Eng Regen Med* 3(8): 655–661.

Kothapalli, C. R. and Ramamurthi, A. 2009c. Biomimetic regeneration of elastin matrices using hyaluronan and copper ion cues. *Tissue Engineering Part A* 15(1): 103–113.

Kothapalli, C. R., Taylor, P. M., Smolenski, R. T., Yacoub, M. H., and Ramamurthi, A. 2009b. Transforming growth factor beta 1 and hyaluronan oligomers synergistically enhance elastin matrix regeneration by vascular smooth muscle cells. *Tissue Eng Part A* 15(3): 501–511.

Kuang, P. P., Zhang, X. H., Rich, C. B. et al. 2007. Activation of elastin transcription by transforming growth factor-beta in human lung fibroblasts. *Am J Physiol Lung Cell Mol Physiol* 292(4): L944–L952.

Kurpinski, K., Lam, H., Chu, J. L. et al. 2010. Transforming growth factor-beta and notch signaling mediate stem cell differentiation into smooth muscle cells. *Stem Cells* 28(4): 734–742.

Kurpinski, K., Park, J., Thakar, R. G., and Li, S. 2006. Regulation of vascular smooth muscle cells and mesenchymal stem cells by mechanical strain. *Mol Cell Biomech* 3(1): 21–34.

Langer, R. and Tirrell, D. A. 2004. Designing materials for biology and medicine. *Nature* 428(6982): 487–492.

Leach, J. B., Wolinsky, J. B., Stone, P. J., and Wong, J. Y. 2005. Crosslinked alpha-elastin biomaterials: Towards a processable elastin mimetic scaffold. *Acta Biomater* 1(2): 155–164.

Lee, K., Silva, E. A., and Mooney, D. J. 2011. Growth factor delivery-based tissue engineering: General approaches and a review of recent developments. *J R Soc Interface* 8(55): 153–170.

Lee, T. H., Song, S. H., Kim, K. L. et al. 2010. Functional recapitulation of smooth muscle cells via induced pluripotent stem cells from human aortic smooth muscle cells. *Circ Res* 106(1): 120–128.

Li, D. Y., Brooke, B., Davis, E. C. et al. 1998a. Elastin is an essential determinant of arterial morphogenesis. *Nature* 393(6682): 276–280.

Li, D. Y., Faury, G., Taylor, D. G. et al. 1998b. Novel arterial pathology in mice and humans hemizygous for elastin. *J Clin Invest* 102(10): 1783–1787.

Losy, F., Dai, J., Pages, C. et al. 2003. Paracrine secretion of transforming growth factor-beta1 in aneurysm healing and stabilization with endovascular smooth muscle cell therapy. *J Vasc Surg* 37(6): 1301–1309.

Lu, L., Stamatas, G. N., and Mikos, A. G. 2000. Controlled release of transforming growth factor beta1 from biodegradable polymer microparticles. *J Biomed Mater Res* 50(3): 440–451.

Luo, Y., Kobler, J. B., Zeitels, S. M., and Langer, R. 2006. Effects of growth factors on extracellular matrix production by vocal fold fibroblasts in 3-dimensional culture. *Tissue Eng* 12(12): 3365–3374.

Lutolf, M. P. and Hubbell, J. A. 2005. Synthetic biomaterials as instructive extracellular microenvironments for morphogenesis in tissue engineering. *Nat Biotechnol* 23(1): 47–55.

Ma, Z., Mao, Z., and Gao, C. 2007. Surface modification and property analysis of biomedical polymers used for tissue engineering. *Colloids Surf B Biointerfaces* 60(2): 137–157.

Maegdefessel, L., Azuma, J., Toh, R. et al. 2012. Inhibition of microRNA-29b reduces murine abdominal aortic aneurysm development. *J Clin Invest* 122(2): 497–506.

Maguire, G. 2013. Stem cell therapy without the cells. *Commun Integr Biol* 6(6): e26631.

Mann, B. K., Schmedlen, R. H., and West, J. L. 2001. Tethered-TGF-beta increases extracellular matrix production of vascular smooth muscle cells. *Biomaterials* 22(5): 439–444.

Manning, M. W., Cassis, L. A., and Daugherty, A. 2003. Differential effects of doxycycline, a broad-spectrum matrix metalloproteinase inhibitor, on angiotensin II-induced atherosclerosis and abdominal aortic aneurysms. *Arterioscler Thromb Vasc Biol* 23(3): 483–488.

Martinon, F. 2010. Signaling by ROS drives inflammasome activation. *Eur J Immunol* 40(3): 616–619.

Mason, C. and Dunnill, P. 2008. A brief definition of regenerative medicine. *Regen Med* 3(1): 1–5.

Mauviel, A., Chen, Y. Q., Kahari, V. M. et al. 1993. Human recombinant interleukin-1 beta up-regulates elastin gene expression in dermal fibroblasts. Evidence for transcriptional regulation in vitro and in vivo. *J Biol Chem* 268(9): 6520–6524.

Mecham, R. P., Lange, G., Madaras, J., and Starcher, B. 1981. Elastin synthesis by ligamentum nuchae fibroblasts: Effects of culture conditions and extracellular matrix on elastin production. *J Cell Biol* 90(2): 332–338.

Mecham, R. P., Levy, B. D., Morris, S. L., Madaras, J. G., and Wrenn, D. S. 1985. Increased cyclic GMP levels lead to a stimulation of elastin production in ligament fibroblasts that is reversed by cyclic AMP. *J Biol Chem* 260(6): 3255–3258.

Mehta, K., Sadeghi, T., McQueen, T., and Lopez-Berestein, G. 1994. Liposome encapsulation circumvents the hepatic clearance mechanisms of all-trans-retinoic acid. *Leuk Res* 18(8): 587–596.

Meinel, L., Zoidis, E., Zapf, J. et al. 2003. Localized insulin-like growth factor I delivery to enhance new bone formation. *Bone* 33(4): 660–672.

Michael, K. E., Vernekar, V. N., Keselowsky, B. G. et al. 2003. Adsorption-induced conformational changes in fibronectin due to interactions with well-defined surface chemistries. *Langmuir* 19(19): 8033–8040.

Mikos, A. G., McIntire, L. V., Anderson, J. M., and Babensee, J. E. 1998. Host response to tissue engineered devices. *Adv Drug Deliv Rev* 33(1–2): 111–139.

Mithieux, S. M., Rasko, J. E., and Weiss, A. S. 2004. Synthetic elastin hydrogels derived from massive elastic assemblies of self-organized human protein monomers. *Biomaterials* 25(20): 4921–4927.

Mitsi, M., Hong, Z., Costello, C. E., and Nugent, M. A. 2006. Heparin-mediated conformational changes in fibronectin expose vascular endothelial growth factor binding sites. *Biochemistry* 45(34): 10319–10328.

Mitts, T. F., Bunda, S., Wang, Y., and Hinek, A. 2010. Aldosterone and mineralocorticoid receptor antagonists modulate elastin and collagen deposition in human skin. *J Invest Dermatol* 130(10): 2396–2406.

Mundargi, R. C., Srirangarajan, S., Agnihotri, S. A. et al. 2007. Development and evaluation of novel biodegradable microspheres based on poly(D,L-lactide-co-glycolide) and poly(epsilon-caprolactone) for controlled delivery of doxycycline in the treatment of human periodontal pocket: In vitro and in vivo studies. *J Control Release* 119(1): 59–68.

Mura, S., Hillaireau, H., Nicolas, J. et al. 2011. Influence of surface charge on the potential toxicity of PLGA nanoparticles towards Calu-3 cells. *Int J Nanomedicine* 6: 2591–2605.

Murphy, G. and Nagase, H. 2008. Progress in matrix metalloproteinase research. *Mol Aspects Med* 29(5): 290–308.

Nguyen, K. T., Shukla, K. P., Moctezuma, M. et al. 2009. Studies of the cellular uptake of hydrogel nanospheres and microspheres by phagocytes, vascular endothelial cells, and smooth muscle cells. *J Biomed Mater Res A* 88(4): 1022–1030.

Noble, P. W. 2002. Hyaluronan and its catabolic products in tissue injury and repair. *Matrix Biol* 21(1): 25–29.

Nuttelman, C. R., Tripodi, M. C., and Anseth, K. S. 2006. Dexamethasone-functionalized gels induce osteogenic differentiation of encapsulated hMSCs. *J Biomed Mater Res A* 76(1): 183–195.

Ohta, K., Yamaguchi, J. I., Akimoto, M. et al. 1996. Retention mechanism of imidazoles in connective tissue. I. Binding to elastin. *Drug Metab Dispos* 24(12): 1291–1297.

Oitate, M., Hirota, T., Takahashi, M. et al. 2007. Mechanism for covalent binding of rofecoxib to elastin of rat aorta. *J Pharmacol Exp Ther* 320(3): 1195–1203.

Ono, R. N., Sengle, G., Charbonneau, N. L. et al. 2009. Latent transforming growth factor beta-binding proteins and fibulins compete for fibrillin-1 and exhibit exquisite specificities in binding sites. *J Biol Chem* 284(25): 16872–16881.

Owens, G. K., Kumar, M. S., and Wamhoff, B. R. 2004. Molecular regulation of vascular smooth muscle cell differentiation in development and disease. *Physiol Rev* 84(3): 767–801.

Panyam, J., Zhou, W. Z., Prabha, S., Sahoo, S. K., and Labhasetwar, V. 2002. Rapid endo-lysosomal escape of poly(DL-lactide-co-glycolide) nanoparticles: Implications for drug and gene delivery. *FASEB J* 16(10): 1217–1226.

Parks, W. C., Pierce, R. A., Lee, K. A., and Mecham, R. P. 1993. Elastin. In *Advances in Molecular and Cell Biology*, edited by E. Edward Bittar, 133–181. Elsevier.

Parthasarathy, R. and Mehta, K. 1998. Altered metabolism of all-trans-retinoic acid in liposome-encapsulated form. *Cancer Lett* 134(2): 121–128.

Patel, P., Mundargi, R. C., Babu, V. R. et al. 2008. Microencapsulation of doxycycline into poly(lactide-co-glycolide) by spray drying technique: Effect of polymer molecular weight on process parameters. *Journal of Applied Polymer Science* 108(6): 4038–4046.

Patel, R. S., Cho, D. Y., Tian, C. et al. 2012. Doxycycline delivery from PLGA microspheres prepared by a modified solvent removal method. *J Microencapsul* 29(4): 344–352.

Piette, M., Castagne, D., Delattre, L., and Piel, G. 2007. Preparation and evaluation of liposomes encapsulating synthetic MMP inhibitor (Ro 28-2653)—Cyclodextrin complexes. *J Incl Phenom Macrocycl Chem* 57(1–4): 101–103.

Popova, A. P., Bozyk, P. D., Goldsmith, A. M. et al. 2010. Autocrine production of TGF-beta1 promotes myofibroblastic differentiation of neonatal lung mesenchymal stem cells. *Am J Physiol Lung Cell Mol Physiol* 298(6): L735–L743.

Rahn, D. D., Acevedo, J. F., and Word, R. A. 2008. Effect of vaginal distention on elastic fiber synthesis and matrix degradation in the vaginal wall: Potential role in the pathogenesis of pelvic organ prolapse. *Am J Physiol Regul Integr Comp Physiol* 295(4): R1351–R1358.

Rich, C. B., Fontanilla, M. R., Nugent, M., and Foster, J. A. 1999. Basic fibroblast growth factor decreases elastin gene transcription through an AP1/cAMP-response element hybrid site in the distal promoter. *J Biol Chem* 274(47): 33433–33439.

Rich, C. B., Goud, H. D., Bashir, M., Rosenbloom, J., and Foster, J. A. 1993. Developmental regulation of aortic elastin gene expression involves disruption of an IGF-I sensitive repressor complex. *Biochem Biophys Res Commun* 196(3): 1316–1322.

Robert, L., Jacob, M. P., and Fulop, T. 1995. Elastin in blood vessels. *Ciba Found Symp* 192: 286–299; discussion 299–303.

Ross, J. J., Hong, Z. G., Willenbring, B. et al. 2006. Cytokine-induced differentiation of multipotent adult progenitor cells into functional smooth muscle cells. *J Clin Invest* 116(12): 3139–3149.

Safran, S. A., Gov, N., Nicolas, A., Schwarz, U. S., and Tlusty, T. 2005. Physics of cell elasticity, shape and adhesion. *Physica A* 352(1): 171–201.

Sahoo, S., Ang, L. T., Goh, J. C., and Toh, S. L. 2010. Growth factor delivery through electrospun nanofibers in scaffolds for tissue engineering applications. *J Biomed Mater Res A* 93(4): 1539–1550.

Salazar, K. D., Lankford, S. M., and Brody, A. R. 2009. Mesenchymal stem cells produce Wnt isoforms and TGF-beta1 that mediate proliferation and pro-collagen expression by lung fibroblasts. *Am J Physiol Lung Cell Mol Physiol* 297(5): L1002–L1011.

Sales, V. L., Engelmayr, G. C., Mettler, B. A. et al. 2006. Transforming growth factor-beta 1 modulates extracellular matrix production, proliferation, and apoptosis of endothelial progenitor cells in tissue-engineering scaffolds. *Circulation* 114: I193–I199.

Sangare, L., Morisset, R., Gaboury, L., and Ravaoarinoro, M. 2001. Effects of cationic liposome-encapsulated doxycycline on experimental Chlamydia trachomatis genital infection in mice. *J Antimicrob Chemother* 47(3): 323–331.

Sen, S., Bunda, S., Shi, J. et al. 2011. Retinoblastoma protein modulates the inverse relationship between cellular proliferation and elastogenesis. *J Biol Chem* 286(42): 36580–36591.

Senior, R. M., Griffin, G. L., and Mecham, R. P. 1980. Chemotactic activity of elastin-derived peptides. *J Clin Invest* 66(4): 859–862.

Sephel, G. C. and Davidson, J. M. 1986. Elastin production in human skin fibroblast cultures and its decline with age. *J Invest Dermatol* 86(3): 279–285.

Shanahan, C. M., Weissberg, P. L., and Metcalfe, J. C. 1993. Isolation of gene markers of differentiated and proliferating vascular smooth muscle cells. *Circ Res* 73(1): 193–204.

Shanley, C. J., Gharaee-Kermani, M., Sarkar, R. et al. 1997. Transforming growth factor-beta 1 increases lysyl oxidase enzyme activity and mRNA in rat aortic smooth muscle cells. *J Vasc Surg* 25(3): 446–452.

Sherratt, M. J., Bax, D. V., Chaudhry, S. S. et al. 2005. Substrate chemistry influences the morphology and biological function of adsorbed extracellular matrix assemblies. *Biomaterials* 26(34): 7192–7206.

Shi, J., Wang, A., Sen, S. et al. 2012. Insulin induces production of new elastin in cultures of human aortic smooth muscle cells. *Am J Pathol* 180(2): 715–726.

Silva, A. K., Richard, C., Bessodes, M., Scherman, D., and Merten, O. W. 2009. Growth factor delivery approaches in hydrogels. *Biomacromolecules* 10(1): 9–18.

Simionescu, A., Philips, K., and Vyavahare, N. 2005. Elastin-derived peptides and TGF-beta1 induce osteogenic responses in smooth muscle cells. *Biochem Biophys Res Commun* 334(2): 524–532.

Sivaraman, B., Bashur, C. A., and Ramamurthi, A. 2012. Advances in biomimetic regeneration of elastic matrix structures. *Drug Deliv Transl Res* 2(5): 323–350.

Sivaraman, B. and Ramamurthi, A. 2013. Multifunctional nanoparticles for doxycycline delivery towards localized elastic matrix stabilization and regenerative repair. *Acta Biomater* 9(5): 6511–6525.

Stephan, S., Ball, S. G., Williamson, M. et al. 2006. Cell-matrix biology in vascular tissue engineering. *J Anat* 209(4): 495–502.

Sugii, S., Kida, Y., Berggren, W. T., and Evans, R. M. 2011. Feeder-dependent and feeder-independent iPS cell derivation from human and mouse adipose stem cells. *Nat Protoc* 6(3): 346–358.

Suyama, K. and Nakamura, F. 1990. Isolation and characterization of new crosslinking amino acid "allodesmosine" from hydrolysate of elastin. *Biochem Biophys Res Commun* 170(2): 713–718.

Swaminathan, G., Gadepalli, V. S., Stoilov, I. et al. 2014. Pro-elastogenic effects of bone marrow mesenchymal stem cell-derived smooth muscle cells on cultured aneurysmal smooth muscle cells. *J Tissue Eng Regen Med* 2014. doi: 10.1002/term.1964.

Swee, M. H., Parks, W. C., and Pierce, R. A. 1995. Developmental regulation of elastin production. Expression of tropoelastin pre-mRNA persists after down-regulation of steady-state mRNA levels. *J Biol Chem* 270(25): 14899–14906.

Tajima, S., Hayashi, A., and Suzuki, T. 1997. Elastin expression is up-regulated by retinoic acid but not by retinol in chick embryonic skin fibroblasts. *J Dermatol Sci* 15(3): 166–172.

Tanaka, H., Sugita, T., Yasunaga, Y. et al. 2005. Efficiency of magnetic liposomal transforming growth factor-beta 1 in the repair of articular cartilage defects in a rabbit model. *J Biomed Mater Res A* 73(3): 255–263.

TeKoppele, J. M., Beekman, B., Verzijl, N. et al. 1998. Doxycycline inhibits collagen synthesis by differentiated articular chondrocytes. *Adv Dent Res* 12(2): 63–67.

Tian, X., Fan, J., Yu, M. et al. 2014. Adipose stem cells promote smooth muscle cells to secrete elastin in rat abdominal aortic aneurysm. *PLoS ONE* 9(9): e108105.

Turnbull, I. C., Hadri, L., Rapti, K. et al. 2011. Aortic implantation of mesenchymal stem cells after aneurysm injury in a porcine model. *J Surg Res* 170(1): e179–e188.

Wada, N., Wang, B., Lin, N. H. et al. 2011. Induced pluripotent stem cell lines derived from human gingival fibroblasts and periodontal ligament fibroblasts. *J Periodontal Res* 46(4): 438–447.

Wagenseil, J. E. and Mecham, R. P. 2007. New insights into elastic fiber assembly. *Birth Defects Res C Embryo Today* 81(4): 229–240.

Wang, X., Xu, H., Zhao, Y. et al. 2012. Poly(lactide-co-glycolide) encapsulated hydroxyapatite microspheres for sustained release of doxycycline. *Mater Sci Eng B* 177(4): 367–372.

Wight, T. N. and Merrilees, M. J. 2004. Proteoglycans in atherosclerosis and restenosis: Key roles for versican. *Circ Res* 94(9): 1158–1167.

Wognum, S., Schmidt, D. E., and Sacks, M. S. 2009. On the mechanical role of de novo synthesized elastin in the urinary bladder wall. *J Biomech Eng* 131(10): 101018.

Wojtowicz-Praga, S. M., Dickson, R. B., and Hawkins, M. J. 1997. Matrix metalloproteinase inhibitors. *Invest New Drugs* 15(1): 61–75.

Wolfe, B. L., Rich, C. B., Goud, H. D. et al. 1993. Insulin-like growth factor-I regulates transcription of the elastin gene. *J Biol Chem* 268(17): 12418–12426.

Xie, C. Q., Huang, H., Wei, S. et al. 2009. A comparison of murine smooth muscle cells generated from embryonic versus induced pluripotent stem cells. *Stem Cells Dev* 18(5): 741–748.

Xie, S. Z., Fang, N. T., Liu, S. et al. 2008. Differentiation of smooth muscle progenitor cells in peripheral blood and its application in tissue engineered blood vessels. *J Zhejiang Univ Sci B* 9(12): 923–930.

Yang, G., Woodhouse, K. A., and Yip, C. M. 2002. Substrate-facilitated assembly of elastin-like peptides: Studies by variable-temperature in situ atomic force microscopy. *J Am Chem Soc* 124(36): 10648–10649.

Yu, J., Du, K. T., Fang, Q. et al. 2010. The use of human mesenchymal stem cells encapsulated in RGD modified alginate microspheres in the repair of myocardial infarction in the rat. *Biomaterials* 31(27): 7012–7020.

Zhang, J., Guan, J., Niu, X. et al. 2015. Exosomes released from human induced pluripotent stem cells-derived MSCs facilitate cutaneous wound healing by promoting collagen synthesis and angiogenesis. *J Transl Med* 13: 49.

Zhang, M., Dang, L., Guo, F. et al. 2012. Coenzyme Q(10) enhances dermal elastin expression, inhibits IL-1alpha production and melanin synthesis in vitro. *Int J Cosmet Sci* 34(3): 273–279.

Zimmermann, D. R., Dours-Zimmermann, M. T., Schubert, M., and Bruckner-Tuderman, L. 1994. Versican is expressed in the proliferating zone in the epidermis and in association with the elastic network of the dermis. *J Cell* 4(5): 817–825.

CHAPTER 5

Scaffold and Biomechanical Transductive Approaches to Elastic Tissue Engineering

Nian Shen, Svenja Hinderer, and
Katja Schenke-Layland

CONTENTS

5.1 INTRODUCTION

Elastin-containing elastic fibers are one of the main components of the extracellular matrix (ECM), endowing dynamic tissues such as lungs, skin, blood vessels, heart valve leaflets, and ligaments with flexibility and elasticity. Previous research efforts suggest that poor recruitment and cross-linking of elastin precursors as well as the need to organize the matrix into functional structures are the main limitations when aiming to develop a tissue-engineered elastic matrix. Scaffolds that mimic the cellular microenvironment in vitro can either be designed to recapitulate the elastic properties of the native ECM or they can be used to induce cell-mediated elastic fiber assembly. Applying defined biophysical signals to further mimic physiological parameters is another potential solution to induce elastic fiber formation and maturation. This chapter provides an overview of scaffolds and biomechanical approaches in elastic matrix engineering and discusses recent advances and prospects for the application of these two strategies.

5.2 SCAFFOLDS IN TISSUE ENGINEERING

Tissue-engineered constructs are generated using cells, biomolecules, and biomaterial scaffolds and aim to support, replace, or regenerate damaged tissues and organs. The scaffolds are designed to provide a three-dimensional (3D), ECM mimicking microenvironment, where cells can attach, migrate, proliferate, and differentiate (Schenke-Layland et al. 2011). Rat aortic smooth muscle cells for example showed an increased proliferation on 3D electrospun scaffolds when compared with two-dimensional (2D) controls (Bashur and Ramamurthi 2011a). It has previously been demonstrated that mechanical properties such as strength, stiffness, and elasticity also significantly impact cell behavior (Kim et al. 2012, Hopkins et al. 2013). Mesenchymal stem cells are able to differentiate into neural, myogenic, or osteogenic tissue when cultured on 3D hydrogels with a stiffness of 0.1, 11, or 34 kPa, respectively (Kim et al. 2012). Therefore, the choices of material as well as the selection of an adequate fabrication method are important parameters in scaffold design.

5.2.1 Scaffolds with Elastic Properties

Scaffolds used for in vivo applications need to resist mechanical forces including high pressure, tension, and compression. Especially in the field of cardiovascular or skin tissue engineering, resilient and highly elastic scaffolds are desired. Therefore, various synthetic and natural polymers have been used in order to generate scaffolds with elastic properties. The degradable elastomer poly(glycerol sebacate) (PGS) has been intensively studied for tissue engineering applications (Chen et al. 2008, Masoumi et al. 2014, Jeffries et al. 2015). To generate 3D PGS scaffolds, processing methods such as electrospinning, foaming, and sheet-forming techniques have been investigated. Interestingly, it has been described that electrospun fibrous PGS shows a higher tensile strength compared to porous PGS foams (Jeffries et al. 2015). Masoumi et al. identified microfabricated PGS in combination with electrospun poly-ε-caprolactone (PCL) as a suitable scaffold to replace heart valves (Masoumi et al. 2014).

Because elastin is a major component of elastic fibers, many studies focus on elastin- or tropoelastin-containing scaffolds. Electrospinning of recombinant tropoelastin with PCL results in a scaffold that matches the mechanical properties of the internal mammary artery (Wise et al. 2011). Other technologies to generate elastic scaffolds with elastin are freeze-drying (Chen et al. 2013) or hydrogel formation (Tu et al. 2010). Tu et al. described an elegant hydrogel-forming method where tropoelastin monomers coalesce and form a porous elastic hydrogel after further chemical cross-linking (Tu et al. 2010).

Elastin is an interesting natural biomaterial, because it exhibits non-thrombogenic properties (Waterhouse et al. 2011). Accordingly, an elastin coating of synthetic scaffolds is highly attractive in order to increase cell adhesion and proliferation (Barenghi et al. 2014). Another material investigated for tissue engineering applications are elastin-like peptides (ELPs). ELPs are engineered biopolymers that contain elastin-based repeat motifs. For tissue engineering applications, they are commonly used in combination with other biomaterials (Yeo et al. 2015). For example, reduced platelet adhesion has been determined in vascular grafts composed of ELPs and collagen (Kumar et al. 2013). In another study, the addition of ELPs to collagen hydrogels significantly increased the tensile strength and the elastic modulus of these hydrogels (Boccafoschi et al. 2015). So far, promising results were obtained by using elastic natural and synthetic 3D scaffolds for tissue engineering. Although it is possible to adjust material properties using different materials and different scaffold fabrication techniques, much more research is necessary in order to completely recapitulate the mechanical and biochemical properties of the native ECM.

5.2.2 Elastic Fibers in Tissue-Engineered Constructs

Recombinant elastin and ELPs were successfully used to generate elastic scaffolds; however, due to the absence of microfibrillar components and elastic fiber-associated proteins, these scaffolds are not able to provide biological stimuli like the native ECM (Bashur et al. 2012). Thus, there is a high interest in developing scaffolds and scaffold fabrication methods that enable elastin synthesis and cell-mediated matrix assembly in tissue-engineered constructs (Bashur et al. 2012). Elastic fibers play a major role in normal tissue development (Votteler et al. 2013) and contribute to approximately 30%–50% of the ECM dry weight of vascular tissues (Bashur et al. 2012). In vitro elastin deposition has been described in 2D cell cultures using neonatal or adult rat vascular smooth muscle cells (SMCs) or human neonatal fibroblasts (Hirai et al. 2007, Kothapalli et al. 2009, Noda et al. 2013). There are also strategies to generate elastic fibers in 3D tissue-engineered constructs, such as decellularized scaffolds or synthetic and natural hydrogel. For example, Keire et al. generated scaffolds using rat arterial SMCs in combination with the cell-sheet technology. Interestingly, not only tropoelastin and elastin-associated protein and gene expression were observed, but also desmosine cross-links, indicating maturation of elastic fibers (Keire et al. 2009). Furthermore, hyaluronic acid (HA)-based scaffolds have been prepared and cultured with rat aortic SMCs in order to induce elastogenesis. A significant upregulation of elastin-stabilizing desmosine cross-links was determined in this study (Joddar and Ramamurthi 2006b). HA seems to be an interesting biomaterial or biomaterial modification agent when aiming for robust cell-mediated elastic matrix deposition. High molecular weight HA stimulates and enhances elastin precursor recruitment and deposition as a matrix through largely electrostatic interactions, whereas the introduction of smaller HA molecules leads to an increased tropoelastin synthesis (Joddar and Ramamurthi 2006a, Joddar et al. 2007). Although there are some approaches using animal-derived cells to generate mature elastic fibers in 3D tissue-engineered constructs, the generation of human-based elastic matrix still remains challenging. Various human studies show (tropo-)elastin upregulation on both, the RNA and protein level (Sommer et al. 2013); however, detailed information on elastic fiber assembly, cross-linking, or maturation is commonly missing. Hinderer et al. used a fibrous and porous polymeric HA-coated scaffold composed of poly(L-lactide) (PLA) and poly(ethylene glycol) dimethacrylate (PEGdma) and seeded human vascular SMCs to induce elastic matrix assembly. Ultrastructural analysis after a dynamic culture revealed microfibril formation as well as elastin deposition (Hinderer et al. 2015). Despite these promising results, developing a tissue-engineered elastic fiber-containing matrix with an appropriate size for clinical use is still an unmet challenge in the field (Bashur et al. 2012).

5.3 BIOMECHANICAL TRANSDUCTION STRATEGIES TOWARD ELASTIC TISSUE ENGINEERING

Previous research efforts suggest that the main limitations to growing elastic tissues in vitro are poor recruitment and cross-linking of elastin precursors and the need to organize the matrix into functional structures (Opitz et al. 2004, Zhang et al. 2009, Bashur and Ramamurthi 2011b, Bashur et al. 2012). These challenges have been addressed via multiple approaches (Kim et al. 1999, Iwasaki et al. 2008, Lee et al. 2011, Lin et al. 2011, Bashur et al. 2012). As discussed before, the scaffold, which provides a 3D microenvironment to the cells, is one potential solution to induce mature elastic fiber formation while at the same time serving to direct the orientation of elastic matrix structures (Patel et al. 2006, Lin et al. 2011). Biomechanical transduction of SMCs and fibroblasts via the application of mechanical stimuli has been shown to modulate the synthesis of almost all major components of the ECM, including elastin, collagen, glycosaminoglycans, proteoglycans, glycoproteins, and various soluble proteins such as growth factors during development and disease (Choe et al. 2006, Gupta and Grande-Allen 2006, Boccafoschi et al. 2013). This section will focus on induction of elastogenesis using biomechanical cues.

5.3.1 Signaling Pathways Activated by Mechanotransduction in Cells

Several biological components, such as ion channels, intergrins, and cell surface receptors, have been proposed to act as cellular mechanosensors and are depicted schematically in Figure 5.1. Such mechanosensors activate signaling pathways, which in turn activate transcription factors and modulate the expression of mechanosensitive genes (Brosig 2011). Many cells and organs are exposed to at least one of these mechanical stimuli: shear stress, stretch, compression, or tension. In general, external stimuli can impact cellular behavior (Brosig 2011, Huang et al. 2004). For example, cardiac cells adapt to high strain by increasing

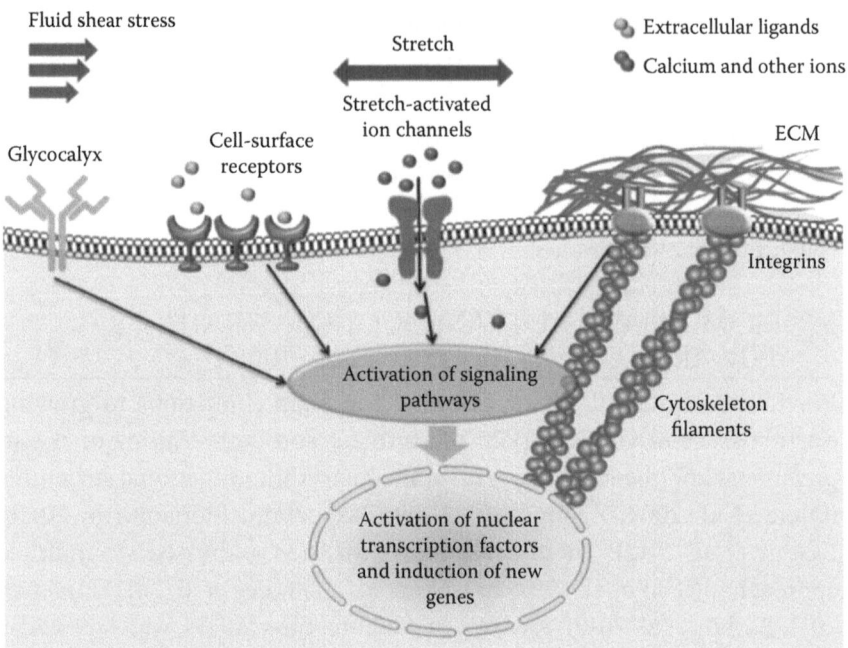

FIGURE 5.1 Schematic depiction of how cells are exposed to various types of mechanical stimuli by their local environment.

their cell size and modifying their surrounding ECM (Huang et al. 2004, Jaalouk and Lammerding 2009). Mechanotransduction is the transduction of mechanical stimuli into biochemical signals, which is crucial for normal organ development and the maintenance of tissues that are under permanent mechanical stress (Jaalouk and Lammerding 2009). As depicted in Figure 5.1, several components such as ion channels, cell surface receptors, and cell adhesion molecules can act as mechanosensors that transmit mechanical changes of the environment to the cell (Haga et al. 2007, Jaalouk and Lammerding 2009, Brosig 2011, Shi and Tarbell 2011). Cells, including SMCs and fibroblasts, respond directly to stretch by opening stretch-activated ion channels in the membranes and allowing the transport of calcium and other ions (Jaalouk and Lammerding 2009). Stretching of cells activates a nonselective cation channel, which is permeable to K^+, Na^+, and Ca^{2+} (Davis et al. 1992). It leads to the activation of the phosphatidylinositol 3 kinase (PI3K)–protein kinase B (Akt) signal transduction pathway (Haga et al. 2003) and p21 (Ras)/extracellular signal regulated kinases

1/2 (ERK1/2) signaling pathway (Iwasaki et al. 2000). Activating these signaling pathways further regulates cell proliferation and apoptosis (Iwasaki et al. 2003). In addition to ion channels, integrins and integrin-associated proteins as well as cell-surface receptors play a significant role in response to mechanotransduction mediated by stretch (Haga et al. 2007, Jaalouk and Lammerding 2009, Qiu et al. 2013). Integrins interact with specific ECM proteins with a variety of focal adhesion kinase (FAK) and tyrosine-protein kinase (c-Src) proteins, which regulate the cell functions via Ras homolog gene family, member A (RhoA)/Rho-associated protein kinase (ROCK) signaling pathway (Gambillara et al. 2008). Additionaly, activated integrins can lead to the initiation of mitogen-activated kinase pathway (MAPK) via FAK and activate nuclear factor-kappaB (NF-κB) and p53 (Wernig et al. 2003, Zampetaki et al. 2005, Qiu et al. 2013). The receptor tyrosine kinase is also involved in mechanotransduction (Katsumi et al. 2004). Stretching of cells induces a rapid phosphorylation of platelet-derived growth factor (PDGF) receptor alpha and epidermal growth factor (EGF) receptor (Hu et al. 1998, Balestreire and Apodaca 2007, Qiu et al. 2013). As a direct response, intracellular ERK1/2 signaling pathway is triggered to regulate ECM synthesis and cell proliferation (Lehoux et al. 2006, Qiu et al. 2013). Nevertheless, it has to be noticed that mechanical stimuli often activate multiple signaling pathways at once. It is rather difficult to perform research on one specific pathway, because signaling pathways can have significant overlap and crosstalk (Jaalouk and Lammerding 2009).

Similar to stretch, ion channels (Ca^{2+} and other ion channels), cell surface receptors, and cell adhesion molecules act as cell mechanosensors when the cells are exposed to fluid shear stress (Chen et al. 1999, Haga et al. 2007, Jaalouk and Lammerding 2009, Shi and Tarbell 2011). It has been reported that exposure to shear stress activates multiple cellular signaling pathways including MAPK, calcium, and Ras/Rho and Akt signaling (Zampetaki et al. 2005, Ingber 2006, Shi and Tarbell 2011). The activation of these pathways controls cell proliferation, migration, apoptosis, and ECM synthesis (Huang et al. 2004, Jaalouk and Lammerding 2009, Shi and Tarbell 2011). Specifically the surface protein glycocalyx can sense fluid shear stress (Kang et al. 2011). The glycocalyx plays a dominant role in controling SMC contraction in vitro and modulating the SMC phenotype by amplifying interstitial flow-mediated mechanotransduction (Kang et al. 2011, Shi and Tarbell 2011).

5.3.2 Impact of Mechanical Signals on Elastogenesis Using Vascular SMCs

Bioreactors have been employed to expose cells to defined mechanical signals in vitro that can mimic the biophysical in vivo environment. There has been an increasing interest in using bioreactor systems to promote elastogenesis in vascular SMC cultures due to its importance for vascular tissue engineering (Patel et al. 2006). Table 5.1 summarizes studies that have been performed utilizing SMCs for elastic fiber formation. In general, applying mechanical forces to SMCs leads to an increased collagen and elastin synthesis (Howard et al. 1998, Gupta and Grande-Allen 2006, Gao et al. 2008, Venkataraman et al. 2014). These responses are highly dependent on parameters such as flow rate, strain magnitude, frequency, and duration (Gupta and Grande-Allen 2006, Gao et al. 2008, Venkataraman et al. 2014). Sumpio et al. seeded porcine SMCs in a flexible culture well and exposed them to high strains (25%) at 0.05 Hz. As a result, a significant increase in total protein and collagen synthesis was detected after 5 days (Sumpio et al. 1988). Another study showed an increased elastin and collagen synthesis by applying 20% strain for 4 to 14 days on rat aortic SMCs (Kim et al. 1999). Additionally, long-term application (4–20 weeks) of cyclic strains upregulated elastin and collagen gene expression. However, it has to be noticed that an extremely high strain can also lead to vascular SMC apoptosis via the endothelin B receptor, which is located in the cell membrane (Cattaruzza et al. 2000). Venkataraman et al. applied a low cyclic strain (2.5%) between 0.5, 1.5, and 3 Hz to human vascular SMCs. The authors determined a significant increase in elastin mRNA expression and total matrix secretion after 21 days of culture when using a frequency of 1.5 Hz (Venkataraman et al. 2014). Although strain was used as one of the important parameters to induce elastin synthesis, many groups did not consider the effect of shear stress due to the fact that vascular SMCs are not directly exposed to the blood flow in vivo. However, Shi and Tarbell demonstrated that shear forces experienced by endothelial cells (ECs) in blood vessels can be transferred to the underlying SMCs (Shi and Tarbell 2011). Furthermore, SMCs are exposed to interstitial flow, which is driven by the transvascular pressure (Figure 5.2). It was estimated that the transmural interstitial shear stress on SMCs is approximately 1 dyne/cm^2, even though the superficial interstitial flow velocity is extremely low (~10^{-6} cm/s) (Shi and Tarbell 2011). According to Qiu et al., high shear stress leads to SMC apoptosis, whereas low shear stress results in the induction of matrix

TABLE 5.1 Summary of Mechanical Stimulation Regimens Used to Regulate Elastin Synthesis

Construct	Cell Type	Mechanical Stimuli Conditions	Duration	Elastogenic Results
Flexible culture plates	Porcine SMCs	25% strain at 0.05 Hz	5d	In total protein ↑ Collagen ↑ (Sumpio et al. 1988)
Collagen I or PLA scaffold	Rat aortic SMCs	0–20% cyclic strain at 0.05–0.25Hz	4–14d 5–20w	Elastin and collagen expression ↑ ELN and COL1;↑ Elastin protein expression ↑ (Kim et al. 1999)
Collagen I	Human vascular SMCs from aorta and FB	10% cyclic strain	4–8d	ELN ↑ (Seliktar et al. 2003)
3D tubular collagen gel	Human vascular SMCs	2.5% cyclic strain at 0.5, 1.5, and 3 Hz	21d	ELN and total matrix elastin↑(Venkataraman et al. 2014)
PGA scaffold	Bovine SMCs and ECs	Pulsatile culture, flow rate: 0.2 to 0.6 l/min	30d static then 2w dynamic	Matrix elastin around regions of high cell densities (Iwasaki et al. 2008)
Electrospun silk fibroin scaffolds	Human coronary artery SMCs and human aortic ECs	Physiological pulsatile flow	15d	ELN ↑ No elastic fiber (Zhang et al. 2009)
PGS tubular scaffold	Baboon arterial SMCs and endothelial progenitor cells	Pulsatile flow from 1 ml/min to 12 dynes/cm^2	7d SMCs and 2w coculture	Circumferentially aligned elastin (Gao et al. 2008)
		Pulsatile flow from 2 ml/min to 14 ml/min	7w SMCs and 2w coculture	

(Continued)

TABLE 5.1 (*Continued*) Summary of Mechanical Stimulation Regimens Used to Regulate Elastin Synthesis

Construct	Cell Type	Mechanical Stimuli Conditions	Duration	Elastogenic Results
PGS scaffold	Baboon SMCs	Pulsatile flow	3w	Mature elastin equivalent to 19% of the native arteries (Lee et al. 2011)
PEG and PLA electrospun scaffold	Human vascular SMCs	Laminar flow 0.74 ml/min first day, then 1.48 ml/min	3d and 6d	Elastin gene and protein expression; ↑ elastic fiber-associated proteins, maturing elastic fibers (Hinderer et al. 2015)

SMC, smooth muscle cells ; d, day; w, week.

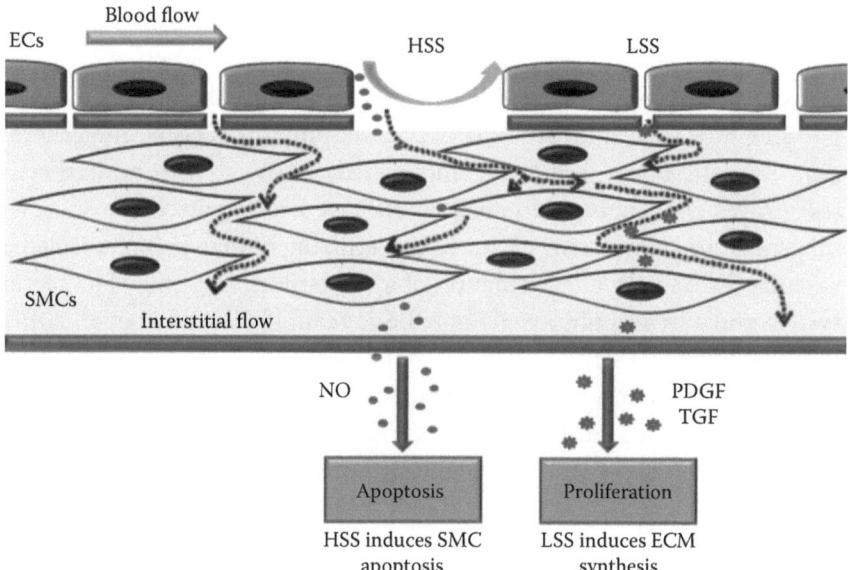

FIGURE 5.2 Schematic depiction of how shear stress regulates vascular SMC activity. In the vasculature, SMCs are exposed to low transmural interstitial flow indicated by the dashed lines. Low shear stress (LSS) upregulates vascular SMC proliferation, migration, and ECM synthesis through the release of platelet-derived growth factor (PDGF) and transforming growth factor (TGF-β) by endothelial cells (ECs). When the endothelium is damaged or injured, the superficial SMCs are exposed to the blood flow. High shear stress (HSS) induces SMC apoptosis through the release of nitric oxide (NO) by ECs. (Adapted from Shi and Tarbell 2011, Qiu et al. 2013, with permission.)

synthesis, including collagen and elastin synthesis (Qiu et al. 2013). Other groups have confirmed that application of low shear stress leads to elastin synthesis (Gao et al. 2008, Iwasaki et al. 2008, Zhang et al. 2009).

Iwasaki et al. seeded bovine aortic SMCs on PGA and PCL sheets, and bovine aortic fibroblasts on PGA sheets. The SMC sheets were then wrapped around a 6 mm silicone tube, cultured for 30 days, subsequently seeded with bovine aortic ECs, and finally exposed to a regulated gradual increased flow and pressure from 0.2 L/min and 20 mm Hg to 0.6 L/min and 100 mm Hg for another 2 weeks. As a result, the engineered vessels showed equivalent elastic characteristics to native arteries in tensile tests (Iwasaki et al. 2008). To stimulate ECM generation, tubular electrospun silk fibroin scaffolds that were seeded with human coronary artery SMCs, and human aortic ECs were exposed to physiological pulsatile flow (Zhang et al. 2009). In this study, an increased elastin gene expression was observed, although no elastic fibers were visualizable using Verhoeff's elastic stain. Lee et al. reported to induce elastin production, which was equivalent to 19% of the native arteries, by using baboon SMCs and a pulsatile flow (Lee et al. 2011). However, despite this success, the generation of elastic fibers in a tissue-engineered construct with human cells still proves challenging. Hinderer et al. have first reported the successful generation of maturing elastic fibers, utilizing human primary isolated vascular SMCs with a combination of a customized fluid-flow bioreactor system and a hybrid fibrous 3D polymeric scaffold (Hinderer et al. 2015). In this study, shear stress between 6×10^{-4} and 11×10^{-4} dyne/cm^2 (equals 6–11×10^{-5} Pa) was applied to the human SMCs. This shear stress differs from the physiological blood luminal flow, but as discussed previously, it corresponds to the in vivo condition, where SMCs are exposed to an extremely low transmural interstitial flow (Hinderer et al. 2015).

5.3.3 Effect of Mechanical Cues on Fibroblasts

Fibroblasts are the most abundant cells in the human body and have been widely used for producing tissue-engineered skin substitutes (Wong et al. 2007). Over the past two decades, various research efforts have focused on the incorporation of elastic fibers into tissue-engineered skin substitutes. Fibroblasts, specifically cardiac, lung, and tendon fibroblasts, were exposed to tension, compression, and shear stress (Chiquet et al. 2009, Shi and Tarbell 2011). Mechanical stimulation of fibroblasts in vitro has been reported to significantly increase proliferation (Yang et al. 2004), modulate cell morphology to an elongated, spindle-like shape (Lee et al. 2005, Wang et al. 2004), and alter ECM deposition (MacKenna et al. 2000, Lee et al. 2005). Exposing human dermal fibroblasts to biophysical signals resulted in an increased expression of 57 genes related to ECM proteins that included collagen types I and VI, fibronectin, as well as elastin (Kessler et al. 2001). In addition, there are reports about an increased elastin protein expression due to mechanical stimulation. For example, Bing et al. subjected rat pelvic ligament fibroblasts to 10% strain (1 Hz and 2 Hz) for 12 hours, followed by a co-culture with bone marrow stromal cells under stretch for an additional 6 to 12 days, after which a significant increase of elastin, LOX, and fibulin-5 was reported (Bing et al. 2012). In contrast, Howard et al. applied biaxial stretch (5%, 0.5Hz, 14 hours) to ligament fibroblasts (Howard et al. 1998). The authors observed that although collagen type I and fibronectin synthesis were increased, tropoelastin production was decreased compared to the static controls. One of the possible reasons for these opposing results is that the parameters of the mechanical stimulation varied between the studies. Fibroblasts are highly sensitive to the flow rate, strain magnitude, frequency, and duration; therefore, different stimuli parameters potentially lead to completely different results and cannot be objectively compared with each other. Another possible reason might be that the fibroblast and bone marrow stromal cell co-culture system in the study performed by Bing et al. led to the increase of elastin. Despite the great promise of such studies, only a few reports have focused on the induction of elastogenesis by fibroblasts utilizing biomechanical cues. Further studies are required to address this complex problem. Our previous study using human vascular SMCs showed the successful generation of maturing elastic fibers in vitro (Hinderer et al. 2015). Therefore, we aimed to identify if the same experimental approach would lead to the production of maturing elastic fibers employing human dermal fibroblasts. For this purpose, foreskin fibroblasts were isolated from patients between 2 and 7 years, and normal adult skin fibroblasts were isolated from patients ranging between 20 and 40 years. All cells were used between passages 3 and 4. To produce the 3D fibrous hybrid scaffolds, we electrospun poly(L-lactide) (PLA) and poly(ethylene glycol) dimethacrylate (PEGdma) as previously described (Hinderer et al. 2015). A fluid flow bioreactor capable of providing laminar shear stress was used in this study. Scaffolds were coated with 1:5 mixture of 1% w/v HA in Dulbecco's phosphate-buffered saline (PBS) 2 hours prior to cell seeding. HA of a molecular weight of ~750,000 Da was used in this study due to its ability to support tropoelastin cross-linking (Joddar and Ramamurthi 2006b, Hinderer et al. 2015). Approximately 3×10^5 cells were seeded onto each scaffold. After 24 hours of preculture, the scaffolds were transferred into the bioreactor system with Dulbecco's modified eagle medium (DMEM) supplemented with 10% v/v fetal bovine serum (FBS) and 1% v/v penicillin/streptomycin as well as 3.2 ng/ml transforming growth factor beta 1 (TGFβ1). TGFβ1 had been reported to play a crucial role in protein binding and elastic fiber assembly (Kothapalli et al. 2009, Hinderer et al. 2015). Furthermore, the combination of TGFβ1 and HA induced much greater assembly of mature elastin fibers (Kothapalli et al. 2009, Hinderer et al. 2015). In order to provide constant medium change without shearing the cells off, the flow rate was initially set at 0.74 ml/min and then adjusted to 1.48 ml/min from the second day on. As a control, cell-seeded scaffolds were statically cultured without applying shear stress. After 6 days of dynamic culture, the scaffolds from the bioreactor and the static controls were harvested and further analyzed. Quantitative real-time polymerase chain reaction (qPCR) was performed as previously described (Hinderer et al. 2015) using elastin (ELN), fibulin-5 (FBLN5), fibrillin-1 (FBN1), fibronectin (FN1), EMILIN1, and glyceraldehyde 3-phosphate dehydrogenase (GAPDH) primers from Qiagen. Immunofluorescence staining (IF staining) was performed according to the previously published protocol in order to detect the secreted proteins (Hinderer et al. 2015). As shown in Figure 5.3, shear stress induced a fivefold upregulation of ELN

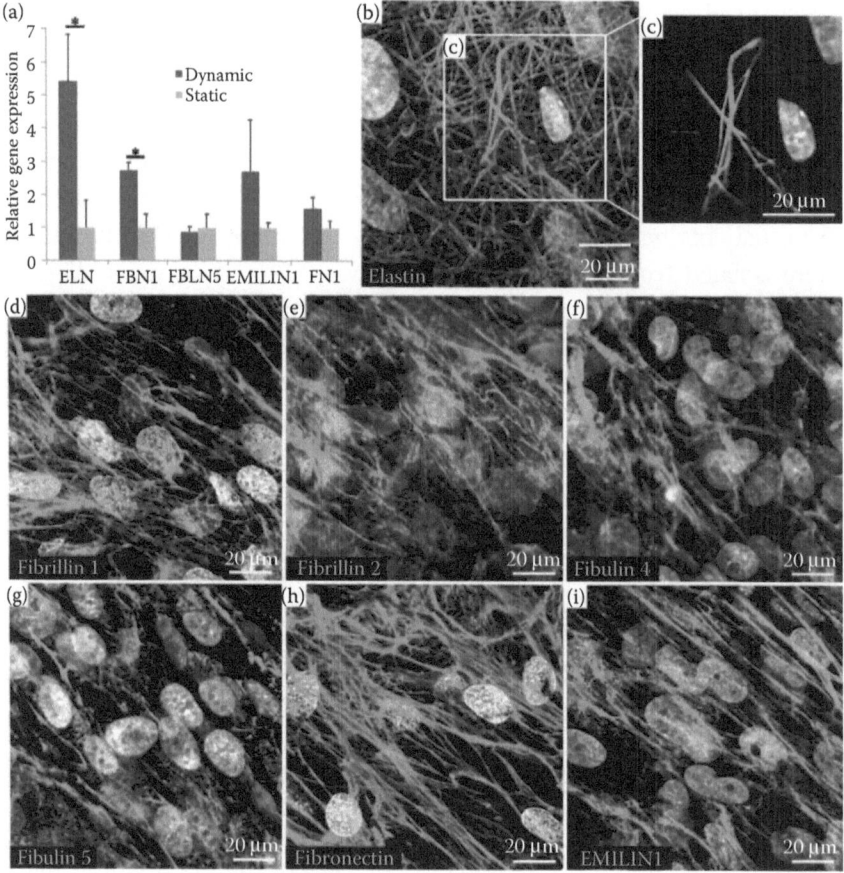

FIGURE 5.3 Impact of shear stress on cultured foreskin fibroblasts. (a) Gene expression of ELN (elastin), FBN1 (fibrillin-1), FBLN5 (fibulin-5), EMILIN-1, and FN1 (fibronectin). (b–i) IF staining of elastin and elastogenesis-associated proteins after a 6-day dynamic culture on 3D HA-coated scaffolds with TGFβ1. Cell nuclei are depicted in white (DAPI). *$p \leq .05$ static versus dynamic (Student's t-test was used for statistics analysis).

and threefold upregulation of FBN1 when compared to the static controls (ELN: 5.41 ± 1.43 (dynamic) vs. 1 ± 0.82 (static), $p = .021$; FBN1: 2.72 ± 0.23 (dynamic) vs. 1 ± 0.41 (static), $p = .01$). An increase in FBLN5, FN1, and EMILIN1 expression was also noticed, although this increase was not statistically significant. IF staining of the six-day dynamically cultured foreskin fibroblasts revealed the presence of elastic fibers (Figure 5.3b,c). In addition, the elastogenesis-associated proteins fibrillin 1 and 2, fibulin 4 and 5, as well as fibronectin and EMILIN-1, which have been proven to be critical for proper matrix assembly and cross-linking (Zanetti et al. 2004, Votteler et al. 2013), were highly expressed (Figure 5.3d–i).

Similar results were seen using normal adult skin fibroblasts. As shown in Figure 5.4a, approximately fourfold upregulation of ELN and two-fold upregulation of FBN1 were determined when comparing dynamic versus static cultures (ELN 3.75 ± 0.29 (dynamic) vs. 1 ± 0.49 (static), $p = .0028$; FBN1 1.94 ± 0.38 (dynamic) vs. 1 ± 0.41 (static), $p = .042$). Elastin and elastogenesis-associated protein expression profiles were also similar to those seen in the 6-day dynamic foreskin fibroblast cultures (Figure 5.4b–i).

It is well established that IF staining utilizing commercially available elastin antibodies cannot discriminate between tropoelastin and cross-linked elastin. For the detection of cross-links, we thus employed Raman microspectroscopy. Raman microspectroscopy is a laser-based technology that is increasingly employed in the field of tissue engineering and regenerative medicine (Movasaghi et al. 2007, Brauchle and Schenke-Layland 2013). With this technology, it is possible to generate individual biochemical fingerprints by detecting molecular vibrations from proteins, lipids, nucleic acids, as well as macromolecular conformations (Chan et al. 2006, Brauchle and Schenke-Layland 2013). Raman spectroscopy has been used to characterize ECM proteins, such as collagen (Gullekson et al. 2011, Nguyen et al. 2012, Votteler et al. 2012b), elastin (Frushour and Koenig 1975, Debelle et al. 1995, Votteler et al. 2012a), and proteoglycans (Pudlas et al. 2013, Gamsjaeger et al. 2014). Frushour and Koenig have investigated the Raman spectra of collagen, gelatin, and elastin. They identified three Raman bands, 529, 966, and 1108 cm^{-1} that can be assigned to desmosine and isodesmosine (Frushour and Koenig 1975). Desmosine and isodesmosine are two elastic fiber-specific amino acids that are involved in cross-linking of elastic fibers (Kielty et al. 2002). In our study, the dynamically cultured dermal fibroblasts were harvested from the bioreactor cultures and placed in glass bottom dishes filled with PBS. Thirty spectra from

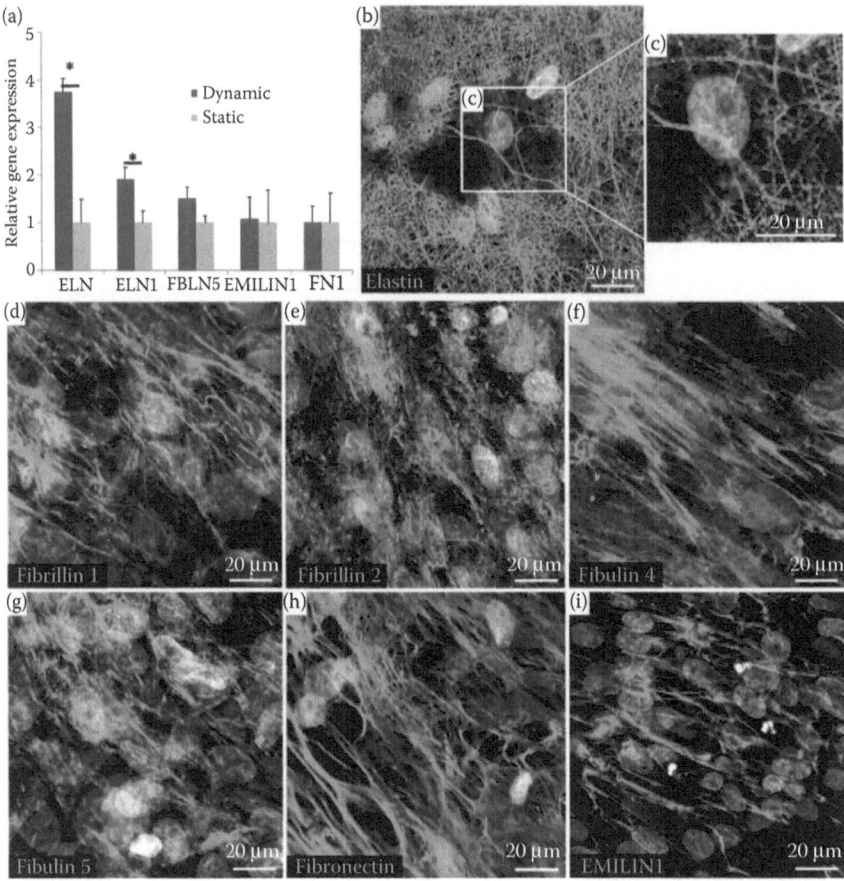

FIGURE 5.4 Impact of shear stress on adult skin fibroblasts. (a) Gene expression of ELN (elastin), FBN1 (fibrillin-1), FBLN5 (fibulin-5), EMILIN-1, and FN1 (fibronectin). (b–i) IF staining of elastin and elastogenesis-associated proteins after a 6-day dynamic culture on 3D HA-coated scaffolds with TGFβ1. Cell nuclei are stained with DAPI (white). $^*p \leq .05$ static versus dynamic (student's t-test was used for statistics analysis).

three samples were measured with a custom-built Raman microspectrometer (Pudlas et al. 2011). In order to exclude background signals from the scaffold, 30 spectra from three different PEGdma and PLA scaffolds were measured as control. All Raman spectra were reduced to the spectral region between 400 and 1800 cm^{-1} and processed as previously described (Pudlas et al. 2011). Figure 5.5 shows the average Raman spectra of the six-day dynamically cultured dermal fibroblasts and the static controls. These two sample groups revealed clearly distinguishable Raman spectra

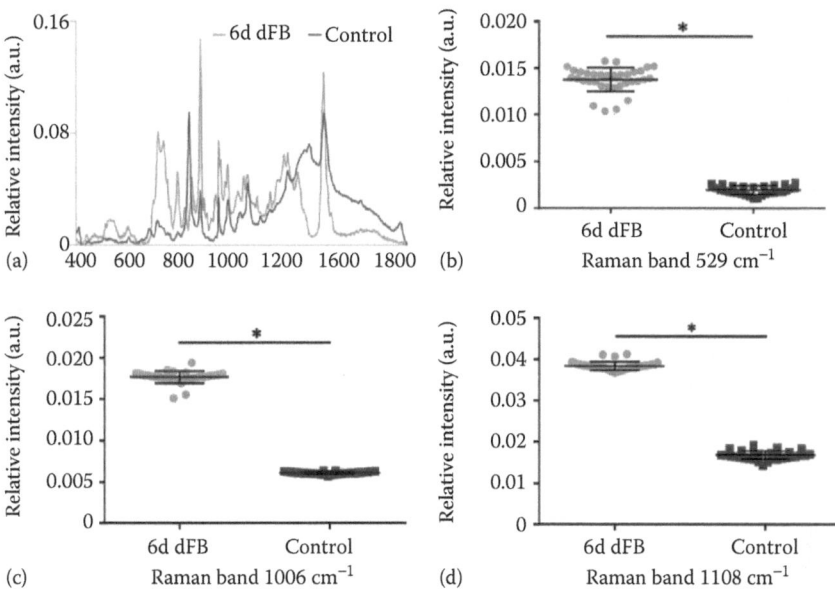

(a) (b) (c) (d)

FIGURE 5.5 Raman spectra analysis of human dermal fibroblasts after 6-day dynamic culture on 3D HA-coated scaffolds with TGFβ1. (a) Mean Raman spectra of dynamically cultured dermal fibroblasts and the corresponding static controls. Raman bands at (b) 529 cm⁻¹ (c) 966 cm⁻¹, and (d) 1108 cm⁻¹ indicate maturation of elastic fibers. *$p \leq .001$.

patterns. When focusing on the previously identified Raman bands at 529, 966, and 1108 cm⁻¹ (Frushour and Koenig 1975), significantly higher intensities were seen in the 6-day dynamic cultures when compared to the static controls (Raman band 529 cm⁻¹, $p = 4.22 \times 10^{-52}$; Raman band 966 cm⁻¹, $p = 4.12 \times 10^{-52}$; Raman band 1108 cm⁻¹, $p = 9.66 \times 10^{-39}$), indicating the presence of properly cross-linked, mature elastic fibers.

5.4 CONCLUSION

In order to provide an optimal environment for cells to synthesize elastin and to assemble it to a functional elastic matrix, several different factors need to be carefully considered. Here, we discussed two parameters in detail that are crucial for elastic tissue engineering: (a) three-dimensionality to mimic the ECM structure and (b) mechanical forces to mimic physiological parameters such as blood flow and the corresponding strains. It has been shown that either factor has a significant impact on cell behavior and elastic fiber maturation. In future studies, the interplay of such factors must be further explored, especially when aiming for the engineering of implants for elastic fiber-rich tissues and organs.

ACKNOWLEDGMENTS

The authors thank Shannon L. Layland (Fraunhofer IGB Stuttgart, Germany) and Marsha W. Rolle (Worchester Polytechnic Institute, the United States) for their thoughtful suggestions. This work was financially supported by the Fraunhofer-Gesellschaft Internal programs (Attract to KSL, Talenta speed up to SH), the BMBF (0316059 to KSL), and the Ministry of Science, Research and the Arts of Baden-Württemberg (33-729.55-3/214 and SI-BW 01222-91 to KSL).

REFERENCES

Balestreire, E. M. and G. Apodaca. 2007. Apical epidermal growth factor receptor signaling: Regulation of stretch-dependent exocytosis in bladder umbrella cells. *Molecular Biology of the Cell* 18(4): 1312–1323.

Barenghi, R., S. Beke, I. Romano et al. 2014. Elastin-coated biodegradable photopolymer scaffolds for tissue engineering applications. *BioMed Research International* 2014: 624–645.

Bashur, C. A. and A. Ramamurthi. 2011a. Aligned electrospun scaffolds and elastogenic factors for vascular cell-mediated elastic matrix assembly. *Journal of Tissue Engineering and Regenerative Medicine* 6(9): 673–686.

Bashur, C. A. and A. Ramamurthi. 2011b. Perspectives on strategies to direct elastic matrix assembly. *Journal of Tissue Science & Engineering* 2: 106e.

Bashur, C. A., L. Venkataraman, and A. Ramamurthi. 2012. Tissue engineering and regenerative strategies to replicate biocomplexity of vascular elastic matrix assembly. *Tissue Engineering Part B Reviews* 18(3): 203–217.

Bing, Z., L. Linlin, Y. Jianguo et al. 2012. Effect of mechanical stretch on the expressions of elastin, LOX and Fibulin-5 in rat BMSCs with ligament fibroblasts co-culture. *Molecular Biology Reports* 39(5): 6077–6085.

Boccafoschi, F., C. Mosca, M. Ramella, G. Valente, and M. Cannas. 2013. The effect of mechanical strain on soft (cardiovascular) and hard (bone) tissues: Common pathways for different biological outcomes. *Cell Adhesion & Migration* 7(2): 165–173.

Boccafoschi, F., M. Ramella, T. Sibillano et al. 2015. Human elastin polypeptides improve the biomechanical properties of three-dimensional matrices through the regulation of elastogenesis. *Journal of Biomedical Materials Research Part A* 103(3): 1218–1230.

Brauchle, E. and K. Schenke-Layland. 2013. Raman spectroscopy in biomedicine–Non-invasive in vitro analysis of cells and extracellular matrix components in tissues. *Biotechnology Journal* 8(3): 288–297.

Brosig, M. 2011. Mechanotransduction in fibroblasts. PhD dissertation, Universität Basel.

Cattaruzza, M., C. Dimigen, H. Ehrenreich, and M. Hecker. 2000. Stretch-induced endothelin B receptor-mediated apoptosis in vascular smooth muscle cells. *FASEB Journal* 14(7): 991–998.

Chan, J. W., D. S. Taylor, T. Zwerdling et al. 2006. Micro-Raman spectroscopy detects individual neoplastic and normal hematopoietic cells. *Biophysical Journal* 90(2): 648–656.

Chen, K. D., Y. S. Li, M. Kim et al. 1999. Mechanotransduction in response to shear stress. Roles of receptor tyrosine kinases, integrins, and Shc. *Journal of Biological Chemistry* 274(26): 18393–18400.

Chen, Q., A. Bruyneel, C. Carr, and J. Czernuszka. 2013. Bio-mechanical properties of novel bi-layer collagen-elastin scaffolds for heart valve tissue engineering. *Procedia Engineering* 59: 247–254.

Chen, Q. Z., A. Bismarck, U. Hansen et al. 2008. Characterisation of a soft elastomer poly(glycerol sebacate) designed to match the mechanical properties of myocardial tissue. *Biomaterials* 29(1): 47–57.

Chiquet, M., L. Gelman, R. Lutz, and S. Maier. 2009. From mechanotransduction to extracellular matrix gene expression in fibroblasts. *Biochimica et Biophysica Acta (BBA)–Molecular Cell Research* 1793(5): 911–920.

Choe, M. M., P. H. Sporn, and M. A. Swartz. 2006. Extracellular matrix remodeling by dynamic strain in a three-dimensional tissue-engineered human airway wall model. *American Journal of Respiratory Cell and Molecular Biology* 35(3): 306–313.

Davis, M. J., G. A. Meininger, and D. C. Zawieja. 1992. Stretch-induced increases in intracellular calcium of isolated vascular smooth muscle cells. *American Journal of Physiology* 263(4 Pt 2): H1292–H1299.

Debelle, L., A. J. Alix, M. P. Jacob et al. 1995. Bovine elastin and κ-elastin secondary structure determination by optical spectroscopies. *Journal of Biological Chemistry* 270(44): 26099–26103.

Frushour, B. G. and J. L. Koenig. 1975. Raman scattering of collagen, gelatin, and elastin. *Biopolymers* 14(2): 379–391.

Gambillara, V., T. Thacher, P. Silacci, and N. Stergiopulos. 2008. Effects of reduced cyclic stretch on vascular smooth muscle cell function of pig carotids perfused ex vivo. *American Journal of Hypertension* 21(4): 425–431.

Gamsjaeger, S., K. Klaushofer, and E. P. Paschalis. 2014. Raman analysis of proteoglycans simultaneously in bone and cartilage. *Journal of Raman Spectroscopy* 45(9): 794–800.

Gao, J., P. Crapo, R. Nerem, and Y. Wang. 2008. Co-expression of elastin and collagen leads to highly compliant engineered blood vessels. *Journal of Biomedical Materials Research Part A* 85(4): 1120–1128.

Gullekson, C., L. Lucas, K. Hewitt, and L. Kreplak. 2011. Surface-sensitive Raman spectroscopy of collagen I fibrils. *Biophysical Journal* 100(7): 1837–1845.

Gupta, V. and K. J. Grande-Allen. 2006. Effects of static and cyclic loading in regulating extracellular matrix synthesis by cardiovascular cells. *Cardiovascular Research* 72(3): 375–383.

Haga, J. H., Y. S. Li, and S. Chien. 2007. Molecular basis of the effects of mechanical stretch on vascular smooth muscle cells. *Journal of Biomechanics* 40(5): 947–960.

Haga, M., A. Yamashita, J. Paszkowiak, B. E. Sumpio, and A. Dardik. 2003. Oscillatory shear stress increases smooth muscle cell proliferation and Akt phosphorylation. *Journal of Vascular Surgery* 37(6): 1277–1284.

Hinderer, S., N. Shen, L. J. Ringuette et al. 2015. In vitro elastogenesis – Instructing human vascular smooth muscle cells to generate an elastic fiber-containing extracellular matrix scaffold. *Biomedical Materials* 10(3): 034102.

Hirai, M., M. Horiguchi, T. Ohbayashi et al. 2007. Latent TGF-[beta]-binding protein 2 binds to DANCE/fibulin-5 and regulates elastic fiber assembly. *EMBO Journal* 26(14): 3283–3295.

Hopkins, A. M., L. De Laporte, F. Tortelli et al. 2013. Silk hydrogels as soft substrates for neural tissue engineering. *Advanced Functional Materials* 23(41): 5140–5149.

Howard, P. S., U. Kucich, R. Taliwal, and J. M. Korostoff. 1998. Mechanical forces alter extracellular matrix synthesis by human periodontal ligament fibroblasts. *Journal of Periodontal Research* 33(8): 500–508.

Hu, Y., G. Böck, G. Wick, and Q. Xu. 1998. Activation of PDGF receptor α in vascular smooth muscle cells by mechanical stress. *The FASEB Journal* 12(12): 1135–1142.

Huang, H., R. D. Kamm, and R. T. Lee. 2004. Cell mechanics and mechanotransduction: Pathways, probes, and physiology. *American Journal of Physiology* 287(1): C1–11.

Ingber, D. E. 2006. Cellular mechanotransduction: Putting all the pieces together again. *The FASEB Journal* 20(7): 811–827.

Iwasaki, H., S. Eguchi, H. Ueno, F. Marumo, and Y. Hirata. 2000. Mechanical stretch stimulates growth of vascular smooth muscle cells via epidermal growth factor receptor. *American Journal of Physiology* 278(2): H521–H529.

Iwasaki, H., T. Yoshimoto, T. Sugiyama, and Y. Hirata. 2003. Activation of cell adhesion kinase β by mechanical stretch in vascular smooth muscle cells. *Endocrinology* 144(6): 2304–2310.

Iwasaki, K., K. Kojima, S. Kodama et al. 2008. Bioengineered three-layered robust and elastic artery using hemodynamically-equivalent pulsatile bioreactor. *Circulation* 118(14 Suppl): S52–57.

Jaalouk, D. E. and J. Lammerding. 2009. Mechanotransduction gone awry. *Nature Reviews Molecular Cell Biology* 10(1): 63–73.

Jeffries, E. M., R. A. Allen, J. Gao, M. Pesce, and Y. Wang. 2015. Highly elastic and suturable electrospun poly(glycerol sebacate) fibrous scaffolds. *Acta Biomaterialia* 18: 30–39.

Joddar, B., S. Ibrahim, and A. Ramamurthi. 2007. Impact of delivery mode of hyaluronan oligomers on elastogenic responses of adult vascular smooth muscle cells. *Biomaterials* 28(27): 3918–3927.

Joddar, B. and A. Ramamurthi. 2006a. Elastogenic effects of exogenous hyaluronan oligosaccharides on vascular smooth muscle cells. *Biomaterials* 27(33): 5698–5707.

Joddar, B. and A. Ramamurthi. 2006b. Fragment size- and dose-specific effects of hyaluronan on matrix synthesis by vascular smooth muscle cells. *Biomaterials* 27(15): 2994–3004.

Kang, H., Y. Fan, and X. Deng. 2011. Vascular smooth muscle cell glycocalyx modulates shear-induced proliferation, migration, and NO production responses. *American Journal of Physiology* 300(1): H76–H83.

Katsumi, A., A. W. Orr, E. Tzima, and M. A. Schwartz. 2004. Integrins in mechanotransduction. *Journal of Biological Chemistry* 279(13): 12001–12004.

Keire, P. A., N. L'Heureux, R. B. Vernon et al. 2009. Expression of versican isoform V3 in the absence of ascorbate improves elastogenesis in engineered vascular constructs. *Tissue Engineering Part A* 16(2): 501–512.

Kessler, D., S. Dethlefsen, I. Haase et al. 2001. Fibroblasts in mechanically stressed collagen lattices assume a "synthetic" phenotype. *The Journal of Biological Chemistry* 276(39): 36575–36585.

Kielty, C. M., M. J. Sherratt, and C. A. Shuttleworth. 2002. Elastic fibres. *Journal of Cell Science* 115(Pt 14): 2817–2828.

Kim, B. S., J. Nikolovski, J. Bonadio, and D. J. Mooney. 1999. Cyclic mechanical strain regulates the development of engineered smooth muscle tissue. *Nature Biotechnology* 17(10): 979–983.

Kim, T. G., H. S. Shin, and D. W. Lim. 2012. Biomimetic scaffolds for tissue engineering. *Advanced Functional Materials* 22(12): 2446–2468.

Kothapalli, C. R., P. M. Taylor, R. T. Smolenski, M. H. Yacoub, and A. Ramamurthi. 2009. Transforming growth factor beta 1 and hyaluronan oligomers synergistically enhance elastin matrix regeneration by vascular smooth muscle cells. *Tissue Engineering Part A* 15(3): 501–511.

Kumar, V. A., J. M. Caves, C. A. Haller et al. 2013. Acellular vascular grafts generated from collagen and elastin analogs. *Acta Biomaterialia* 9(9): 8067–8074.

Lee, C. H., H. J. Shin, I. H. Cho et al. 2005. Nanofiber alignment and direction of mechanical strain affect the ECM production of human ACL fibroblast. *Biomaterials* 26(11): 1261–1270.

Lee, K. W., D. B Stolz, and Y. Wang. 2011. Substantial expression of mature elastin in arterial constructs. *Proceedings of the National Academy of Sciences* 108(7): 2705–2710.

Lehoux, S., Y. Castier, and A. Tedgui. 2006. Molecular mechanisms of the vascular responses to haemodynamic forces. *Journal of Internal Medicine* 259(4): 381–392.

Lin, S., M. Sandig, and K. Mequanint. 2011. Three-dimensional topography of synthetic scaffolds induces elastin synthesis by human coronary artery smooth muscle cells. *Tissue Engineering Part A* 17(11–12): 1561–1571.

MacKenna, D., S. R. Summerour, and F. J. Villarreal. 2000. Role of mechanical factors in modulating cardiac fibroblast function and extracellular matrix synthesis. *Cardiovascular Research* 46(2): 257–263.

Masoumi, N., N. Annabi, A. Assmann et al. 2014. Tri-layered elastomeric scaffolds for engineering heart valve leaflets. *Biomaterials* 35(27): 7774–7785.

Movasaghi, Z., S. Rehman, and I. U. Rehman. 2007. Raman spectroscopy of biological tissues. *Applied Spectroscopy Reviews* 42(5): 493–541.

Nguyen, T. T., C. Gobinet, J. Feru et al. 2012. Characterization of type I and IV collagens by Raman microspectroscopy: Identification of spectral markers of the dermo-epidermal junction. *Spectroscopy: An International Journal* 27(5–6): 7.

Noda, K., B. Dabovic, K. Takagi et al. 2013. Latent TGF-β binding protein 4 promotes elastic fiber assembly by interacting with fibulin-5. *Proceedings of the National Academy of Sciences of the United States of America* 110(8): 2852–2857.

Opitz, F., K. Schenke-Layland, T. U. Cohnert et al. 2004. Tissue engineering of aortic tissue: Dire consequence of suboptimal elastic fiber synthesis in vivo. *Cardiovascular Research* 63(4): 719–730.

Patel, A., B. Fine, M. Sandig, and K. Mequanint. 2006. Elastin biosynthesis: The missing link in tissue-engineered blood vessels. *Cardiovascular Research* 71(1): 40–49.

Pudlas, M., E. Brauchle, T. J. Klein, D. W. Hutmacher, and K. Schenke-Layland. 2013. Non-invasive identification of proteoglycans and chondrocyte differentiation state by Raman microspectroscopy. *Journal of Biophotonics* 6(2): 205–211.

Pudlas, M., D. A. C Berrio, M. Votteler et al. 2011. Non-contact discrimination of bone marrow mesenchymal stem cells and fibroblasts using Raman microspectroscopy. *Medical Laser Application* 26(3): 119–125.

Qiu, J., Y. Zheng, J. Hu et al. 2013. Biomechanical regulation of vascular smooth muscle cell functions: From in vitro to in vivo understanding. *Interface* 11(90).

Schenke-Layland, K., A. Nsair, B. Van Handel et al. 2011. Recapitulation of the embryonic cardiovascular progenitor cell niche. *Biomaterials* 32(11): 2748–2756.

Seliktar, D., R. M. Nerem, and Z. S. Galis. 2003. Mechanical strain-stimulated remodeling of tissue-engineered blood vessel constructs. *Tissue Eng* 9(4): 657–666.

Shi, Z. D. and J. M. Tarbell. 2011. Fluid flow mechanotransduction in vascular smooth muscle cells and fibroblasts. *Annals of Biomedical Engineering* 39(6): 1608–1619.

Sommer, N., M. Sattler, J. M. Weise et al. 2013. A tissue-engineered human dermal construct utilizing fibroblasts and transforming growth factor β1 to promote elastogenesis. *Biotechnology Journal* 8(3): 317–326.

Sumpio, B. E., A. J. Banes, W. G. Link, and G. Johnson, Jr. 1988. Enhanced collagen production by smooth muscle cells during repetitive mechanical stretching. *Archives of Surgery* 123(10): 1233–1236.

Tu, Yi., S. G. Wise, and A. S. Weiss. 2010. Stages in tropoelastin coalescence during synthetic elastin hydrogel formation. *Micron* 41(3): 268–272.

Venkataraman, L., C. A. Bashur, and A. Ramamurthi. 2014. Impact of cyclic stretch on induced elastogenesis within collagenous conduits. *Tissue Engineering Part A* 20(9–10): 1403–1415.

Votteler, M., D. A. Carvajal Berrio, A. Horke et al. 2013. Elastogenesis at the onset of human cardiac valve development. *Development* 140(11): 2345–2353.

Votteler, M., D. A. Carvajal Berrio, M Pudlas, H Walles, and K Schenke-Layland. 2012a. Non-contact, label-free monitoring of cells and extracellular matrix using Raman spectroscopy. *Journal of Visualized Experiments* 29(63): 3977.

Votteler, M., D. A. Carvajal Berrio, M. Pudlas et al. 2012b. Raman spectroscopy for the non-contact and non-destructive monitoring of collagen damage within tissues. *Journal of Biophotonics* 5(1): 47–56.

Wang, J. H., G. Yang, Z. Li, and W. Shen. 2004. Fibroblast responses to cyclic mechanical stretching depend on cell orientation to the stretching direction. *Journal of Biomechanics* 37(4): 573–576.

Waterhouse, A., S. G. Wise, M. K. Ng, and A. S. Weiss. 2011. Elastin as a non-thrombogenic biomaterial. *Tissue Engineering Part B Reviews* 17(2): 93–99.

Wernig, F., M. Mayr, and Q. Xu. 2003. Mechanical stretch-induced apoptosis in smooth muscle cells is mediated by β1-integrin signaling pathways. *Hypertension* 41(4): 903–911.

Wise, S. G., M. J. Byrom, A. Waterhouse et al. 2011. A multilayered synthetic human elastin/polycaprolactone hybrid vascular graft with tailored mechanical properties. *Acta Biomaterialia* 7(1): 295–303.

Wong, T., J. A. McGrath, and H. Navsaria. 2007. The role of fibroblasts in tissue engineering and regeneration. *The British journal of dermatology* 156(6): 1149–1155.

Yang, G., R. C. Crawford, and J. H. Wang. 2004. Proliferation and collagen production of human patellar tendon fibroblasts in response to cyclic uniaxial stretching in serum-free conditions. *Journal of Biomechanics* 37(10): 1543–1550.

Yeo, G. C., B. Aghaei-Ghareh-Bolagh, E. P. Brackenreg et al. 2015. Fabricated elastin. *Advanced Healthcare Materials* 4(16): 2530–2556.

Zampetaki, A., Z. Zhang, Y. Hu, and Q. Xu. 2005. Biomechanical stress induces IL-6 expression in smooth muscle cells via Ras/Rac1-p38 MAPK-NF-κB signaling pathways. *American Journal of Physiology* 288(6): H2946–H2954.

Zanetti, M., P. Braghetta, P. Sabatelli et al. 2004. EMILIN-1 deficiency induces elastogenesis and vascular cell defects. *Molecular and Cellular Biology* 24(2): 638–650.

Zhang, X., X. Wang, V. Keshav et al. 2009. Dynamic culture conditions to generate silk-based tissue-engineered vascular grafts. *Biomaterials* 30(19): 3213–3223.

CHAPTER 6

Pharmacologic Strategies for Preserving Elastic Matrix

Nasim Nosoudi, Vaideesh Parasaram,
Saketh R. Karamched, Aniqa Chowdhury,
and Naren Vyavahare

CONTENTS

6.1 INTRODUCTION

Elastin is a physiologically important protein present in the extracellular matrix (ECM) that renders elastic properties to some of the vital tissues such as arteries, skin, and lungs. Majority of elastin deposition occurs during embryonic and childhood stages, and with a half-life period of 74 years it rarely remodels in adults (Cleary et al. 1967, Shapiro et al. 1991). Elastin synthesis has been documented in fibroblasts, smooth muscle cells (SMCs), chondrocytes, and endothelial cells (Burke and Ross 1979, Quintarelli et al. 1979, Cantor et al. 1980, Mecham et al. 1981). Briefly, cells secrete tropoelastin monomers that are then anchored on microfibrillar scaffold already present in the ECM. Tropoelastin molecules are cross-linked to each other with their lysine residues by lysyl oxidase (LOX) enzyme (Davis and Mecham 1993). Degradation of elastic fibers under inflammatory conditions results in permanent loss of elastin, and it leads to loss of elasticity in the organs.

Damage to the elastin fibers can either be due to genetic disorder or acquired during disease process. Arterial tortuosity syndrome, *cutis laxa, pseudoxanthoma elasticum*, and supravalvular aortic stenosis are some of the genetic disorders of elastin, while Marshall syndrome, solar lactinic elastosis, abdominal aortic aneurysm (AAA), chronic obstructive pulmonary disease (COPD), calcification of arteries, and aging of skin are some of the acquired elastin disorders (Baldwin et al. 2013). Elastin is degraded by enzymes called *elastases*. Depending on the mechanism of catalysis, few members of serine (*e.g.* neutrophil elastase, pancreatic elastase), cysteine (Cathepsin K), and metalloproteinases (MMP-2, MMP-9, and MMP-12) can cleave elastin (Werb et al. 1982, Mecham et al. 1997, Neurath 1999, Houghton et al. 2011, Lu et al. 2011). In diseases such as AAA and COPD, inflammation and oxidative damage initiate and aggravate the elastin degradation, while in skin elastin loss can occur due to aging and photooxidation (Thompson et al. 2006, Uitto 2008, Tuder and Petrache 2012). In this chapter, we will discuss some of the major acquired elastin degradation disorders in various organs and pharmacological treatments available to either prevent or repair elastin degradation.

6.2 PHARMACOLOGICAL APPROACHES FOR ELASTIN PRESERVATION IN AAA

Aneurysms are an abnormal widening or ballooning of a portion of an artery that creates structural weakness in the blood vessel wall, which are typically located in the abdominal and thoracic aortae and brain arteries, where early stages of growth are asymptomatic. In the United States, AAA is the tenth leading cause of death in men over age 55 (Go et al. 2013). Ruptured AAAs are 75%–90% fatal if immediate hospitalization is delayed. The increasing awareness of AAA disease and an ultrasound screening benefit offered by Medicare (SAAVE act) for elderly patients who have smoked at least 100 cigarettes in their lifetime has dramatically increased the pool of patients with small-AAA seeking treatment options for early-stage disease (Lee et al. 2009). In fact, the majority of AAA are detected at an early stage of the disease. However, current imaging methods do not provide enough information about the progression of the disease, and no pharmacological method is available to prevent aneurysmal growth. Clinicians face a dilemma when deciding whether risk of AAA rupture justifies risks associated with surgery, especially because these mostly elderly patients typically have comorbidities. Two pharmacological approaches have shown positive results in animals to inhibit AAA growth: (1) rendering the ECM resistant to further proteolytic damage by inhibition of enzymes, or (2) regenerating ECM proteins to repair aneurysmal tissue. Some of the treatments have been tested clinically but none have so far shown statistical improvement in the disease in humans. Elastin degradation occurs due to release of elastases by inflammatory cells and vascular cells under inflammatory conditions, and due to free radical damage. Many strategies that are presented below that reduce inflammation, prevent oxidative free radical damage, or inhibit elastase type enzymes can most probably halt elastin degradation. The published data are not directly showing elastin stabilization except our work presented later, but these strategies may be indirectly preventing further elastin degradation in arteries.

6.3 ACE INHIBITORS AND ATII RECEPTOR INHIBITORS

Angiotensin II (Ang II) is an octapeptide hormone that plays an important role in cardiovascular homeostasis (Castro-Chaves and Leite-Moreira 2004). It regulates blood pressure by inducing vasoconstriction and the release of aldosterone that exists in the adrenal cortex. In experiments with animals, the administration of Ang II decreases the content of elastin in the aortic wall and in an AAA (Tham et al. 2002). Additionally, it has been shown that Ang II has a role in AAA development in a hyperlipidimic mouse model (Lu et al. 2008, Cassis et al. 2009). Angiotensin I (Ang I) converting enzyme (ACE) catalyzes Ang I to Ang II conversion (Crisan and Carr 2000) and degrades bradykinin, a potent endothelium-dependent vasodilator (Hecker et al. 1994, Sasamura and Itoh 2011) and therefore raises the blood pressure. AT1 and AT2 receptors, both have the same affinity to bind to Ang II. Naturally, the inhibition of ATR (angiotensin receptor) and ACE shows strong potential for pharmacological approaches to prevent the hypertension, heart failure, diabetic nephropathy, and postmyocardial infarction (Ferrario 2006). A few studies have investigated their potential in treating AAA. Lisinopril, an ACE inhibitor, and candesartan, an ATR inhibitor, were used in an Ang II/ApoE$^{-/-}$ AAA mice model. Lisinopril group showed 18% and candesartan group showed a 23% reduction in the aortic diameter after 40 weeks when these drugs were administered by subcutaneous injections (Inoue et al. 2009). In another study, administration of ACE inhibitor (enalapril) or an Ang II receptor blocker (losartan) in deoxycorticosterone acetate and salt-induced aneurysms were studied. It resulted in a significant reduction in blood pressure due to active blockage of the renin–angiotensin system. But, none of them reduced aortic diameters of suprarenal abdominal aorta (Liu et al. 2013). Another study investigated the effects of ACE inhibitors on 3426 human patients including 665 patients with ruptured aneurysms and 2761 of those with intact aortas. It showed a significant (18%) lower risk of aortic rupture in those who received ACE inhibitors compared with patients not treated with an ACE inhibitor (Hackam et al. 2006).

Others have also looked at blocking AT1 receptor. An AT1 inhibitor, losartan, has shown favorable results *in vivo*, as the subcutaneous delivery of it successfully inhibited the AAAs formation (Tsui 2010). In another study, an alternative AT1 receptor antagonist, valsartan, significantly reduced aneurysm development in elastase-infused rats without affecting blood pressure (Fujiwara et al. 2008).

6.4 TETRACYCLINES

Tetracycline antibiotics exhibit matrix metalloproteinase (MMP)-inhibiting properties (Curci et al. 1998). One specific tetracycline antibiotic, doxycycline, has been extensively studied in AAA treatment. It has been shown that subcutaneous injection of doxycycline (25 mg/day) in rat-elastase model of AAA significantly reduced AAA development (Petrinec et al. 1996), although there was no apparent elastic lamellae preservation. Oral administration of doxycycline in the Ang II mice model of AAA showed a 50% lower rate of AAA formation (Manning et al. 2003). It should be noted that the mice received doxycycline a week before the infusion of Ang II, which suggested a protective role for the drug in formation of AAA. Doxycycline treatment has also been tested clinically. There was a 5.5-fold decrease in MMP-9 mRNA and 2.5-fold decrease in activity compared to the control group, for eight patients treated with doxycycline a week before the repair (Curci et al. 2000). In another study, 60 patients who elected to go for aneurysmal repair received doxycycline (50, 100, or 300 mg/dL) or no medication (control) showed reduced aortic wall inflammation. Aortic wall neutrophils and cytotoxic T cells were reduced by 72% and 95%, respectively (Lindeman et al. 2009). In contrast, in another study, 286 patients with small AAAs were studied with daily dose of 100 mg of doxycycline ($n = 144$) or placebo ($n = 142$) for a time period of 18 months. This trial concluded that doxycycline therapy did not result in aneurysm growth reduction and the incidence of surgical repair was similar in both groups (Meijer et al. 2014).

Long-term administration studies of doxycycline have reported some side effects such as nonspecific gastrointestinal symptoms and tooth discoloration (Baxter et al. 2002). In an effort to limit the side effects resulting from systemic doxycycline delivery, continuous periaortic delivery of doxycycline was shown to be effective in the prevention of AAA in rats (Sho et al. 2004). Because of this, the targeted delivery procedure of doxycycline shows a lot of promise in AAA treatment, potentially as a pharmacological adjunct to endovascular aneurysm repair. A recent study has shown that poly (lactic-co-glycolic acid) nanoparticles (NPs) can be developed with positive charge on the surface that can bind to elastin via hydrophobic interactions and can deliver doxycycline in a controlled fashion in cell cultures (Sivaraman and Ramamurthi 2013).

6.5 STATINS

Statins are hydroxyl methyl glutamyl-coenzyme A inhibitors that are broadly used because of their lipid-lowering effects. Reducing lipid levels is a well-documented treatment for preventing progression of atherosclerosis, although there are additional unrelated effects of statins that have been demonstrated and termed "pleiotropic statins effects." Anti-inflammatory effects, antioxidant effects, and reduction of MMP secretion are all possible pleiotropic effects of statins (Ducajú et al. 2011). There have been a number of both animal and clinical studies undertaken to study the effect of statins on AAA development. ApoE$^{-/-}$ mice perfused with porcine elastase were treated with simvastatin (2 mg/kg subcutaneously), resulted in the suppression of AAA development (Steinmetz et al. 2005). In another study, simvastatin group showed a 20-fold reduction in MMP-9 gene expression and 9-fold increase in TIMP-1 mRNA expression as compared to the vehicle-treated controls. The statin appeared to preserve smooth muscle alpha actin in the medial layer (Lee et al. 2012). Simvastatin did not alter inflammatory cells infiltration into AAA; however, atorvastatin has been shown to suppress macrophage recruitment through inhibition of intercellular adhesion molecule-1 expression in the vascular wall, resulting in MMP-12 inhibition (Ducajú et al. 2011).

It has been shown in patients receiving statins for cholesterol reduction therapy that the rate of aneurysm growth was reduced (4.5 ± 0.6 cm for statin group and 5.3 ± 0.6 cm in patients not treated with statins at 24-month follow-up [$p < .001$]) and mortality was decreased (5% in statin group vs. 16% in nonstatin group after 44 months of follow-up [Sukhija et al. 2006]). Administration of simvastatin in patients who were to undergo open surgical repair prior to the surgery showed a significant decrease in MMP-9 activity (Evans et al. 2007). Overall, statins may be useful in controlling AAA growth, although the exact molecular mechanisms have yet to be determined. It appears that statins therapy leads to a reduction of the inflammation in the aneurysmal wall, in addition to diminishing MMP expression and/or enhancing the synthesis of their inhibitors, TIMPs (Ducajú et al. 2011).

6.6 β-BLOCKERS

Catecholamines (norepinephrine, epinephrine) are hormones that activate a specific type of receptors on cell surfaces known as adrenergic receptors. These receptors allow drugs and hormones to bind to it through their specific structure. This system closely resembles a lock-and-key phenomenon. The sympathetic nervous system nerve endings release the catecholamines. The sympathetic nervous system specializes in helping the body to withstand stress, anxiety, and exercise. β-Adrenergic receptors, found in the heart, blood vessels, and the lungs, can be stimulated by catecholamine binding, which increases the activity of cells in the body. The stimulation of the β-adrenergic receptor causes an increase in heart rate, heart muscle contraction, blood pressure, and relaxation of smooth muscle in the bronchial tubes in the lung, all of which improve the body's ability to perform cardiovascular activity by improving lung expansion.

Beta-adrenergic blockers (β-blockers) are a key class of drugs for several heart diseases treatments. They can be ingested or injected and prevent catecholamines from interacting with receptors, reducing blood pressure and heart rate. By making the heart pump less intensely, the oxygen need of the heart is decreased (Frishman 2003).

Propranolol, a beta-blocker, has been examined for use in AAA treatment. So far, it has been delivered to aneurysm prone turkeys and blotchy mice, and it has yielded a 150% increase in insoluble elastin and 54% increase in insoluble collagen. These results suggest that the drug directly affects the cross-linking of matrix proteins (Boucek et al. 1983, Brophy et al. 1989). Slaiby et al. also used a hypertensive rat model to demonstrate the inhibitory effects of propranolol with regard to AAAs. An AAA was created by perfusing elastase in genetically hypertensive Wistar–Kyoto rats and delivering propranolol subcutaneously for 2 weeks. Two drug doses were used (10 and 30 mg/kg by subcutaneous injection). Control rats received same volume of saline solution. The results yielded a 50% reduction in diameter in normotensive rats and a 25% reduction in hypertensive rats (Slaiby et al. 1994, Ricci et al. 1996). A randomized trial for propranolol on 548 small aneurysm patients was conducted to further examine these promising results; however, there was a thorough failure of propranolol to inhibit AAA development in patients (Propranolol Aneurysm Trial Investigators 2002). Additionally, no significant difference in the rate of arterial expansion and mortality between the groups was found. In fact, the propranolol actually caused side effects and a subsequent discontinuation of medication by several patients because of poor tolerance to the treatment. Dyspnea is one of the reported side effect in human studies that could not be tolerated (Lindholt et al. 1999). In a double-blind study, patients with AAA (diameter between 3.0 and 5.0 cm) received either a placebo ($n = 272$) or propranolol ($n = 276$). The growth rate was equal annually in both groups and there was no difference in death rate (Propranolol Aneurysm Trial Investigators 2002).

6.7 ANTIOXIDANT THERAPY

It is known that local oxidative stress (reactive oxygen species [ROS]) is high in aneurysmal tissue, so reducing this stress appears to have potential therapeutic effects for AAAs. Using a hyperlipidimic Ang II mice model, Gavrila et al. showed for the first time that supplemental vitamin E decreases aortic diameter and decreases elastin degradation. They showed that fatal rupture can be decreased by 44% and macrophage infiltration can be reduced (Gavrila et al. 2005). The benefits of vitamin E cannot be clearly determined from these studies, but it must be noted that the vitamin E dosage given to humans (50 IU/day) was notably less than that given to the rodents (2 IU/g). In a more recent study, failure of antioxidant (vitamin E and vitamin C) therapy was reported for protecting against Ang II-induced aortic rupture in aged apolipoprotein (E)-deficient mice (Jiang et al. 2007).

6.8 ANTI-INFLAMMATORY AGENTS

Inflammation is a major part of AAAs; therefore, anti-inflammatory agents have been investigated to determine their potential effect on AAAs. Nonsteroidal anti-inflammatory drugs (NSAIDs) are common to inhibit cyclooxegenase (COX), which converts to prostaglandin, in turn inducing inflammation and MMP production. A recent study tested 63 control patients and 15 patients taking NSAIDs (treated group) and found a 50% reduction in AAA growth rate for the treated group in comparison to the control (Walton et al. 1999). In another trial with 447 patients taking NSAID orally caused a significant increase in aortic wall stiffness (Claridge et al. 2013).

In a study using elastase-induced AAA rat models, the ability of prednisolone and cyclosporine as inhibitors in AAA progression was shown. Treated rats showed a ~30% reduction in arterial diameter compared to the control groups 9 days after perfusion, and infiltration of cells was significantly reduced in the aortas of treated rats (Dobrin et al. 1996). A few other studies also found that blocking proinflammatory cytokine tumor necrosis factor-α (TNF-α) inhibited AAA progression in elastase rat models (Hingorani et al. 1998, Xiong et al. 2009). Hingorani et al. investigated the effect of TNF-α and IL-1 antagonists on the development of AAA in a rat model. TNF-α binding protein was able to block post elastase dilation, while IL-1RA had no effect on post elastase dilation. Xiong et al. found that both mRNA and protein level of TNF-α were increased in aneurysmal tissue samples. They also tested mice lacking expression of TNF-α and found that they were resistant to AAA formation.

6.9 SYNTHETIC INHIBITORS OF MMPs

MMPs are very important in aneurysm development, in particular MMP-2, -9, and -12, are shown to degrade elastin, and are essential for aneurysm growth (Longo et al. 2002). The use of synthetic MMP inhibitors has been tested to slow AAA growth. Hydroxamate group of inhibitors contain a hydroxamate (-CONHOH) group that chelates the zinc atom in the active site of the MMP enzyme, thus they are called "hydroxamate-based MMP inhibitors" (Brown 1997). The first two MMP inhibitors to be tested in patients were ilomastat (GM6001) and batimastat (BB-94) (Millar et al. 1998).

BB-94 (Batimastat) is a broad-spectrum inhibitor of metalloproteinases. It has been effectively used to prevent AAA in animals by controlling inflammatory responses. In a rat study, treatment with BB-94 (6 days with a daily intraperitoneal injection of 15 mg) showed significantly less aneurysmal dilatation (113% increase in aortic size), as compared with the control rats (157% increase in aortic size) (Bigatel et al. 1999). Another MMP inhibitor, XL784, was administered via gavage in different doses (50–500 mg/kg daily) in elastase-perfused mice model of AAA. Control mice all developed aneurysms while treatment with all doses of XL784 were effective in inhibiting aortic dilatation in a dose-dependent manner (Ennis et al. 2012). In another study, with RS 132908 (100 mg/kg/day subcutaneous injection) a 50% reduction in aneurysmal development was observed in elastase-perfused male Wistar rat model of AAA. Moreover, aortic wall desmosine content in treated group was significantly higher than that in control group (Moore et al. 1999). Because of low bioavailability of previous generation of MMP inhibitors, a second generation of hydroxamate-based MMP inhibitor marimastat was developed. It is active orally but it has musculoskeletal side effects (Bramhall et al. 2001). In a study, saphenous vein samples were obtained from bypass surgery patients. Segments were cultured with and without marimastat for 14 days. Results from histology showed that marimastat reduced neointimal thickening significantly and can be a therapeutic target for intimal hyperplasia (Porter et al. 1998). The second generation of MMP inhibitors has not been investigated as a potential treatment of AAA as of yet.

6.10 INHIBITOR OF c-JUN N TERMINAL KINASE

In the past few years, pharmacological inhibition of c-Jun N terminal kinase (JNK) has shown a promise to slow AAA development. It has been shown that overexpressed phosphorylated JNK in human AAA samples lead to the activation of MMP-9 and proinflammatory signaling in vascular SMC (VSMC). Furthermore, by using a specific inhibitor to selectively inhibit JNK, AAA formation was prevented in $CaCl_2$ and Ang II-induced ApoE$^{-/-}$ mouse models (Miyake and Morishita 2009). Yoshimura et al. (2005) identified JNK as a proximal signaling molecule in the AAA pathogenesis because AAA tissue showed a high level of phosphorylated JNK. The inhibition of JNK did more than just suppression of MMP activation and migration of inflammatory cells; it also regenerated the structure of aortic tissue. This study highlighted the role of the ECM protein synthesis upregulation toward AAA treatment (Miyake and Morishita 2009).

6.11 GENE THERAPY APPROACHES

Gene therapy is an ambitious approach to resist and regress aneurysm formation by transfer of genes directly to the aneurysmal site with the aim of gene incorporation and continued expression by host cells.

Xiong et al. (2008) performed both *in vitro* and *in vivo* trials using recombinant tropoelastin gene with an adenovector tagged with green fluorescent protein (AdTE-GFP) as the transfection vehicle. The expression of recombinant tropoelastin was quantified by mRNA levels in a 5-day-cell culture experiment. The *in vivo* study was performed using an elastase perfused rat model for AAA. Two weeks post AAA induction, rats were transfected with AdTE-GFP or an adeno vector containing no recombinant gene. Aortic diameters of the transfected group showed a significant reduction, better elastin structure, and higher mRNA levels of tropoelastin. Tropoelastin mRNA levels were not as elevated as the *in vitro* study. Also, the expression levels were reduced drastically by the end of 4 weeks. Transient gene expression is one of the drawbacks of adenoviral gene therapy, nevertheless the technology is highly sophisticated and could have a lot of potential in the future for AAA treatment (Xiong et al. 2008).

Yoshimura et al. (2006) studied the effect of gene transfer of *Lox* that is an enzyme crucial for the cross-linking of tropoelastin to form elastin fibers. In a AAA rat model, adenovirus transfer of *Lox* gene was performed in one group while Lac Z was transferred to another group. Reduction in aneurysm formation in the Lox transfected group not only indicated the importance of the enzyme in preserving aortic wall strength but also demonstrated the possibility of using such means to slow down aneurysm progression (Yoshimura et al. 2006). Nakashima et al. experimented the use of decoy oligonucleotides against transcription factors such as NFKβ in rat AAA model. Decreased aortic dilatation, lowered MMP levels, and better elastin preservation were achieved (Nakashima et al. 2004).

Each aforementioned approach was tested as a systemic therapy and targeted cellular products. In most of the animal studies showing positive results, pharmacological inhibition was initiated at the onset of an aneurysm to prevent its formation (Table 6.1), which is not clinically relevant. Patients when diagnosed will have already developed an aneurysm. The therapy to halt and reverse already formed aneurysm is needed.

TABLE 6.1 Pharmacological Inhibition of ECM Degradation in Animal Models of AAA

Author	Year	Animal Model	Treatment Protocol	Results
Slaiby et al.	1994	Hypertensive rats elastase	Propranolol injections were begun on the first postoperative day and continued for 14 days.	Propranolol-treated rats had significantly smaller AAA than placebo-treated controls ($p < .05$).
Petrinec et al.	1996	Normotensive rats elastase	Doxycycline injections were given twice daily from the first postoperative day and aorta were harvested after 0, 2, 7, and 14 days.	Doxycyclcine-treated rats did not have aneurysm while saline controls showed dilation after 7 days (aortic diameter of >3 mm).
Curci et al.	1998	Normotensive rats elastase	Doxycycline injections were begun 8 hours after perfusion on the first postoperative day and continued for 7 days.	Doxycycline-treated rats showed significantly lower aortic dilation when compared to the saline group.
Bigatel et al.	1999	Normotensive rats elastase	Batimastat injections were begun postoperatively and continued daily for 7 days.	Batimastat-treated rats showed significantly lower AAA when compared to the saline group.
Moore et al.	1999	Normotensive rats elastase	RS 132908 injections were started on the first postoperative day and continued for 14 days.	RS 132908-treated rats showed significantly lesser dilation compared to the saline control group.
Liao et al.	2001	Normotensive rats elastase	Drinking water supplemented with captopril (CP), lisinopril (LP), enalapril (EP), or losartan (LOS) was given to the animals beginning on the first postoperative day and continued for 14 days.	All the three ACE inhibitors prevented aortic dilation in treated rats compared to control group.
Johanning et al.	2001	Normotensive rats elastase	Aminoguanidine (200 mg/kg) injections were begun on the morning of first postoperative day and continued for 7 days. One group received the injections 3 days prior to surgery and continued through 7 days postoperatively.	Aminoguanidine administration in elastase-infused aortas significantly reduced aortic dilation compared to the control group.

(Continued)

TABLE 6.1 (*Continued*) Pharmacological Inhibition of ECM Degradation in Animal Models of AAA

Author	Year	Animal Model	Treatment Protocol	Results
Manning et al.	2003	Normotensive mice Apo E⁻/⁻ Ang II	Doxycycline administered daily in the drinking water 1 week before pump implantation and continued throughout.	Doxycycline administration reduced the formation of AAA but showed no effect on atherosclerotic formation.
Nakashima et al.	2004	Normotensive rats elastase	Chimeric decoy oligodeoxynucleotide (ODN) was transfected at the same time as surgery.	Novel strategy with chimeric decoy ODN achieved inhibition of AAA progression.
Steinmetz et al.	2005	Hypercholesterolemic Apo E⁻/⁻ mice elastase	Subcutaenous injections of simvastatin were given per day or vehicle on the first postoperative day perfusion and kept for 14 days.	Simvastatin-treated mice exhibited reduction in AAAs compared with vehicle-treated controls.
Kalyanasundaram et al.	2006	Normotensive rats elastase	Simvastatin was administered by gastric lavage daily starting the day before surgery and continued for 7 days.	Simvastatin significantly suppressed aneurysm expansion compared to placebo group.
Fujiwara et al.	2008	Normotensive rats elastase	Valsartan was administered daily, via osmotic minipumps implanted, from the day of operation and continued for 4 weeks.	Valsartan treatment significantly prevented the progression of AAA.
Tomita et al.	2008	Normotensive rats elastase	Nifedipine was administered via osmotic mini pump from the day of surgery and continued for 4 weeks.	Treatment with nifedipine showed significant inhibition of the progression of AAA at 14 and 28 days compared to the control.
Shang et al.	2012	Normotensive rats elastase	Tan IIA was administered daily by intraperitoneal injection starting 1 day prior to the operation and continued till the end of the study.	Tan IIA treatment inhibitedthe development of AAA compared to control group. Sham rats were also used to prove that the inhibition was successful.

(*Continued*)

TABLE 6.1 (*Continued*) Pharmacological Inhibition of ECM Degradation in Animal Models of AAA

Author	Year	Animal Model	Treatment Protocol	Results
Xiong et al.	2014	Normotensive rats elastase perfusion and extraluminal CaCl$_2$ application	Perindopril was fed orally on a daily basis beginning on the first postoperative day and continued for 28 days.	Perindopril inhibited the aortic degeneration and AAA formation compared to the control group.
Shang et al.	2014	Normotensive rats elastase	Vitamin C was intraperitoneally injected, starting 1 week before surgery and continued throughout the study.	Vitamin C attenuated AAA progression when compared to control groups.

6.12 PHARMACOLOGICAL APPROACHES FOR ELASTIN PRESERVATION IN COPD

COPD is characterized by narrowing of air ways and thus decreasing the capacity of gas exchange in lungs. Emphysema is one of the pathological conditions associated with COPD. Elastic fibers in lung tether the alveolar walls to keep them open. Emphysema progresses by the action of elastases that fragment the elastin fibers. Loss of this elastin network causes alveoli to enlarge and decrease gas exchange capacity. Physiologically, the lungs will lose their elastic recoil in COPD which cannot be reversed fully.

6.12.1 Elastin Damage in COPD

Emphysema refers to air way disease in which inflammation-mediated elastin damage occurs over a long period of time. Smoking has been identified as a major contributor of COPD while alpha-1 antitrypsin deficiency (AATD) and exposure to particulate matter also contribute toward the disease (Fletcher and Peto 1977, Mahadeva and Lomas 1998, Hnizdo et al. 2003, 2004, Laurell and Eriksson 2013). Currently, widely accepted hypothesis about emphysema is that chronic exposure to cigarette smoke and particulate matter causes irritation in the alveoli and this triggers an inflammatory response. This response attracts many types of inflammatory cells such as macrophages, neutrophils, and lymphocytes. Cytokines, ROS, prostaglandins, leukotrienes, proteases, and so on mediate the progression of the disease. This leads to a protease/antiprotease imbalance in the lungs that causes the breakdown of elastin (Wright and Churg 2007). The pathology of emphysema consists of phenotypic change in fibroblasts (Zhang et al. 2012). In the first step, the degradation products of elastin fibers act as chemoattractants (Houghton et al. 2006). Subsequently, the inflammatory response shifts to chronic phase, alveoli tend to enlarge, and small air ways constrict allowing less air to escape during exhalation. Finally, the irreparable loss of elastin network leaves macroscopically visible holes in the lungs (Cotran et al. 1999) (Figure 6.1). MMPs have been attributed a central role in the degradation of elastin fibers in addition to the neutrophil elastase (Churg et al. 2012).

The elastin loss associated with COPD is irreversible. The reason being that elastic fiber assembly requires the production and interplay of multitudes of the molecules (fibrillin and fibulin microfibrils, LOX, microfibril-associated glycoproteins, and latent TGF-β binding protein) in temporal sequence. The adult cells are unable to reactivate the many required genes in

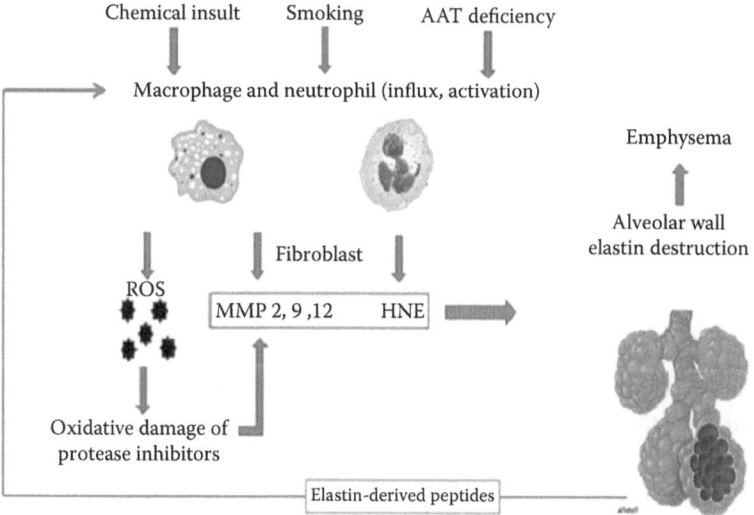

FIGURE 6.1   Schematic diagram showing the pathological mechanisms of elastin degradation in emphysema.

the appropriate ratios and in the sequence required (Shifren and Mecham 2006). The loss of elastin in the alveolar walls results in decreased surface area for gas exchange. Unfortunately, there is no pharmacological treatment available that can specifically prevent the elastin from degradation and regenerate lost elastin. All of the available treatments for COPD have been directed majorly toward providing short-term relief for breathing and halting the active inflammation in the lungs. Decreasing the inflammation does not necessarily restore the lung capacity that has been lost in terms of elastic recoil but it may serve the purpose of indirectly halting further elastin degradation and therefore the progression of COPD.

6.12.2 Anti-Inflammatory Drugs

Because corticosteroids have proven to be ineffective in reducing inflammation in COPD, new drugs like phosphodiesterase 4 (PDE) inhibitors, TNF-α inhibitors, NF-kB inhibitors, p38 mitogen-activated protein kinase (MAPK) inhibitors, adhesion molecule inhibitors, PI-3 K inhibitors, anti-inflammatory cytokines, leukotriene B4 inhibitors, and chemokine inhibitors are being evaluated for their respective anti-inflammatory efficacies. Many reviews have presented these pharmacologic approaches in a detailed fashion (Barnes 2003, 2004, Molfino and Jeffery 2007,

TABLE 6.2   Examples of Anti-Inflammatory Class of Drugs Used in Emphysema

Drug Class	Examples
Bronchodilator/PDE inhibitors	Theophylline (Zhou et al. 2006, Ford et al. 2010)
PDE4 inhibitors	Cilomilast, Roflumilast, Tetomilast (Compton et al. 2001, Gamble et al. 2003, Grootendorst et al. 2007)
MAPK inhibitors	SD-282 (Smith et al. 2006)
PI3K γ/δ inhibitors	Small molecule inhibitors of PI3Kγ/δ (Ameriks and Venable 2009)
Macrolide antibiotics	Azithromycin (Friedlander and Albert 2010, Sugawara et al. 2011)

Dunsmore 2008, Barnes 2013). Few of them are presented in Table 6.2. Recently, inhalable powder of a flower *Lonicera japonica* has also exhibited some interesting results from the anti-inflammatory view of disease (Park et al. 2014).

6.12.3 MMP Inhibitors

Another approach that is closer to the aim of preserving elastin is to inhibit MMPs that are involved in degrading elastin protein and shown to play a vital role in COPD as discovered recently (Churg et al. 2012). In a guinea pig study involving cigarette smoke exposure, an MMP9/12 inhibitor AZ11557272 has ameliorated the emphysema conditions (Churg et al. 2007). In a mouse study, an MMP inhibitor ilomastat reduced macrophage levels and air space enlargement (~96% of reduction) (Pemberton et al. 2005). In another study using a broad spectrum MMP inhibitor CP-471,474 delayed the emphysema induced by cigarette smoke in guinea pigs (Selman et al. 2003). Vandenbroucke et al. (2011) discussed other MMP inhibitors that are being evaluated for various lung diseases. But none of the documented research either evaluated elastin loss with such treatments or aim to target elastin specific therapy to improve the mechanical function of the lung.

6.12.4 Elastase Inhibitors

Another class of drugs that are being used in research are elastase inhibitors. Inhibiting human neutrophil elastase (HNE) can be a direct treatment to prevent further deterioration of mechanical function of lungs. Several elastase inhibitors have been developed and tested as a possible therapeutic treatment for emphysema in animal models (Kleinerman et al. 1980, Lungarella et al. 1986, Williams et al. 1991, Herbert et al. 1992). A study with succinyl-alanyl-alanyl-prolyl-valine-chloromethyl ketone

(CMK) in hamsters showed CMK protection against emphysema when instilled 1 hour before HNE instillation (Lucey et al. 1989). Pretreatment of hamsters with FR901277, an elastase inhibitor, has been reported to significantly reduce the pulmonary emphysema caused by instillation of porcine pancreatic elastase intratracheally. It also protected elastin from damage due to HNE in paw edema in mice (Fujie et al. 1999). ZD0892, a synthetic serine elastase inhibitor, showed reduction in inflammation levels and desmosine levels were also returned to control values (Wright et al. 2002). So far sivelestat sodium hydrate (ONO-5046) is the only HNE inhibitor that is in use, but its use is highly limited owing to its organ toxicity and irreversible inhibition of HNE (Kuraki et al. 2002, Ohbayashi 2002, Stevens et al. 2011, Lucas et al. 2013). In this perspective, a potential neutrophil elastase inhibitor can definitely have a key role in preserving elastin in lungs.

6.12.5 Alpha-1 Antitrypsin Delivery

AATD is a minor cause of emphysema. Its main role is to maintain a balance between protease and antiprotease activity by inhibiting the proteolytic enzymes such as neutrophil elastase (Janoff 1972, Gadek et al. 1981, American Thoracic Society/European Respiratory Society 2003, Schluchter et al. 1998). In the absence of this protein, elastase activity increases and causes elastin breakdown in lungs. For people with AATD, delivery of this protein has been investigated as a possible option to ameliorate the lung physiological function. Purified alpha-1 antitrypsin (AAT) can come from sources such as plasma derived from healthy individuals and recombinant protein (Sandhaus 2004). Prolastin is a pioneer product of purified AAT from serum of healthy individuals (Sandhaus 1993). Early trials conducted in the late 1990s have all reported that patients who received Prolastin had lower mortality and reduced decline in lung function (Seersholm et al. 1997, Wencker et al. 1998). With the recent advances in gene delivery, it has been made possible to deliver AAT using this method using various vectors (Mueller and Flotte 2013). Murine model of cigarette smoke-induced emphysema has shown improvement with the usage of inhaled recombinant AAT. When treated for 6 months, the animals showed a 73% reduction in air space enlargement and also had lower neutrophil levels in the broncheoalveolar lavage fluid (Pemberton et al. 2006). Delivery of AAT may be considered as a useful treatment for preserving elastin by inhibiting neutrophil elastase activity in patients with emphysema.

6.13 PHARMACOLOGICAL APPROACHES FOR ELASTIN PRESERVATION IN SKIN

Aging of the skin occurs as a result of the breakdown of the ECM components, collagen and elastin. As we age, elastin and collagen in the skin are degraded by enzymes such as MMPs and photo- and oxidative damage. Several genetic disorders are also related to the breakdown of ECM proteins. Skin loses the ability to produce new elastin fibers as we age, leading to loss of elasticity and subsequent aging of the skin. Treatments exist in the market to preserve mostly collagen. However, regeneration of all ECM proteins is essential for reversing the aging of the skin. Several approaches have been tested to preserve and regenerate ECM proteins in skin but very few target elastin repair.

6.13.1 ACE Inhibitors

The ACE inhibitors reduce scarring of the skin by reducing inflammation that occurs as a result of injury to the skin. ACE inhibitors have been shown to inhibit cyclooxygenase-2 (COX-2) inhibitors and fibrogenesis, thereby reducing inflammation. This has been shown to result in scar reduction (Kim et al. 2012). ACE inhibitors may also be effective in reducing aging of skin. A study showed that photoaging of the skin of hairless mice by exposure to UV-B irradiation resulted in the increased expression of ACE and Ang II receptors, resulting in excessive skin scarring and aging. Treatment with ACE inhibitors improved skin wrinkles (Matsuura-Hachiya et al. 2013). It has also been shown that enalapril, an ACE inhibitor, results in increased collagen biosynthesis in human skin fibroblasts (Szoka et al. 2015).

6.13.2 Tetracyclines

Skin and soft tissue infections (SSTIs) occur due to the invasion of skin and soft tissues by microbial agents. Antibiotics, such as doxycycline, are used to treat SSTIs (Ki and Rotstein 2008). Doxycycline is used for methicillin-resistant staphylococcus aureus infections on the skin (Bhambri and Kim 2009). Doxycycline has been shown to inhibit MMPs (Castro et al. 2011). Thus, doxycycline may be effective for inhibiting MMPs in the skin to prevent aging; however, the safety and efficacy of this treatment on the skin have not been explored.

6.13.3 Antioxidants

Antioxidants are substances that prevent the oxidation of other molecules. Antioxidants work to combat free radicals, which are formed as a result of oxygen use in the body. Free radicals have an unpaired valence electron; thus, free radicals are highly chemically reactive. Free radicals attempt to form an octet by gaining an electron from proteins in the skin. This leads to damage to the structure of the skin and alters the DNA, leading to aging. Free radicals lead to the activation of MMPs (Gu et al. 2011). It has been shown that ultraviolet (UV) exposure leads to free radical formation in the skin (Jurkiewicz and Buettner 1994). Aging is caused by the slow cumulative oxidation of ECM proteins in the skin over a lifetime according to the free radical theory of aging (Biesalski 2002). Thus, antioxidants can protect ECM proteins in the skin from oxidation and prevent ECM damage caused by MMPs.

Polyphenols such as epigallocatechin-3-gallate (EGCG) and reservatol are chemicals characterized by the presence of large number of phenol groups, which contribute to the unique properties of these compounds. EGCG is the most abundant polyphenol found in tea. The treatment with EGCG hinders collagen destruction in human dermal fibroblasts that have been damaged by UV-B irradiation by inhibiting activation of collagenases, MMP-1, MMP-8, and MMP-13 (Bae et al. 2008). The anti-aging effect of EGCG was examined in male Fischer 344 rats through dietary administration, and it was found that high dose EGCG (500 mg/kg/day over 6 months) provided protection against oxidative stress (Meng et al. 2008). In a separate study, administration of EGCG through diet to male rats was found to significantly decrease the levels of ROS, a free radical, and malondialdehyde, a marker for oxidative stress (Niu et al. 2013). EGCG has also been shown to inhibit MMP-1 expression in heat-shocked human dermal fibroblasts; thus, EGCG may be an effective treatment for thermal skin aging (Kim et al. 2013). Extracts of pomace from Riesling grapes containing polyphenols were analyzed for inhibition of collagenase and elastase activity. It was found that the extract showed dose-dependent inhibition against collagenase with an IC50 value of 20.3 μg/mL and elastase with an IC50 value of 14.7 μg/mL. Thus, EGCG functions as an antioxidant to prevent free radicals from activating MMPs, which subsequently degrade ECM proteins in the skin, leading to loss of structure. Reservatol, a polyphenol, has also been shown to reduce ROS in UV-B exposed keratinocytes (Park and Lee 2008).

Tocopherols, or vitamin E, are composed of a hydrophobic side chain and a chromanol ring and possess antioxidant properties due to the hydroxyl group on the chromanol ring, which reduces free radicals by donating a hydrogen atom (Masaki 2010). In a study, 12-O-tetradecanoylphorbol-13-acetate was used to induce oxidative stress in skin. Tocopherol was applied 30 minutes prior to treatment with 12-O-tetradecanoylphorbol-13-acetate, and it was found to inhibit xanthine oxidase activity, myeloperoxidase activity, the induction of H_2O_2, and lipid peroxidation, which are all signs of oxidative stress (Rahman et al. 2008). α-Tocopherol has been studied with aging fibroblasts, and it was shown to downregulate MMP-1 through AP-1 DNA binding (Ricciarelli et al. 1999).

Ascorbic acid, a form of vitamin, has antioxidant properties and has studied for use on the skin to prevent aging. ROS are eliminated by ascorbic acid due to the oxidation of ascorbate to form a radical cation, which is subsequently oxidized to form dehydroascorbate (Masaki 2010). Dehydroascorbate reacts with the oxidants of ROS. Additionally, prolyl hydroxylase, an enzyme in the skin which hydroxylates prolyl residues in elastin and procollagen, requires ascorbic acid as a cofactor; this process is necessary for efficient collagen production (Myllylä et al. 1984, Davidson et al. 1997). However, ascorbic acid has poor skin penetration; thus, several derivatives have been analyzed, such as 2-O-α-glucoside, 6-acylated ascorbic acid 2-O-α-glucoside, and tetra-isopalmitoyl ascorbic acid (Masaki 2010).

Conenzyme Q10 (CoQ10) is an intracellular antioxidant that has been shown to reduce DNA damage caused by UV irradiation. CoQ10 has been shown to inhibit MMP-1 production in human dermal fibroblasts. This is due to the downregulation of IL-6 expression in keratinocytes after UV-B exposure (Inui et al. 2008). CoQ10 has also been shown to accelerate the production of basement membrane components in keratinocytes and fibroblasts, such as type IV and VII collagens, indicating possible anti-aging effects (Muta-Takada et al. 2009).

Ergothioneine is a natural amino acid containing sulfur that appears to act as an antioxidant. Ergothioneine suppressed the expression on MMP-1 in UV-A irradiated fibroblasts (Obayashi et al. 2005).

6.13.4 Retinoic Acid

Retinoic acid, a metabolite of vitamin A, is frequently used as a topical treatment for skin. Retinoids are a class of compounds that are forms of vitamin A. There are the three generations of retinoids. The first generation of retinoids includes retinol, retinal, isotretinoin, treinoin, and alitretinoin. The second generation of retinoids includes etretinate and acitretin. The third generation of retinoids includes tazaroten, bexarotene, and adapalene.

Retinol has been shown to increase dermal collagen production and elastin fiber formation in human dermal fibroblasts *in vitro* (Rossetti et al. 2011). It has been shown that retinoid derivatives, retinol and retinoic acid, cause a two fold increase in the concentration of elastin in chick embryonic skin fibroblasts after 24 hours of treatment (Tajima et al. 1997). Tropoelastin, the monomer of elastin, mRNA expression was found to be upregulated in human skin after treatment with topical retinoic acid (Chen et al. 2009). The application of trans-retinoic acid prior to UV-B irradiation of human skin substantially reduced MMP induction (Fisher et al. 1996). Thus, retinoic acid may be applied to preserve collagen and elastin in the skin.

6.14 STRATEGIES TO REGENERATE LOST ELASTIN IN TISSUES

All the aforementioned treatments for vascular, lung, and skin have shown to either stop inflammation or inhibit enzymes that degrade elastin. To date, there is no actual treatment to regenerate lost elastin. Ours is the one of the few groups that has been working specifically on elastin preservation and regeneration. We focused on three different polyphenols for comparing and investigating their interactions with elastin. The structures of pentagalloyl glucose (PGG), (–)-epigallocatechin-3-O-gallate, and (+)-catechin are shown in Figure 6.2.

PGG is a polyphenol, derivative of tannic acid found in green tea and wine. We have found that PGG can stabilize elastin and protect elastin fiber from further damage. It binds to elastin by hydrophobic interactions and makes it resistant to degradation by elastases (Isenburg et al. 2006). We have shown that periadventitial administration of PGG inhibits the development and further progression of already developed AAA in a calcium chloride injury rat model (Isenburg et al. 2007). Polyphenols not only protect elastin from degradation but also increase insoluble elastin production in healthy and aneurysmal VSMCs *in vitro* as shown recently by us. Polyphenols including PGG, EGCG, and catechin were shown to increase coacervation of tropoelastin and LOX activity and thus increase insoluble cross-linked elastin deposition (Figure 6.3). Additionally, polyphenol treatments also decreased cellular MMP-2 activity as detected by zymography (Sinha et al. 2014a).

We also tested if polyphenols can increase elastin production by pulmonary fibroblasts as a treatment for emphysema. We treated rat pulmonary fibroblasts with TNF-α to mimic the inflammatory conditions of emphysema and then treated cells with PGG to investigate elastin deposition by

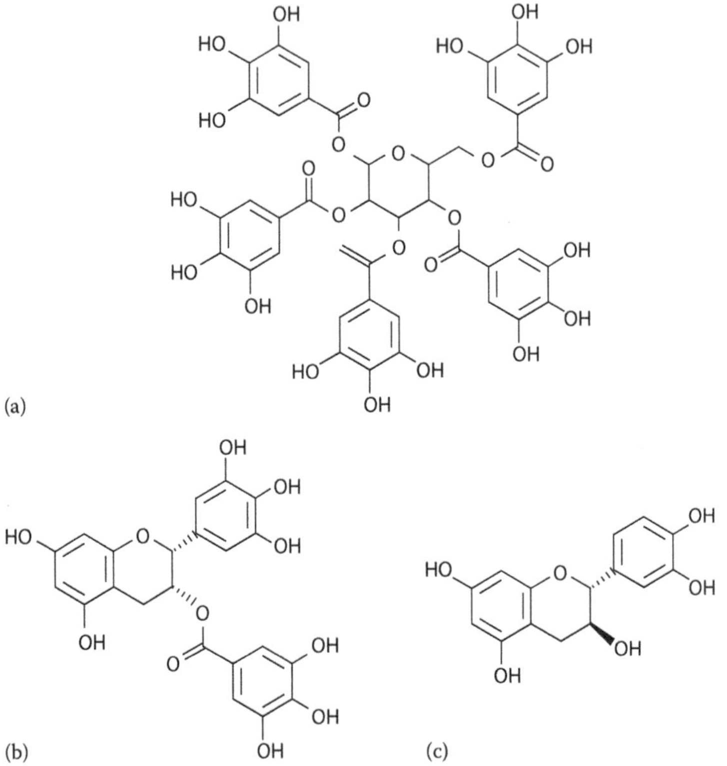

FIGURE 6.2   Structure of (a) PGG, (b) EGCG, and (c) catechin. (From Sinha, A., *Vascular nanomedicine: Site specific delivery of elastin stabilizing therapeutics to damaged arteries*, PhD, Bioengineering, Clemson University, Clemson, SC, 2013, with permission.)

fibroblasts. PGG was effective in reducing the MMP-2 and MMP-9 activity in the spent medium of cell cultures and showed a significant increase in deposited elastin (Parasaram et al. 2014).

As we discovered that polyphenols can increase elastin deposition, we wanted to deliver these polyphenols to the sites of elastin degradation. In a healthy elastic fiber, amorphous elastin is surrounded by microfibrillar proteins. Lack of microfibrils covering elastin is one of the characteristics of degrading elastin (Figure 6.4). Taking advantage of this characteristic of damaged elastin, we have developed a novel targeting strategy of coating the NPs with anti-elastin antibody that recognizes exposed amorphous core elastin.

This elastin antibody-coated NPs have been demonstrated to target only degraded elastin while sparing healthy elastin (Figure 6.5). We have

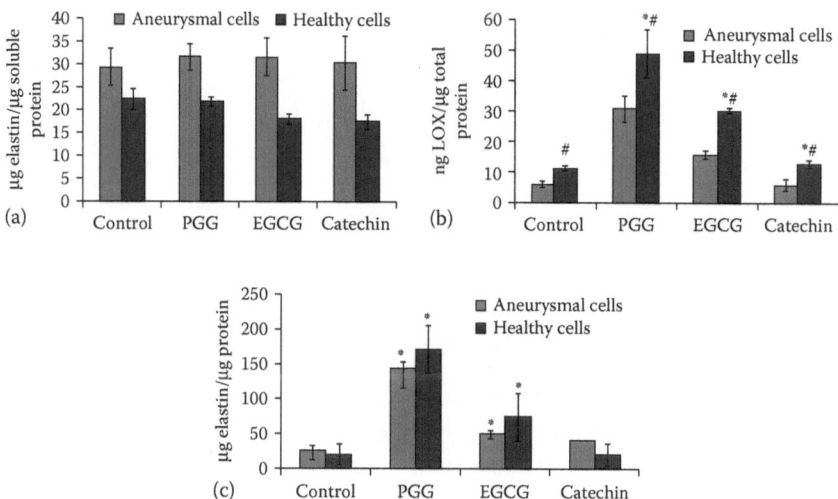

FIGURE 6.3 (a) Tropoelastin, (b) LOX, and (c) insoluble elastin production in PGG, EGCG, and catechin treated cell. (Reprinted with permission from Sinha, A. et al., *Biochem. Biophys. Res. Commun.*, 444, 205, 2014a.)

shown precise targeting of NPs to degraded vascular elastic lamina when NPs were delivered systemically in three different animal models of vascular disease (Sinha et al. 2014b). These NPs have been used to deliver batimastat (BB-94), a synthetic MMP inhibitor to successfully inhibit local MMP activity in AAA site $CaCl_2$ rat model (Nosoudi 2014). It significantly inhibited aneurysm expansion in a 4-week study at a very low dose (a 580-fold lower BB-94 concentration than others used systemically) (Bigatel et al. 1999).

We are currently working on delivery of PGG to the site of AAA by using targeted NPs as a treatment option to prevent further disease progression and regenerate lost elastin. Toward this aim, we are optimizing NPs loaded with PGG in terms of loading, release, particle size, and other characteristics.

Ramamurthi et al. have also been working on alternate treatments for regenerating elastin. They showed that combination of transforming growth factor beta 1 (TGF-β1) and HA oligomers improves elastin regeneration in VSMCs. This combination enhances the synthesis of tropoelastin by 8-fold and matrix elastin protein by 5.5-fold (Kothapalli et al. 2009b). Subsequently, they examined whether these cues likewise enhance elastin matrix synthesis and assembly by TNF-α-stimulated SMCs;

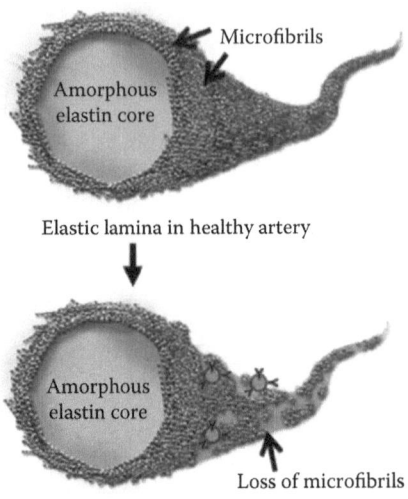

FIGURE 6.4 Elastic lamina fibers schematic. In healthy elastic lamina, core amorphous elastin is coated on the surface with microfibrills such as fibrillins and fibulins. In the diseased state, the microfibrillar proteins degrade along with amorphous elastin, thus exposing core elastin. NPs coated with antibodies that are specific to core elastin are used to target degraded elastic lamina in diseased artery while sparing healthy vessel with native elastic lamina. (Reprinted with permission from Sinha, A. et al., *Nanomedicine,* 10, 1003, 2014b.)

TNF-α-activated SMCs simulate the events within vascular aneurysms *in vivo.* Inflammation caused by these cells was ameliorated by the addition of TGF-β1 and HA oligomer cues, also resulting in enhanced tropoelastin and collagen production, improved yield of matrix elastin, and crosslinking (Kothapalli and Ramamurthi 2010). Rat aneurysmal SMCs isolated from CaCl₂ injury induced/elastase perfused AAA segments showed significantly higher amounts of collagen/elastin protein synthesis and crosslinking when supplemented with TGF-β1 and HA cues. Therefore, it was suggested that TGF-β1 and HA oligomers are potentially useful in suppressing SMC activation by TNF-α and inducing regenerative elastin repair within aneurysms (Kothapalli et al. 2009a, Gacchina et al. 2011).

In a three-dimensional (3D) cell culture study, Venkataraman et al. have shown that TGF-β1 and HA synergistically enhance elastic matrix deposition by adult rat aortic SMCs (RASMCs) seeded within nonelastogenic, statically loaded 3D gels (Venkataraman and Ramamurthi 2011). To test the delivery and efficacy of these cues in a local environment, NPs

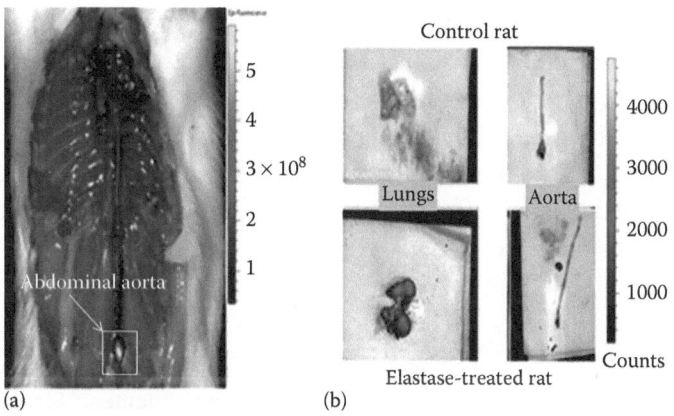

FIGURE 6.5 Anti-elastin antibody-coated NPs targeting damaged elastin in aorta (a) and lungs (b). (a) Male SD rats abdominal aorta distal to kidneys were injured locally by periadventitial application of calcium chloride (area marked with a square) and were allowed to develop aneurysm over a period of 10 days. (b) Male SD rats were instilled intratracheally with porcine pancreatic elastase and were allowed to develop elastin damage over a period of 4 weeks. Targeting was observed using DiR-loaded NPs coated with anti-elastin antibody to target damaged elastin in both cases. Fluorescence signal could be seen in (a) only at the site of elastin damage and in (b) in elastase-treated rat lungs while the healthy elastin in aorta has been spared by the NPs.

were developed for localized, controlled, and sustained delivery of DOX and TGF-β1 to human aortic SMCs within 3D gels; these gels resemble arterial tissue microenvironment. DOX and TGF-β1 released from these NPs influenced elastogenic outcomes positively over 21 days of culture, which were comparable to that induced by exogenous supplementation of DOX and TGF-β1 at a much lower dosage (Venkataraman et al. 2014). Further, Ramamurthi et al. have developed NPs for targeted, controlled, and sustained delivery of HA-o toward the elastogenic induction of aneurysmal RASMCs, resulting in dose-dependent increases in elastic matrix synthesis, recruitment and activity of LOX (Sylvester et al. 2013). They successfully developed an NP-based system for controlled and sustained delivery of the two elastogenic cues *in vitro*.

We would like to summarize this chapter by noting the importance of elastin network in some of the very important organs of our body and stress the requirement for preserving the same. The increasing need for stabilizing elastin in AAA comes from the observation that the ruptures are fatal and that there is no treatment for small AAA. Even in COPD, we believe that restoration of lung recoil by regenerating elastin in the lungs will be more helpful for patients than just using short-term relief treatments. New cosmetic treatments coming up every day remind us of the importance of regenerating elastin and other ECM molecules of skin. We believe that with the increased awareness and ongoing research on elastin and its preservation strategies will point us toward a new direction in treating human diseases and make us live a better life.

REFERENCES

American Thoracic Society/European Respiratory Society. 2003. American Thoracic Society/European Respiratory Society statement: Standards for the diagnosis and management of individuals with alpha-1 antitrypsin deficiency. *Am J Respir Crit Care Med* 168(7): 818–900.

Ameriks, M. K. and J. D. Venable. 2009. Small molecule inhibitors of phosphoinositide 3-kinase (PI3K) delta and gamma. *Curr Top Med Chem* 9(8): 738–753.

Bae, J.-Y., Jung-Suk, C., Yean-Jung, C., Seung-Yong, S., Sang-Wook, K., Seoung, J. H., and Young-Hee, K. 2008. Epigallocatechin gallate hampers collagen destruction and collagenase activation in ultraviolet-B-irradiated human dermal fibroblasts: Involvement of mitogen-activated protein kinase. *Food Chem Toxicol* 46(4): 1298–1307.

Baldwin, A. K., A. Simpson, R. Steer, S. A. Cain, and C. M. Kielty. 2013. Elastic fibres in health and disease. *Expert Rev Mol Med* 15: e8.

Barnes, P. J. 2003. Chronic obstructive pulmonary disease * 12: New treatments for COPD. *Thorax* 58(9): 803–808.

Barnes, P. J. 2004. COPD: Is there light at the end of the tunnel? *Curr Opin Pharmacol* 4(3): 263–272.

Barnes, P. J. 2013. Anti-Inflammatory therapeutics in COPD: Past, present, and future. In *Smoking and Lung Inflammation*, edited by Thomas J. Rogers, Gerard J. Criner and William D. Cornwell, pp. 191–213. Springer, New York.

Baxter, B. T., W. H. Pearce, E. A. Waltke, F. N. Littooy, J. W. Hallett, Jr., K. C. Kent, G. R. Upchurch, Jr. et al. 2002. Prolonged administration of doxycycline in patients with small asymptomatic abdominal aortic aneurysms: Report of a prospective (Phase II) multicenter study. *J Vasc Surg* 36(1): 1–12.

Bhambri, S. and G. Kim. 2009. Use of oral doxycycline for community-acquired methicillin-resistant staphylococcus aureus (CA-MRSA) infections. *J Clin Aesthet Dermatol* 2(4): 45–50.

Biesalski, H. K. 2002. Free radical theory of aging. *Curr Opin Clin Nutr Metab Care* 5(1): 5–10.

Bigatel, D. A., J. R. Elmore, D. J. Carey, G. Cizmeci-Smith, D. P. Franklin, and J. R. Youkey. 1999. The matrix metalloproteinase inhibitor BB-94 limits expansion of experimental abdominal aortic aneurysms. *J Vasc Surg* 29 (1): 130–138.

Boucek, R. J., Z. Gunja-Smith, N. L. Noble, and C. F. Simpson. 1983. Modulation by propranolol of the lysyl cross-links in aortic elastin and collagen of the aneurysm-prone Turkey. *Biochem Pharmacol* 32(2): 275–280.

Bramhall, S. R., A. Rosemurgy, P. D. Brown, C. Bowry, J. A. C. Buckels, and Marimastat Pancreatic Cancer Study Group. 2001. Marimastat as first-line therapy for patients with unresectable pancreatic cancer: A randomized trial. *J Clin Oncol* 19(15): 3447–3455.

Brophy, C. M., J. E. Tilson, and M. D. Tilson. 1989. Propranolol stimulates the crosslinking of matrix components in skin from the aneurysm-prone Blotchy mouse. *J Surg Res* 46(4): 330–332.

Brown, P. D. 1997. Matrix metalloproteinase inhibitors in the treatment of cancer. *Med Oncol* 14(1): 1–10.

Burke, J. M. and R. Ross. 1979. Synthesis of connective tissue macromolecules by smooth muscle. *Int Rev Connect Tissue Res* 8: 119–157.

Cantor, J. O., S. Keller, M. S. Parshley, T. V. Darnule, A. T. Darnule, J. M. Cerreta, G. M. Turino, and I. Mandl. 1980. Synthesis of crosslinked elastin by an endothelial cell culture. *Biochem Biophys Res Commun* 95(4): 1381–1386.

Cassis, L. A., M. Gupte, S. Thayer, X. Zhang, R. Charnigo, D. A. Howatt, D. L. Rateri, and A. Daugherty. 2009. ANG II infusion promotes abdominal aortic aneurysms independent of increased blood pressure in hypercholesterolemic mice. *Am J Physiol Heart Circ Physiol* 296(5): H1660–H1665.

Castro, M. M., A. D. Kandasamy, N. Youssef, R. Schulz, and Tetracyclines Clinical Applications of Non-Antibacterial. 2011. Matrix metalloproteinase inhibitor properties of tetracyclines: Therapeutic potential in cardiovascular diseases. *Pharmacol Res* 64(6): 551–560.

Castro-Chaves, P. and A. F Leite-Moreira. 2004. Renin-angiotensin system and its role in cardiovascular physiopathology and therapy. *Rev Port Cardiol* 23: II61–II77.

Chen, Z., M. H. Shin, Y. J. Moon, S. R. Lee, Y. K. Kim, J. E. Seo, J. E. Kim, K. H. Kim, and J. H. Chung. 2009. Modulation of elastin exon 26A mRNA and protein expression in human skin in vivo. *Exp Dermatol* 18(4): 378–386.

Churg, A., R. Wang, X. Wang, P. O. Onnervik, K. Thim, and J. L. Wright. 2007. Effect of an MMP-9/MMP-12 inhibitor on smoke-induced emphysema and airway remodelling in guinea pigs. *Thorax* 62(8): 706–713.

Churg, A., S. Zhou, and J. L. Wright. 2012. Series "Matrix Metalloproteinases in lung health and disease" Matrix Metalloproteinases in Copd. *Eur Respir J* 39(1): 197–209.

Claridge, M., S. Hobbs, C. Quick, N. Day, A. Bradbury, and T. Wilmink. 2013. Nonsteroidal antiinflammatory drugs are associated with increased aortic stiffness. *Int J Nanomedicine* 8: 4361–4369.

Cleary, E. G., L. B. Sandberg, and D. S. Jackson. 1967. The changes in chemical composition during development of the bovine nuchal ligament. *J Cell Biol* 33(3): 469–479.

Compton, C. H., J. Gubb, R. Nieman, J. Edelson, O. Amit, A. Bakst, J. G. Ayres, J. P. Creemers, G. Schultze-Werninghaus, C. Brambilla, N. C. Barnes, and Group International Study. 2001. Cilomilast, a selective phosphodiesterase-4 inhibitor for treatment of patients with chronic obstructive pulmonary disease: A randomised, dose-ranging study. *Lancet* 358(9278): 265–270.

Cotran, R. S., V. Kumar, T. Collins, and S. L. Robbins. 1999. *Robbins Pathologic Basis of Disease*. Philadelphia, PA: Saunders.

Crisan, D. and J. Carr. 2000. Angiotensin I-converting enzyme: Genotype and disease associations. *J Mol Diagn* 2(3): 105–115.

Curci, J. A., D. Mao, D. G. Bohner, B. T. Allen, B. G. Rubin, J. M. Reilly, G. A. Sicard, and R. W. Thompson. 2000. Preoperative treatment with doxycycline reduces aortic wall expression and activation of matrix metalloproteinases in patients with abdominal aortic aneurysms. *J Vasc Surg* 31(2): 325–342.

Curci, J. A., D. Petrinec, S. Liao, L. M. Golub, and R. W Thompson. 1998. Pharmacologic suppression of experimental abdominal aortic aneurysms: A comparison of doxycycline and four chemically modified tetracyclines. *J Vasc Surg* 28(6): 1082–1093.

Davidson, J. M., P. A. LuValle, O. Zoia, D. Quaglino, Jr., and M. Giro. 1997. Ascorbate differentially regulates elastin and collagen biosynthesis in vascular smooth muscle cells and skin fibroblasts by pretranslational mechanisms. *J Biol Chem* 272(1): 345–352.

Davis, E. C. and R. P Mecham. 1993. Elastic fiber organization. In *Tissue Engineering*, edited by Eugene Bell, pp. 26–34. Boston, MA: Birkhäuser.

Dobrin, P. B., N. Baumgartner, S. Anidjar, G. Chejfec, and R. Mrkvicka. 1996. Inflammatory aspects of experimental aneurysms. *Ann N Y Acad Sci* 800(1): 74–88.

Ducajú, G. M., A. L. Farré, J. Modrego, and J. Serrano. 2011. *Actual Pharmacological Treatment to Reduce Growth of Small Abdominal Aneurysm*: Rijeka, Croatia: INTECH Open Access Publisher.

Dunsmore, S. E. 2008. Treatment of COPD: A matrix perspective. *Int J Chron Obstruct Pulmon Dis* 3(1): 113–122.

Ennis, T., J. Jin, S. Bartlett, B. Arif, K. Grapperhaus, and J. A Curci. 2012. Effect of novel limited-spectrum MMP inhibitor XL784 in abdominal aortic aneurysms. *J Cardiovasc Pharmacol Ther* 17(4): 417–426.

Evans, J., J. T. Powell, E. Schwalbe, I. M. Loftus, and M. M. Thompson. 2007. Simvastatin Attenuates the Activity of Matrix Metalloprotease-9 in Aneurysmal Aortic Tissue. *Eur J Vasc Endovasc Surg* 34(3): 302–303.

Ferrario, C. M. 2006. Role of angiotensin II in cardiovascular disease therapeutic implications of more than a century of research. *J Renin Angiotensin Aldosterone Syst* 7(1): 3–14.

Fisher, G. J., S. C. Datta, H. S. Talwar, Z. Q. Wang, J. Varani, S. Kang, and J. J. Voorhees. 1996. Molecular basis of sun-induced premature skin ageing and retinoid antagonism. *Nature* 379(6563): 335–330.

Fletcher, C. and R. Peto. 1977. The natural history of chronic airflow obstruction. *Br Med J* 1(6077): 1645–1648.

Ford, P. A., A. L. Durham, R. E. Russell, F. Gordon, I. M. Adcock, and P. J. Barnes. 2010. Treatment effects of low-dose theophylline combined with an inhaled corticosteroid in COPD. *Chest* 137(6): 1338–1344.

Friedlander, A. L. and R. K. Albert. 2010. Chronic macrolide therapy in inflammatory airways diseases. *Chest* 138(5): 1202–1212.

Frishman, W. H. 2003. Beta-adrenergic blockers. *Circulation* 107(18): e117–e119.

Fujie, K., Y. Shinguh, A. Yamazaki, H. Hatanaka, M. Okamoto, and M. Okuhara. 1999. Inhibition of elastase-induced acute inflammation and pulmonary emphysema in hamsters by a novel neutrophil elastase inhibitor FR901277. *Inflamm Res* 48(3): 160–167.

Fujiwara, Y., S. Shiraya, T. Miyake, S. Yamakawa, M. Aoki, H. Makino, M. Nishimura, and R. Morishita. 2008. Inhibition of experimental abdominal aortic aneurysm in a rat model by the angiotensin receptor blocker valsartan. *Int J Mol Med* 22(6): 703–708.

Gacchina, C. E., P. Deb, J. L. Barth, and A. Ramamurthi. 2011. Elastogenic inductability of smooth muscle cells from a rat model of late stage abdominal aortic aneurysms. *Tissue Eng Part A* 17(13–14): 1699–1711.

Gadek, J. E., G. A. Fells, R. L. Zimmerman, S. I. Rennard, and R. G. Crystal. 1981. Antielastases of the human alveolar structures. Implications for the protease-antiprotease theory of emphysema. *J Clin Invest* 68(4): 889–898.

Gamble, E., D. C. Grootendorst, C. E. Brightling, S. Troy, Y. Qiu, J. Zhu, D. Parker et al. 2003. Antiinflammatory effects of the phosphodiesterase-4 inhibitor cilomilast (Ariflo) in chronic obstructive pulmonary disease. *Am J Respir Crit Care Med* 168(8): 976–982.

Gavrila, D., W. G. Li, M. L. McCormick, M. Thomas, A. Daugherty, L. A. Cassis, F. J. Miller, L. W. Oberley, K. C. Dellsperger, and N. L. Weintraub. 2005. Vitamin E inhibits abdominal aortic aneurysm formation in angiotensin II–infused apolipoprotein E-deficient mice. *Arterioscler Thromb Vasc Biol* 25(8): 1671–1677.

Go, A. S., D. Mozaffarian, V. L. Roger, E. J. Benjamin, J. D. Berry, W. B. Borden, D. M. Bravata et al. 2013. Heart disease and stroke statistics – 2013 update: A report from the American Heart Association. *Circulation* 127(1): e6–e245.

Grootendorst, D. C., S. A. Gauw, R. M. Verhoosel, P. J. Sterk, J. J. Hospers, D. Bredenbroker, T. D. Bethke, P. S. Hiemstra, and K. F. Rabe. 2007. Reduction in sputum neutrophil and eosinophil numbers by the PDE4 inhibitor roflumilast in patients with COPD. *Thorax* 62(12): 1081–1087.

Gu, Y., C. M. Dee, and J. Shen. 2011. Interaction of free radicals, matrix metalloproteinases and caveolin-1 impacts blood-brain barrier permeability. *Front Biosci* 3: 1216–1231.

Hackam, D. G., D. Thiruchelvam, and D. A. Redelmeier. 2006. Angiotensin-converting enzyme inhibitors and aortic rupture: A population-based case-control study. *Lancet* 368(9536): 659–665.

Hecker, M., I. Pörsti, and R. Busse. 1994. Mechanisms involved in the angiotensin II-independent hypotensive action of ACE inhibitors. *Braz J Med Biol Res* 27(8): 1917–1921.

Herbert, J. M., D. Frehel, M. P. Rosso, E. Seban, C. Castet, O. Pepin, J. P. Maffrand, and G. Le Fur. 1992. Biochemical and pharmacological activities of SR 26831, a potent and selective elastase inhibitor. *J Pharmacol Exp Ther* 260(2): 809–816.

Hingorani, A., E. Ascher, M. Scheinman, W. Yorkovich, P. DePippo, C. T. Ladoulis, and S. Salles-Cunha. 1998. The effect of tumor necrosis factor binding protein and interleukin-1 receptor antagonist on the development of abdominal aortic aneurysms in a rat model. *J Vasc Surg* 28(3): 522–526.

Hnizdo, E., P. A. Sullivan, K. M. Bang, and G. Wagner. 2004. Airflow obstruction attributable to work in industry and occupation among US race/ethnic groups: A study of NHANES III data. *Am J Ind Med* 46(2): 126–135.

Houghton, A. M., P. A. Quintero, D. L. Perkins, D. K. Kobayashi, D. G. Kelley, L. A. Marconcini, R. P. Mecham, R. M. Senior, and S. D. Shapiro. 2006. Elastin fragments drive disease progression in a murine model of emphysema. *J Clin Invest* 116(3): 753–759.

Houghton, A. M., M. Mouded, and S. D. Shapiro. 2011. Consequences of elastolysis. In *Extracellular Matrix Degradation*, edited by William C. Parks and Robert P. Mecham, pp. 217–249. Berlin/Heidelberg, Germany: Springer.

Inoue, N., M. Muramatsu, D. Jin, S. Takai, T. Hayashi, H. Katayama, Y. Kitaura, H. Tamai, and M. Miyazaki. 2009. Involvement of vascular angiotensin II-forming enzymes in the progression of aortic abdominal aneurysms in angiotensin II- infused ApoE-deficient mice. *J Atheroscler Thromb* 16(3): 164–171.

Inui, M., M. Ooe, K. Fujii, H. Matsunaka, M. Yoshida, and M. Ichihashi. 2008. Mechanisms of inhibitory effects of CoQ10 on UVB-induced wrinkle formation in vitro and in vivo. *BioFactors (Oxford, England)* 32(1–4): 1–4.

Isenburg, J. C., N. V. Karamchandani, D. T. Simionescu, and N. R. Vyavahare. 2006. Structural requirements for stabilization of vascular elastin by polyphenolic tannins. *Biomaterials* 27(19): 3645–3651.

Isenburg, J. C., D. T. Simionescu, B. C. Starcher, and N. R. Vyavahare. 2007. Elastin stabilization for treatment of abdominal aortic aneurysms. *Circulation* 115(13): 1729–1737.

Janoff, A. 1972. Inhibition of human granulocyte elastase by serum alpha-1-antitrypsin. *Am Rev Respir Dis* 105(1): 121–122.

Jiang, F., G. T. Jones, and G. J. Dusting. 2007. Failure of antioxidants to protect against angiotensin II-induced aortic rupture in aged apolipoprotein (E)-deficient mice. *Br J Pharmacol* 152(6): 880–890.

Johanning, J. M, D. P. Franklin, D. C. Han, D. J. Carey, and J. R. Elmore. 2001. Inhibition of inducible nitric oxide synthase limits nitric oxide production and experimental aneurysm expansion. *J Vasc Surg* 33(3): 579–586.

Jurkiewicz, B. A. and G. R. Buettner. 1994. Ultraviolet light-induced free radical formation in skin: An electron paramagnetic resonance study. *Photochem Photobiol* 59(1): 1–4.

Kalyanasundaram, A., J. R. Elmore, J. R. Manazer, A. Golden, D. P. Franklin, S. W. Galt, E. M. Zakhary, and D. J. Carey. 2006. Simvastatin suppresses experimental aortic aneurysm expansion. *J Vasc Surg* 43(1): 117–117. e39.

Ki, V. and C. Rotstein. 2008. Bacterial skin and soft tissue infections in adults: A review of their epidemiology, pathogenesis, diagnosis, treatment and site of care. *Can J Infect Dis Med Microbiol* 19(2): 173–184.

Kim, D. Y., Y. S. Han, S. R. Kim, J. H. Park, and B. K. Chun. 2012. Effects of a topical angiotensin-converting enzyme inhibitor and a selective COX-2 inhibitor on the prevention of hypertrophic scarring in the skin of a rabbit ear. *Wounds* 24(12): 356–364.

Kim, J. E., M. H. Shin, and J. H. Chung. 2013. Epigallocatechin-3-gallate prevents heat shock-induced MMP-1 expression by inhibiting AP-1 activity in human dermal fibroblasts. *Arch Dermatol Res* 305(7): 595–602.

Kleinerman, J., V. Ranga, D. Rynbrandt, J. Sorensen, and J. C. Powers. 1980. The effect of the specific elastase inhibitor, alanyl alanyl prolyl alanine chloromethylketone, on elastase-induced emphysema. *Am Rev Respir Dis* 121(2): 381–387.

Kothapalli, C. R., C. E. Gacchina, and A. Ramamurthi. 2009a. Utility of hyaluronan oligomers and transforming growth factor-beta1 factors for elastic matrix regeneration by aneurysmal rat aortic smooth muscle cells. *Tissue Eng Part A* 15(11): 3247–3260.

Kothapalli, C. R. and A. Ramamurthi. 2010. Induced elastin regeneration by chronically activated smooth muscle cells for targeted aneurysm repair. *Acta Biomater* 6(1): 170–178.

Kothapalli, C. R., P. M. Taylor, R. T. Smolenski, M. H. Yacoub, and A. Ramamurthi. 2009b. Transforming growth factor beta 1 and hyaluronan oligomers synergistically enhance elastin matrix regeneration by vascular smooth muscle cells. *Tissue Eng Part A* 15(3): 501–511.

Kuraki, T., M. Ishibashi, M. Takayama, M. Shiraishi, and M. Yoshida. 2002. A novel oral neutrophil elastase inhibitor (ONO-6818) inhibits human neutrophil elastase-induced emphysema in rats. *Am J Respir Crit Care Med* 166(4): 496–500.

Laurell, C. B. and S. Eriksson. 2013. The electrophoretic alpha1-globulin pattern of serum in alpha1-antitrypsin deficiency. 1963. *COPD* 10 (Suppl 1): 3–8.

Lee, B. -S., J. Y. Choi, J. Y. Kim, S. H. Han, and J. E. Park. 2012. Simvastatin and losartan differentially and synergistically inhibit atherosclerosis in apolipoprotein E$^{-/-}$ mice. *Korean Circ J* 42(8): 543–550.

Lee, E. S., E. Pickett, N. Hedayati, D. L. Dawson, and W. C. Pevec. 2009. Implementation of an aortic screening program in clinical practice: Implications for the screen for abdominal aortic aneurysms very efficiently (SAAAVE) Act. *J Vasc Surg* 49(5): 1107–1111.

Liao, S., M. Miralles, B. J. Kelley, J. A. Curci, M. Borhani, and R. W. Thompson. 2001. Suppression of experimental abdominal aortic aneurysms in the rat by treatment with angiotensin-converting enzyme inhibitors. *J Vasc Surg* 33(5): 1057–1064.

Lindeman, J. H. N, H. Abdul-Hussien, J. H. van Bockel, R. Wolterbeek, and R. Kleemann. 2009. Clinical trial of doxycycline for matrix metalloproteinase-9 inhibition in patients with an abdominal aneurysm doxycycline selectively depletes aortic wall neutrophils and cytotoxic t cells. *Circulation* 119(16): 2209–2216.

Lindholt, J. S., E. W. Henneberg, S. Juul, and H. Fasting. 1999. Impaired results of a randomised double blinded clinical trial of propranolol versus placebo on the expansion rate of small abdominal aortic aneurysms. *Int Angiol* 18(1): 52–57.

Liu, S., Z. Xie, A. Daugherty, L. A. Cassis, K. J. Pearson, M. C. Gong, and Z. Guo. 2013. Mineralocorticoid receptor agonists induce mouse aortic aneurysm formation and rupture in the presence of high salt. *Arterioscler Thromb Vasc Biol* 33(7): 1568–1579.

Longo, G. M., W. Xiong, T. C. Greiner, Y. Zhao, N. Fiotti, and B. T. Baxter. 2002. Matrix metalloproteinases 2 and 9 work in concert to produce aortic aneurysms. *J Clin Invest* 110(5): 625–632.

Lu, H., D. L. Rateri, L. A. Cassis, and A. Daugherty. 2008. The role of the renin-angiotensin system in aortic aneurysmal diseases. *Curr Hypertens Rep* 10(2): 99–106.

Lu, P., K. Takai, V. M. Weaver, and Z. Werb. 2011. Extracellular matrix degradation and remodeling in development and disease. *Cold Spring Harb Perspect Biol* 3(12): pii: a005058.

Lucas, S. D., E. Costa, R. C. Guedes, and R. Moreira. 2013. Targeting COPD: Advances on low-molecular-weight inhibitors of human neutrophil elastase. *Med Res Rev* 33(Suppl 1): E73–E101.

Lucey, E. C., P. J. Stone, J. C. Powers, and G. L. Snider. 1989. Amelioration of human neutrophil elastase-induced emphysema in hamsters by pretreatment with an oligopeptide chloromethyl ketone. *Eur Respir J* 2(5): 421–427.

Lungarella, G., C. Gardi, L. Fonzi, L. Comparini, N. N. Share, M. Zimmerman, and P. A. Martorana. 1986. Effect of the novel synthetic protease inhibitor furoyl saccharin on elastase-induced emphysema in rabbits and hamsters. *Exp Lung Res* 11(1): 35–47.

Mahadeva, R. and D. A. Lomas. 1998. Alpha(1)-antitrypsin deficiency, cirrhosis and emphysema. *Thorax* 53(6): 501–505.

Manning, M. W., L. A. Cassis, and A. Daugherty. 2003. Differential effects of doxycycline, a broad-spectrum matrix metalloproteinase inhibitor, on angiotensin II–induced atherosclerosis and abdominal aortic aneurysms. *Arterioscler Thromb Vasc Biol* 23(3): 483–488.

Masaki, H. 2010. Role of antioxidants in the skin: Anti-aging effects. *J Dermatol Sci* 58(2): 85–90.

Matsuura-Hachiya, Y., K. Y. Arai, R. Ozeki, A. Kikuta, and T. Nishiyama. 2013. Angiotensin-converting enzyme inhibitor (enalapril maleate) accelerates recovery of mouse skin from UVB-induced wrinkles. *Biochem Biophys Res Commun* 442(1–2): 38–43.

Mecham, R. P., T. J. Broekelmann, C. J. Fliszar, S. D. Shapiro, H. G. Welgus, and R. M. Senior. 1997. Elastin degradation by matrix metalloproteinases. Cleavage site specificity and mechanisms of elastolysis. *J Biol Chem* 272(29): 18071–18076.

Mecham, R. P., G. Lange, J. Madaras, and B. Starcher. 1981. Elastin synthesis by ligamentum nuchae fibroblasts: Effects of culture conditions and extracellular matrix on elastin production. *J Cell Biol* 90(2): 332–338.

Meijer, CA, T Stigmen, and Pharmaceutical Aneurysm Stabilization Trial Study Group. 2014. Doxycycline for stabilization of abdominal aortic aneurysms: A Randomized trial. *J Vasc Surg* 59(4): 1175–1176.

Meng, Q., C. N. Velalar, and R. Ruan. 2008. Regulating the age-related oxidative damage, mitochondrial integrity, and antioxidative enzyme activity in Fischer 344 rats by supplementation of the antioxidant epigallocatechin-3-gallate. *Rejuvenation Res* 11(3): 649–660.

Millar, A. W., P. D. Brown, J. Moore, W. A. Galloway, A. G. Cornish, T. J. Lenehan, and K. P. Lynch. 1998. Results of single and repeat dose studies of the oral matrix metalloproteinase inhibitor marimastat in healthy male volunteers. *Br J Clin Pharmacol* 45(1): 21–26.

Miyake, T. and R. Morishita. 2009. Pharmacological treatment of abdominal aortic aneurysm. *Cardiovasc Res* 83(3): 436–443.

Molfino, N. A. and P. K. Jeffery. 2007. Chronic obstructive pulmonary disease: Histopathology, inflammation and potential therapies. *Pulm Pharmacol Ther* 20(5): 462–472.

Moore, G., S. Liao, J. A. Curci, B. C. Starcher, R. L. Martin, R. T. Hendricks, J. J. Chen, and R. W. Thompson. 1999. Suppression of experimental abdominal aortic aneurysms by systemic treatment with a hydroxamate-based matrix metalloproteinase inhibitor (RS 132908). *J Vasc Surg* 29(3): 522–532.

Mueller, C. and T. R. Flotte. 2013. Gene-based therapy for alpha-1 antitrypsin deficiency. *COPD* 10 (Suppl 1): 44–49.

Muta-Takada, K., T. Terada, H. Yamanishi, Y. Ashida, S. Inomata, T. Nishiyama, and S. Amano. 2009. Coenzyme Q10 protects against oxidative stress-induced cell death and enhances the synthesis of basement membrane components in dermal and epidermal cells. *BioFactors (Oxford, England)* 35(5): 435–441.

Myllylä, R., K. Majamaa, V. Günzler, H. M. Hanauske-Abel, and K. I. Kivirikko. 1984. Ascorbate is consumed stoichiometrically in the uncoupled reactions catalyzed by prolyl 4-hydroxylase and lysyl hydroxylase. *J Biol Chem* 259(9): 5403–5405.

Nakashima, H., M. Aoki, T. Miyake, T. Kawasaki, M. Iwai, N. Jo, M. Oishi, K. Kataoka, S. Ohgi, and T. Ogihara. 2004. Inhibition of experimental abdominal aortic aneurysm in the rat by use of decoy oligodeoxynucleotides suppressing activity of nuclear factor κB and ets transcription factors. *Circulation* 109(1): 132–138.

Neurath, H. 1999. Proteolytic enzymes, past and future. *Proc Natl Acad Sci USA* 96(20): 10962–10963.

Niu, Y., L. Na, R. Feng, L. Gong, Y. Zhao, Q. Li, Y. Li, and C. Sun. 2013. The phytochemical, EGCG, extends lifespan by reducing liver and kidney function damage and improving age-associated inflammation and oxidative stress in healthy rats. *Aging Cell* 12(6): 1041–1049.

Nosoudi, N., A. Sinha, P. Nahar, N. Vyavahare. 2014. inhibition of MMPs in abdominal aortic aneurysm rat model using anti-elastin decorated nanoparticles loaded with batimastat. *BMES 2014 Annual Meeting*, San Antonio, TX.

Obayashi, K., K. Kurihara, Y. Okano, H. Masaki, and D. B. Yarosh. 2005. L-Ergothioneine scavenges superoxide and singlet oxygen and suppresses TNF-alpha and MMP-1 expression in UV-irradiated human dermal fibroblasts. *J Cosmet Sci* 56(1): 17–27.

Ohbayashi, H. 2002. Neutrophil elastase inhibitors as treatment for COPD. *Expert Opin Investig Drugs* 11(7): 965–980.

Parasaram, V., N. Nosoudi, and N. Vyavahare. 2014. Enhanced matrix elastin production and organization using pentagalloyl glucose in pulmonary fibroblast cultures. *Presented at the annual meeting of BioMedical Engineering Society,* San Antonio, TX.

Park, K. and J. H. Lee. 2008. Protective effects of resveratrol on UVB-irradiated HaCaT cells through attenuation of the caspase pathway. *Oncol Rep* 19(2): 413–417.

Park, Y. C., M. Jin, S. H. Kim, M. H. Kim, U. Namgung, and Y. Yeo. 2014. Effects of inhalable microparticle of flower of Lonicera japonica in a mouse model of COPD. *J Ethnopharmacol* 151(1): 123–130.

Pemberton, P. A., J. S. Cantwell, K. M. Kim, D. J. Sundin, D. Kobayashi, J. B. Fink, S. D. Shapiro, and P. J. Barr. 2005. An inhaled matrix metalloprotease inhibitor prevents cigarette smoke-induced emphysema in the mouse. *COPD* 2(3): 303–310.

Pemberton, P. A., D. Kobayashi, B. J. Wilk, J. M. Henstrand, S. D. Shapiro, and P. J. Barr. 2006. Inhaled recombinant alpha 1-antitrypsin ameliorates cigarette smoke-induced emphysema in the mouse. *COPD* 3(2): 101–108.

Petrinec, D., S. Liao, D. R. Holmes, J. M. Reilly, W. C. Parks, and R. W. Thompson. 1996. Doxycycline inhibition of aneurysmal degeneration in an elastase-induced rat model of abdominal aortic aneurysm: Preservation of aortic elastin associated with suppressed production of 92 kD gelatinase. *J Vasc Surg* 23(2): 336–346.

Porter, K. E., I. M. Loftus, M. Peterson, P. R. F. Bell, N. J. M. London, and M. M. Thompson. 1998. Marimastat inhibits neointimal thickening in a model of human vein graft stenosis. *Br J Surg* 85(10): 1373–1377.

Propranolol Aneurysm Trial Investigators. 2002. Propranolol for small abdominal aortic aneurysms: Results of a randomized trial. *J Vasc Surg* 35(1): 72–79.

Quintarelli, G., B. C. Starcher, A. Vocaturo, F. Di Gianfilippo, L. Gotte, and R. P. Mecham. 1979. Fibrogenesis and biosynthesis of elastin in cartilage. *Connect Tissue Res* 7(1): 1–19.

Rahman, S., K. Bhatia, A. Q. Khan, M. Kaur, F. Ahmad, H. Rashid, M. Athar, F. Islam, and S. Raisuddin. 2008. Topically applied vitamin E prevents massive cutaneous inflammatory and oxidative stress responses induced by double application of 12-O-tetradecanoylphorbol-13-acetate (TPA) in mice. *Chem-Biol Interact* 172(3): 195–205.

Ricci, M. A., J. M. Slaiby, G. R. Gadowski, E. D. Hendley, P. Nichols, and D. B. Pilcher. 1996. Effects of hypertension and propranolol upon aneurysm expansion in the Anidjar/Dobrin aneurysm modela. *Ann N Y Acad Sci* 800(1): 89–96.

Ricciarelli, R., P. Maroni, N. Ozer, J. M. Zingg, and A. Azzi. 1999. Age-dependent increase of collagenase expression can be reduced by alpha-tocopherol via protein kinase C inhibition. *Free Radic Biol Med* 27(7–8): 7–8.

Rossetti, D., M. G. Kielmanowicz, S. Vigodman, Y. P. Hu, N. Chen, A. Nkengne, T. Oddos, D. Fischer, M. Seiberg, and C. B. Lin. 2011. A novel anti-ageing mechanism for retinol: Induction of dermal elastin synthesis and elastin fibre formation. *Int J Cosmet Sci* 33(1): 62–69.

Sandhaus, R. A. 1993. Alpha 1-antitrypsin augmentation therapy. *Agents Actions Suppl* 42: 97–102.

Sandhaus, R. A. 2004. Alpha1-antitrypsin deficiency. 6: New and emerging treatments for alpha1-antitrypsin deficiency. *Thorax* 59(10): 904–909.

Sasamura, H. and H. Itoh. 2011. Hypertension and arteriosclerosis. *Nippon Rinsho* 69(1): 125–130.

Schluchter, M. D., A. F. Barker, R. G. Crystal, R. A. Robbins, J. M. Stocks, J. K. Stoller, and M. C. Wu. 1998. Survival and FEV1 decline in individuals with severe deficiency of alpha1-antitrypsin. The Alpha-1-Antitrypsin Deficiency Registry Study Group. *Am J Respir Crit Care Med* 158(1): 49–59.

Seersholm, N., M. Wencker, N. Banik, K. Viskum, A. Dirksen, A. Kok-Jensen, and N. Konietzko. 1997. Does alpha1-antitrypsin augmentation therapy slow the annual decline in FEV1 in patients with severe hereditary alpha1-antitrypsin deficiency? Wissenschaftliche Arbeitsgemeinschaft zur Therapie von Lungenerkrankungen (WATL) alpha1-AT study group. *Eur Respir J* 10(10): 2260–2263.

Selman, M., J. Cisneros-Lira, M. Gaxiola, R. Ramirez, E. M. Kudlacz, P. G. Mitchell, and A. Pardo. 2003. Matrix metalloproteinases inhibition attenuates tobacco smoke-induced emphysema in guinea pigs. *Chest* 123(5): 1633–1641.

Shang, T., Z. Liu, and C.-j. Liu. 2014. Antioxidant vitamin C attenuates experimental abdominal aortic aneurysm development in an elastase-induced rat model. *J Surg Res* 188(1): 316–325.

Shang, T., Z. Liu, M. Zhou, C. K. Zarins, C. Xu, and C.-j. Liu. 2012. Inhibition of experimental abdominal aortic aneurysm in a rat model by way of tanshinone IIA. *J Surg Res* 178(2): 1029–1037.

Shapiro, S. D., S. K. Endicott, M. A. Province, J. A. Pierce, and E. J. Campbell. 1991. Marked longevity of human lung parenchymal elastic fibers deduced from prevalence of D-aspartate and nuclear weapons-related radiocarbon. *J Clin Invest* 87(5): 1828–1834.

Shifren, A. and R. P. Mecham. 2006. The stumbling block in lung repair of emphysema: Elastic fiber assembly. *Proc Am Thorac Soc* 3(5): 428–433.

Sho, E., J. Chu, M. Sho, B. Fernandes, D. Judd, P. Ganesan, H. Kimura, and R. L. Dalman. 2004. Continuous periaortic infusion improves doxycycline efficacy in experimental aortic aneurysms. *J Vasc Surg* 39(6): 1312–1321.

Sinha, A. 2013. Vascular nanomedicine: Site specific delivery of elastin stabilizing therapeutics to damaged arteries. PhD, Bioengineering, Clemson University, Clemson, SC.

Sinha, A., N. Nosoudi, and N. Vyavahare. 2014a. Elasto-regenerative properties of polyphenols. *Biochem Biophys Res Commun* 444(2): 205–211.

Sinha, A., A. Shaporev, N. Nosoudi, Y. Lei, A. Vertegel, S. Lessner, and N. Vyavahare. 2014b. Nanoparticle targeting to diseased vasculature for imaging and therapy. *Nanomedicine* 10(5): 1003–1012.

Sivaraman, B. and A. Ramamurthi. 2013. Multifunctional nanoparticles for doxycycline delivery towards localized elastic matrix stabilization and regenerative repair. *Acta Biomater* 9(5): 6511–6525.

Slaiby, J. M., M. A. Ricci, G. R. Gadowski, E. D. Hendley, and D. B. Pilcher. 1994. Expansion of aortic aneurysms is reduced by propranolol in a hypertensive rat model. *J Vasc Surg* 20(2): 178–183.

Smith, S. J., P. S. Fenwick, A. G. Nicholson, F. Kirschenbaum, T. K. Finney-Hayward, L. S. Higgins, M. A. Giembycz, P. J. Barnes, and L. E. Donnelly. 2006. Inhibitory effect of p38 mitogen-activated protein kinase inhibitors on cytokine release from human macrophages. *Br J Pharmacol* 149(4): 393–404.

Steinmetz, E. F., C. Buckley, L. M. Shames, L. T. Ennis, J. S. Vanvickle-Chavez, D. Mao, L. A. Goeddel, C. J. Hawkins, and R. W. Thompson. 2005. *Treatment with Simvastatin Suppresses the Development of Experimental Abdominal Aortic Aneurysms in Normal and Hypercholesterolemic Mice.* Vol. 241. Hagerstown, MD, ETATS-UNIS: Lippincott Williams & Wilkins.

Stevens, T., K. Ekholm, M. Granse, M. Lindahl, V. Kozma, C. Jungar, T. Ottosson et al. 2011. AZD9668: Pharmacological characterization of a novel oral inhibitor of neutrophil elastase. *J Pharmacol Exp Ther* 339(1): 313–320.

Sugawara, A., A. Sueki, T. Hirose, K. Nagai, H. Gouda, S. Hirono, H. Shima, K. S. Akagawa, S. Omura, and T. Sunazuka. 2011. Novel 12-membered non-antibiotic macrolides from erythromycin A; EM900 series as novel leads for anti-inflammatory and/or immunomodulatory agents. *Bioorg Med Chem Lett* 21(11): 3373–3376.

Sukhija, R., W. S. Aronow, R. Sandhu, P. Kakar, and S. Babu. 2006. Mortality and size of abdominal aortic aneurysm at long-term follow-up of patients not treated surgically and treated with and without statins. *Am J Cardiol* 97(2): 279–280.

Sylvester, A., B. Sivaraman, P. Deb, and A. Ramamurthi. 2013. Nanoparticles for localized delivery of hyaluronan oligomers towards regenerative repair of elastic matrix. *Acta Biomater* 9(12): 9292–302.

Szoka, L., E. Karna, R. P. Morka, and J. A. Palka. 2015. Enalapril stimulates collagen biosynthesis through prolidase-dependent mechanism in cultured fibroblasts. *Naunyn-Schmiedeberg's Arch Pharmacol* 388(6): 677–683.

Tajima, S., A. Hayashi, and T. Suzuki. 1997. Elastin expression is up-regulated by retinoic acid but not by retinol in chick embryonic skin fibroblasts. *J Dermatol Sci* 15(3): 166–172.

Tham, D. M., B. Martin-McNulty, Yi-Xin Wang, V. Da Cunha, D. W. Wilson, C. N. Athanassious, A. F. Powers, M. E. Sullivan, and J. C. Rutledge. 2002. Angiotensin II injures the arterial wall causing increased aortic stiffening in apolipoprotein E-deficient mice. *Am J Physiol Regul Integr Comp Physiol* 283(6): R1442–R1449.

Thompson, R. W., J. A. Curci, T. L. Ennis, D. Mao, M. B. Pagano, and C. T. Pham. 2006. Pathophysiology of abdominal aortic aneurysms: Insights from the elastase-induced model in mice with different genetic backgrounds. *Ann N Y Acad Sci* 1085: 59–73.

Tomita, N., K. Yamasaki, K. Izawa, Y. Kunugiza, T. Ogihara, and R. Morishita. 2008. Inhibition of experimental abdominal aortic aneurysm progression by nifedipine. *Int J Mol Med* 21(2): 239–244.

Tsui, J. C. 2010. Experimental models of abdominal aortic aneurysms. *Open Cardiovasc Med J* 4: 221.

Tuder, R. M. and I. Petrache. 2012. Pathogenesis of chronic obstructive pulmonary disease. *J Clin Invest* 122(8): 2749–2755.

Uitto, J. 2008. The role of elastin and collagen in cutaneous aging: Intrinsic aging versus photoexposure. *J Drugs Dermatol* 7(2 Suppl): s12–s16.

Vandenbroucke, R. E., E. Dejonckheere, and C. Libert. 2011. A therapeutic role for matrix metalloproteinase inhibitors in lung diseases? *Eur Respir J* 38(5): 1200–1214.

Venkataraman, L. and A. Ramamurthi. 2011. Induced elastic matrix deposition within three-dimensional collagen scaffolds. *Tissue Eng Part A* 17(21–22): 2879–2889.

Venkataraman, L., B. Sivaraman, P. Vaidya, and A. Ramamurthi. 2014. Nanoparticulate delivery of agents for induced elastogenesis in three-dimensional collagenous matrices. *J Tissue Eng Regen Med* 10.

Walton, L. J., I. J. Franklin, T. Bayston, L. C. Brown, R. M. Greenhalgh, G. W. Taylor, and J. T. Powell. 1999. Inhibition of prostaglandin E2 synthesis in abdominal aortic aneurysms: Implications for smooth muscle cell viability, inflammatory processes, and the expansion of abdominal aortic aneurysms. *Circulation* 100(1): 48–54.

Wencker, M., N. Banik, R. Buhl, R. Seidel, and N. Konietzko. 1998. Long-term therapy of alpha 1-antitrypsin-deficiency-associated pulmonary emphysema with human alpha 1-antitrypsin. *Pneumologie* 52(10): 545–552.

Werb, Z., M. J. Banda, J. H. McKerrow, and R. A. Sandhaus. 1982. Elastases and elastin degradation. *J Invest Dermatol* 79 (Suppl 1): 154s–159s.

Williams, J. C., R. C. Falcone, C. Knee, R. L. Stein, A. M. Strimpler, B. Reaves, R. E. Giles, and R. D. Krell. 1991. Biologic characterization of ICI 200,880 and ICI 200,355, novel inhibitors of human neutrophil elastase. *Am Rev Respir Dis* 144(4): 875–883.

Wright, J. L. and A. Churg. 2007. Current concepts in mechanisms of emphysema. *Toxicol Pathol* 35(1): 111–115.

Wright, J. L., S. G. Farmer, and A. Churg. 2002. Synthetic serine elastase inhibitor reduces cigarette smoke-induced emphysema in guinea pigs. *Am J Respir Crit Care Med* 166(7): 954–960.

Xiong, F., J. Zhao, G. Zeng, B. Huang, D. Yuan, and Y. Yang. 2014. Inhibition of AAA in a rat model by treatment with ACEI perindopril. *J Surg Res* 189(1): 166–173.

Xiong, J., S. M. Wang, L. H. Chen, Y. Lin, Y. F. Zhu, and C. S. Ye. 2008. Elastic fibers reconstructed using adenovirus-mediated expression of tropoelastin and tested in the elastase model of abdominal aortic aneurysm in rats. *J Vasc Surg* 48(4): 965–973.

Xiong, W., J. MacTaggart, R. Knispel, J. Worth, Y. Persidsky, and B. T. Baxter. 2009. Blocking TNF-α attenuates aneurysm formation in a murine model. *J Immunol* 183(4): 2741–2746.

Yoshimura, K., H. Aoki, M. Onoda, Y. Ikeda, H. Aoyama, N. Morikage, A. Furutani, K. Hamano, and M. Matsuzaki. 2006. Stabilization of extracellular matrix antagonizes proinflammatory signaling and prevents progression of aortic aneurysm in vivo. *Circulation* 114(18): 281–281.

Yoshimura, K., H. Aoki, Y. Ikeda, K. Fujii, N. Akiyama, A. Furutani, Y. Hoshii, N. Tanaka, R. Ricci, and T. Ishihara. 2005. Regression of abdominal aortic aneurysm by inhibition of c-Jun N-terminal kinase. *Nature Med* 11(12): 1330–1338.

Zhang, J., L. Wu, J. M. Qu, C. X. Bai, M. J. Merrilees, and P. N. Black. 2012. Proinflammatory phenotype of COPD fibroblasts not compatible with repair in COPD lung. *J Cell Mol Med* 16(7): 1522–1532.

Zhou, Y., X. Wang, X. Zeng, R. Qiu, J. Xie, S. Liu, J. Zheng, N. Zhong, and P. Ran. 2006. Positive benefits of theophylline in a randomized, double-blind, parallel-group, placebo-controlled study of low-dose, slow-release theophylline in the treatment of COPD for 1 year. *Respirology* 11(5): 603–610.

CHAPTER 7

Sourcing and Manipulating Stem Cells for Elastin Regeneration Applications

Brian M. Balog, Anand Ramamurthi, and
Margot S. Damaser

CONTENTS

7.1 INTRODUCTION

Cell-based tissue regeneration has been shown to have the potential to treat many pathological conditions involving breakdown of the extracellular matrix (ECM) of soft connective tissues, including myocardial infarction, pelvic organ prolapse, and aortic aneurysms (Budatha et al. 2011, Zhuang et al. 2011, Kishore et al. 2013, Swaminathan et al. 2014). More specifically, stem cells including mesenchymal stem cells (MSCs), hematopoietic stem cells (HSCs), fibroblasts, induced pluripotent stem cells (iPSCs), and embryonic stem cells (ESCs) can all variously influence and modulate elastin biology and homeostasis depending on the tissue type and disease context. For example, stem cells are known to generate both proelastogenic factors, such as insulin-like growth factor 1 (IGF-1) that promotes new elastic fiber formation, and anti-elastogenic factors, such as basic fibroblast growth factor (bFGF) (Gogly et al. 2007, Oskowitz et al. 2011). The choice of cells for regeneration of elastic matrix structures (e.g., discrete fibers, fiber meshes, sheets) is thus motivated by the tissue or organ to be regenerated and the disease to be targeted. For example, growth of aortic aneurysms involves progressive and natural irreversible breakdown of elastic fibers that requires buildup of intact elastic fibers for restoring tissue structure and function. In contrast, fibrosis involves accumulation of disorganized collagen that must be tempered to prevent excessive tissue stiffening. Studies with HSCs, fibroblasts, and MSCs have all shown promise in regenerating vascular and cardiac tissues through upregulation of elastogenesis (Kobayashi et al. 2008, Sekiya et al. 2009, Chen et al. 2014). ESCs have also been shown to differentiate into cell types useful for repair of elastin-containing tissues, such as ligaments (Yang et al. 2013). iPSCs may also be useful for this purpose, although they still require extensive characterization prior to use in therapy, due to their relatively recent discovery.

7.2 MECHANISMS UNDERLYING MATRIX REGENERATIVE EFFECTS OF STEM CELLS

Stem cells have the unique ability to self-renew and differentiate into cells of several lineages. There are two major types of stem cells: embryonic stem cell (ESCs) and adult (Gilbert 2010). ESCs have the potential to differentiate into tissues of all three germ layers (Thomson et al. 1998, Tanabe et al. 2014) and are thus termed totipotent. iPSCs are very similar to ESCs in their properties and can form most cell types. They are therefore categorized as pluripotent. Multipotent adult stem cells, which are present in mature tissues, can only generate a subset of cell types compared to ESCs and iPSCs, but are known to actively participate in tissue repair processes (Gilbert 2010). Progenitor cells are similar to stem cells, but have the capacity to undergo only a few cycles of self-renewal, and demonstrate lineage commitment to even fewer cell types than do adult stem cells (Gilbert 2010).

Lineage-directed differentiation was originally considered to be the mechanistic basis for the therapeutic regenerative benefits of stem cells (Gnecchi et al. 2008, Tran and Damaser 2015). For some cell types this is indeed the case. For example, HSCs are used to treat blood diseases, such as myeloma and sickle cell anemia, because they can differentiate into the different types of cells present in blood (Orkin and Zon 2008, Benkerrou 2014). The idea of stem cell differentiation as the mechanism of action has also led researchers to induce stem cell differentiation toward tissue-specific cell lineages prior to administration of cell therapy (Xu et al. 2002, Arikawa et al. 2009, Ayatollahi et al. 2011). For example, ESCs differentiated into neural progenitors have been shown to improve recovery from spinal cord injury in rats (All et al. 2012). Other studies have directed MSCs into cells of an osteogenic lineage for treating bone injury (Amantea et al. 2008). Similarly, MSCs can provide regenerative effects in elastolytic disorders such as aortic aneurysms or chronic obstructive pulmonary disease (Hashizume et al. 2011, Yamawaki-Ogata et al. 2014, Zhang et al. 2014).

Although there is evidence that after injury, endogenous adult stem cells and progenitor cells initiate repair of the injured tissue by replicating and differentiating, in some situations, such as within myocardial infarcts, endogenous stem cells are incapable or insufficient to completely repair the injured tissue (Gnecchi et al. 2008, Kishore et al. 2013). In contrast, studies that have delivered autologous or allografted mulitpotent stem cells to the heart after myocardial infarction have shown functional tissue recovery even with low cell engraftment, leading to broadening of the understanding of the mechanism of cell-based tissue repair (Orlic et al. 2003, Balsam et al. 2004, Murry et al. 2004, Gnecchi et al. 2008, Makridakis et al. 2013). Recent studies have shown that the secretions of stem cells (secretome) facilitate matrix regeneration to a greater extent than replication and differentiation of physically engrafted stem cells (Caplan and Dennis 2006, Gnecchi et al. 2008, Shabbir et al. 2009). Also, secretions from differentiated cells can differ significantly from their parent cell types. For example, Kubal et al. found that the anti-ischemic effects of MSCs were not present when tissues were cocultured with MSC-derived keratinocytes or endothelial cells (Kubal et al. 2006), showing that cells differentiated from stem cells do not secrete the same range of factors as their parent cell types.

7.2.1 Proelastogenic Stem Cell Secretions

Elastic fiber assembly is a highly complex and regulated process, as discussed in greater detail in early chapters of this book. It requires the robust cellular synthesis and bioavailability of essential structural elements, that is, elastin precursor molecules (tropoelastin), prescaffolding glycoprotein microfibrils (e.g., fibrillins), and cross-linking enzymes, such as lysyl oxidase (LOX) and lysyl oxidase like 1 (LOXL1), that catalyze the formation of molecules that interlink adjoining elastin molecules (e.g., desmosine, isodesmosine) and link the elastic fibers of adjoining cells (e.g., fibulin) (Kielty et al. 2002, Sivaraman et al. 2012). Importantly, elastic fiber assembly involves a precise spatiotemporal pattern of organization of each of these components and requires their bioavailability in predetermined proportions for proper elastic fiber formation to occur. The few studies that have investigated the regenerative benefits of stem cell secretome have broadly identified proteins that could be responsible for stimulating elastogenesis *in vitro* and *in vivo* (Bendall et al. 2009, Harvey et al. 2013, Yousef et al. 2013, Zhao et al. 2015).

It is known that mutations in genes coding for elastic fiber assembly proteins can result in life-threatening disorders; for example, a mutation in the elastin gene (ELN) is the basis for development of supravalvular aortic stenosis (SVAS) and heart failure (Milewicz et al. 2000). Differently, a mutation in the fibrillin-1 gene (FBN1) underlies the etiology of Marfan syndrome (Milewicz et al. 2000). Therefore, supplying nonmutated forms of elastin or fibrillin generated robustly by stem cells or their derivatives toward enabling cell-mediated elastic fiber assembly could be a therapeutic modality for alleviation of these disorders. In this context, it has been shown that the medium conditioned by human MSCs contains both soluble and insoluble forms of fibrillin-1 protein, suggesting prospective use of MSCs to restore elastic tissue structure and function in Marfan and other syndromic conditions (Harvey et al. 2013). Elastin-binding protein (EBP), which is cell membrane bound and binds to tropoelastin transported outside of the cell to prevent it from being degraded, has also been detected in the secretome of MSCs (Harvey et al. 2013). In light of previous findings, exogenous elastin precursors—for example, those produced by exogenous stem cells—can be recruited by these, and the parenchymal cell within the intended site of tissue repair and assembled into elastic matrix structures, thus offering promise for further studies (Deng et al. 2015).

LOX and its homologue, LOXL1 are important for cross-linking tropoelastin to form elastic fibers during development and during elastin remodeling (Hayashi et al. 2004, Sivaraman et al. 2012). Mutation and decreased expression of LOXL1 genes have been implicated in the pathophysiology of pelvic organ prolapse and Stickler syndrome (Milewicz et al. 2000, Budatha et al. 2011, Shynlova et al. 2013). In these disease scenarios, making available exogenous LOX and LOXL1 could overcome their decreased bioavailability to be able to potentially affect regenerative repair of the elastic matrix. Recent evidence that MSCs isolated from dental pulp produce LOX, LOXL1, as well as LOXL 2, 3, and 4 (Kim et al. 2013) holds promise toward use of these and MSCs from other sources, besides adult and other stem cell types in treating the above diseases.

Fibulins interface between the cell surface and the elastic fibers and other ECM components such as constituents of the basement membrane (Kielty et al. 2002). They act both as intermolecular bridges within the ECM to form supramolecular structures, and as mediators for cellular processes and tissue remodeling (Kielty et al. 2002). Fibulin-1 (FBLN1) has been found at low concentrations in human MSC secretome and in human ESC secretome (Kielty et al. 2002, Harvey et al. 2013, Halper and Kjaer 2014, Zhao et al. 2015). Additional research is needed to determine if other fibulins are present in the secretome of stem cells and if these can be recruited by parenchymal cells in de-elasticized tissues, on secretome treatment to improve elastic fiber assembly (Wagenseil and Mecham 2007, Yanagisawa and Davis 2010). Additional proteins associated with elastic fibers found in the conditioned media of MSCs are perlecan (PLC), elastin microfibril interface 1 (EMILIN1), and microfibrillar-associated protein 2 (MFAP2) (Harvey et al. 2013).

In addition to the proteins that participate in elastin matrix formation, cell secretions can include biomolecules such as tissue inhibitor of metalloproteinase 1 (TIMP1), an inhibitor of elastolytic matrix metalloproteinases 2 and 9 (MMPs2, 9), which are overexpressed in proteolytically disrupted tissues such as in aortic aneurysms (Lau et al. 2008). It is possible that excessive elastin degradation and insufficient elastin remodeling can lead to disorders such as pelvic organ prolapse (Shynlova et al. 2013). Such biomolecules can contribute to preservation of elastic fiber integrity, a key requirement in seeking to augment net accumulation of newly regenerated elastic matrix in a proteolytically active tissue space. MMP inhibitors such as TIMP1 and TIMP2 have been detected in the medium conditioned by fibroblasts and MSCs (Mias et al. 2009). Inhibited or slowed growth of aortic aneurysms treated with MSCs has been at least in part attributed to generation of these antiproteolytic biomolecules by MSCs (Hashizume et al. 2011, Yamawaki-Ogata et al. 2014).

Stem cells are also known to secrete many proteins and hormones with documented benefits to elastic fiber assembly such as hepatocyte growth factor (HGF), IGF-1, and IGF-binding protein 1 (IGFBP-1) (Sivaraman et al. 2012, Qa'aty et al. 2015). HGF upregulates production of elastin precursor synthesis and is generated by human ESCs (Hirano et al. 2003, Yousef et al. 2013). IGF-1, which increases production of tropoelastin and stimulates elastic matrix deposition, is secreted by human MSCs when cultured under serum-free conditions (Wolfe et al. 1993, Kothapalli and Ramamurthi 2008, Oskowitz et al. 2011). Human ESCs and mouse fibroblasts produce IGFBP-1 (Bendall et al. 2009), an IGF-1-associated protein that increases the half-life of IGF-1 (Baxter 2000). IGF-2 is similar to IGF-1, activates many of the same pathways, and has been found in the conditioned media of ESCs and fibroblasts (Baxter 2000, Bendall et al. 2009). There are additional potential therapeutic aspects of stem cell secretome for elastolytic disorders, such as glucagon-like peptide 1 (GLP-1), which stimulates new elastic fiber production in human cardiac fibroblasts, but these have not yet been identified in the secretome of stem cells (Qa'aty et al. 2015).

7.2.2 Elastin Degrading Factors in Stem Cell Secretions

Homeostasis of the elastic matrix is maintained through a balance between elastogenesis and elastolysis. In a proteolytically active tissue microenvironment, enzymes targeting elastic matrix (e.g., elastases and MMPs) are chronically overexpressed, resulting in continual breakdown and etching of pre-existing fibers. The unavailability of intact pre-existing elastic fibers can present an impediment to assembly of new elastic fibers by cells (Sivaraman et al. 2012). This can result in elastolysis greatly exceeding elastogenesis, resulting in net loss of elastic matrix. While stem cell secretome components provide attractive prospects to enhance the regenerative aspect over matrix breakdown, due consideration must be given to the fact that stem cells can simultaneously generate other biological factors that may have contradictory effects of decreasing elastin synthesis and fiber formation, or increasing degradation of existing fibers (Sivaraman et al. 2012).

Although several factors can inhibit synthesis, only a few are known to be produced by stem cells, that is, bFGF, and versican (Sivaraman et al. 2012). BFGF decreases elastin mRNA synthesis, resulting in decreased generation of elastin fibers. It has been detected in the concentrated conditioned media (CCM) of multiple cell types including human ESCs and mouse fibroblasts (Yousef et al. 2013, Qa'aty et al. 2015).

Versican has been detected in the medium conditioned by MSCs (Harvey et al. 2013). It decreases elastic fiber assembly by releasing EBP from the cell membrane, resulting in a decreased amount of tropoelastin available for nucleation prior to release from the surface of the cell. In addition, MMPs 2 and 9, elastolytic proteinases, are also present in the media of MSCs (Okada et al. 1990, Fulcher and Van Doren 2011, Shen et al. 2015), and culturing MSCs in 3D spheroid culture increases production of MMPs 2 and 9 (Santos et al. 2015). These considerations must be taken into account in utilizing MSCs or the MSC-conditioned medium for stimulating elastin regenerative repair.

Transforming growth factor beta 1 (TGF-β1) can both promote and inhibit elastin synthesis (Kothapalli et al. 2009, Sivaraman et al. 2012). It has been shown to upregulate synthesis of tropoelastin and improve elastic fiber formation by even abnormal vascular SMCs (Losy et al. 2003, Gacchina and Ramamurthi 2011). However, TGF-β1 in combination with elastin peptides can incite matrix mineralization (Simionescu et al. 2005). TGF-β1 is secreted by ESCs, MSCs, and fibroblasts (Bendall et al. 2009, Santos et al. 2015), and these secretions by MSCs are increased under serum-free or hypoxic conditions (Hung et al. 2012, Tsai et al. 2012). TGF-β1 is also stored in the ECM by latent-TGF-β binding proteins 1 and 2, which have also been detected at low levels of MSC secretome (Harvey et al. 2013). The secretome of these cells therefore has the potential to facilitate TGF-β1 storage in the ECM, for subsequent timely release to restore normal signaling and elastin regeneration.

More research needs to be conducted to systematically determine the presence or absence of many of the elastin-associated proteins, elastogenesis promoting factors, and elastin degrading factors, in the secretome of ESCs, iPSCs, MSCs, HSCs, and fibroblasts, the specific conditions under which they are secreted, and the absolute concentrations and relative expression of each needed to influence various aspects of elastic matrix assembly toward being able to restore elastin homeostasis in specific disease states.

7.3 PHYSICAL DELIVERY OF CELLS FOR ELASTIC MATRIX ENGINEERING AND REGENERATIVE REPAIR

7.3.1 Embryonic Stem Cells

The ability of ESCs in culture and *in vivo* to differentiate to generate all three germ layers (endoderm, ectoderm, and mesoderm) has led researchers to investigate their use for regenerative therapy (Loebel et al. 2003, Ginis et al. 2004), as illustrated in Figure 7.1. To harvest either mouse or human ESCs, the blastocyst's outer layer is removed and the inner cell mass is plated onto γ-irradiated or mitomycin-c treated mouse embryonic fibroblasts with high serum content (Thomson and Marshall 1998, Reubinoff et al. 2000). Within a week, ESC colonies will begin to form. To maintain their undifferentiated state, the cells must be transferred to a new mouse embryonic fibroblast feeder layer every few days (Conley et al. 2004). The factors required to be released from the mouse embryonic fibroblast feeder layer to maintain the ESC state are not fully understood. Mouse embryonic fibroblast-conditioned media has been shown to have the same effect as mouse embryonic fibroblasts, but without either the media or feeder layer, the ESCs will spontaneously differentiate into all three germ layers. The xenogeneic source of the feeding layer for human ESCs has prompted efforts to develop new feeder layers, because human ESCs cultured with mouse feeder cells or mouse cell-conditioned media could lead to a xenobiotic pathogen transfer from mouse to humans (Conley et al. 2004). As a result, human ESCs cultured with mouse fibroblasts cannot be used therapeutically (Conley et al. 2004). Defined media that contains no animal proteins could also be more appropriate (Xu et al. 2001). One possible alternative for undifferentiated propagation of human ESCs would be to use human MSCs as the feeder layer (Cheng et al. 2003). Researchers have also differentiated human ESCs into fibroblasts to use them as a feeder layer in human ESC culture (Chen et al. 2009). The labor-intensive nature of ESC culturing makes large-scale clinical ESC therapies difficult (Conley et al. 2004).

Some of the major differences between human and mouse ESCs are their different biochemical features due to differences in gene expression in early development between mice and humans. A number of studies have shown that human ESCs express stage-specific embryonic antigen 4 (SSEA-4), tumor rejection antigen-1-81 (TRA-1-81), TRA-1-60, and vimentin (Kaufman et al. 2001, Conley et al. 2004), whereas mouse ESCs express SSEA-1 and forkhead box d3 (FOXD3) (Loebel et al. 2003).

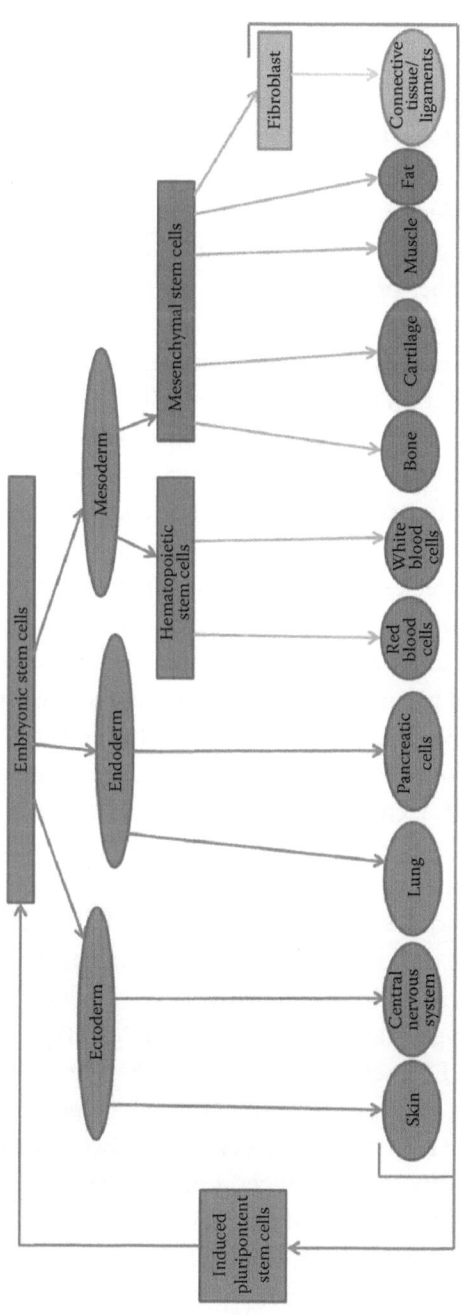

FIGURE 7.1 Schematic showing the different tissues that could be derived from stem cells. The diagram is representational and not entirely inclusive. ESCs can potentially be differentiated into all three germ layers. MSCs can differentiate into muscle, fat, bone, and cartilage. HSCs can differentiate into red and white blood cells. Fibroblasts can differentiate into connective tissue. iPSCs can potentially be generated from any adult cell type, and thereafter be directed to differentiate into multiple cell types, as with ESCs.

Nonetheless, both mouse and human ESCs express octamer-binding transcription factor 3 and 4 (OCT3/4), sex determining region box 2 (SOX-2), undifferentiated embryonic cell transcript factor 1 (UTF-1), REX-1, telomerase reverse transcriptase (TERT), telomeric repeat binding factor (TRF1), fibroblast growth factor receptor 4 (FGFR-4), nonog, and glucose transport 1 (Glut-1), with there being some disagreement on whether they both express SSEA-3 or not (Conley et al. 2004, Ginis et al. 2004). FGFR4 has been demonstrated to contribute to elastic fiber production in mice lungs, suggesting that stimulation of FGFR4 could cause ESCs to increase elastic fiber production and have potential as a proelastogenic therapy (Srisuma et al. 2010). Mouse ESCs are known to remain undifferentiated in a medium containing leukemia inhibitory factor (LIF), but human ESC differentiation is not suppressed with LIF supplements in the media (Burdon et al. 2002). Additionally, mouse ESCs form embryoid bodies (EB): spheroid colonies reminiscent of early embryogenesis, more easily than human ESCs do (Itskovitz-Eldor et al. 2000, Conley et al. 2004). Growth time and subsequent growth factor treatments vary between studies within the same species (Schuldiner et al. 2000). Nonetheless, specific lineage differentiation has not been achieved using the EB method in either species (Conley et al. 2004). On the basis of all the above differences between mouse and human ESCs, studies seeking to investigate ESC use for elastin regenerative repair applications must necessarily focus on human ESCs to avoid poor future clinical translatability of outcomes.

The addition of growth factors to non-EB cultures has been shown to be a useful approach to differentiate ESCs along specific lineages. The addition of bFGF and epidermal growth factor can differentiate ESCs into neuroepithelial progenitor cells (Reubinoff et al. 2001). ESCs can be differentiated into smooth muscle cells (SMCs), but first must be differentiated into MSCs, followed by the addition of TGF-β1 to the media to differentiate them to an SMC lineage (Boyd et al. 2009, Guo et al. 2013). SMCs can also be produced by an EB method, as shown by Ferreira et al. (2007). These SMCs are positive for alpha-actin-2 (ACTA2), calponin 1 (Cnn1), and myosin heavy chain 11 (Myh11) (Guo et al. 2013). Because neither the EB nor the growth factor method produces a pure differentiated population, flow cytometry sorting is required to obtain pure populations of differentiated cells (Levenberg et al. 2002, Conley et al. 2004).

A study using a porcine model of periodontal furcation found that ESCs implanted on a collagen matrix regenerated periodontal ligaments, which are composed primarily of elastin (Yang et al. 2013). ESC-derived SMCs and endothelial cells implanted together in nude mice can produce new microvessels and could represent a possible method to regenerate the elastic matrix in aneurysms (Ferreira et al. 2007), demonstrating that ESCs are also capable of differentiating into SMCs. Differentiation is not the only method by which ESCs could facilitate elastogenesis, as shown in Table 7.1. ESCs are also known to produce HGF and TGF-β1, which stimulate elastic fiber production (Bendall et al. 2009, Yousef et al. 2013).

ESCs have been well characterized, but further research is needed in the area of directed differentiation. They have great potential for the treatment of many diseases, not just elastin dysfunction disorders, but there are concerns that need to be taken into account if selecting them for a study. The type of feeder cells used to culture the ESCs and the method of differentiation are the two major considerations, in addition to ethical concerns regarding the use of ESCs in research and therapy.

7.3.2 Induced Pluripotent Stem Cells

iPSCs are derived from mature differentiated cell types, such as skin, which are then cultured under specific conditions to induce a stem cell-like phenotype. One of the advantages of iPSCs over ESCs is that iPSCs are derived from adult differentiated cells, and are dedifferentiated to a pluripotent state, removing the controversy of using embryonic cells (Takahashi and

TABLE 7.1 Examples of Elastic Matrix Molecules, Proelastic Factors, and Antiproteolytic Factors Produced by Cells, as well as differentiation of Cells into either SMCs or Fibroblasts

	Elastic Matrix Molecules	Proelastic Factors	Antiproteolytic Factors	Differentiation to Smooth Muscle Cells	Differentiation to Fibroblasts
ESC	FBLN1	HGF, TGF-β1	Not Currently Known	Guo et al. (2013), Ferreira et al. (2007)	Chen et al. (2009)
iPSC	Not Currently Known	HGF	Not Currently Known	Wanjare et al. (2013)	N/A
HSC	Not Currently Known	HGF, IGF-1, TGF-β1	Not Currently Known	Sreerekha et al. (2006)	Cossu and Bianco (2003)
MSC	ELN, FBLN1, FBN1, LOX, LOXL1,2,3,4	IGF-1, IGFBP-1, TGF-β1	TIMP1, TIMP2	Swaminathan et al. (2014)	Chang et al. (2014)
Fibroblast	ELN, FBN1	TGF-β1	TIMP1, TIMP2	Watson et al. (2014)	N/A

N/A is used for iPSCs because fibroblasts are the most commonly used cell to create iPSCs.

Yamanaka 2006), as illustrated in Figure 7.1. iPSCs are biochemically and morphologically similar to ESCs, and can differentiate into all three germ layers, as well as express the same cell surface markers as ESCs (humans: SSEA-4, TRA-1-81, TRA1-60; mouse: SSEA-1) (Novosadova and Grivennikov 2014). Additionally, there have been no chromosomal abnormalities reported with iPSCs (Novosadova and Grivennikov 2014). iPSCs can additionally be used autologously (Novosadova and Grivennikov 2014), so that the mature differentiated cells (e.g., dermal fibroblast) isolated from a donor tissue can then be used to derive iPSCs, which can then be differentiated to generate cell types for cell therapy.

Methods of deriving iPSCs from terminally differentiated cell types include viral, microRNA, and small molecule techniques (Mallanna et al. 2010, Subramanyam et al. 2011, Novosadova and Grivennikov 2014). All methods activate four transcription factors: OCT3, SOX-2, cellular myelocytomatosis oncogene homolog (c-Myc), and Kruppel-like family 4 (Klf4) to induce pluripotency (Takahashi Yamanaka 2006 and Nakagawa et al. 2008). OCT3, SOX-2, c-Myc, and Klf4 have all been shown to be important in controlling cell differentiation and are required to induce pluripotency experimentally (Dang et al. 2000, 2006, Boiani and Scholer 2005, Cheng et al. 2007). It is important to note that Klf4 is also key to the phenotypic switch to SMC differentiation that affects iPSC-derived SMCs and their use in elastogenic regeneration (Salmon et al. 2013).

The first technique to be used to induce pluripotency was viral transduction (Takahashi and Yamanaka 2006). However, with viral transduction there is a concern regarding genomic integration of the virus, so an episomal plasmid system that does not integrate into the genome has been used as an alternative method. The effectiveness of these methods is 0.1%–1.0% so only very few iPSCs are produced initially, although more can be created through expansion of relatively few starter cells (Fusaki et al. 2009, Novosadova and Grivennikov 2014).

Nonviral methods have been utilized to try to increase the efficiency of iPSC generation by using additional genes in combination with the above four transcription factors to induce pluripotency. The addition of liver receptor homolog-1 (LRH-1) and retinoic acid receptor gamma (Rarg) has improved efficiency, because LRH-1 and Rarg act together to promote OCT4 expression (Novosadova and Grivennikov 2014). MicroRNAs in addition to transcription factors can also facilitate induction of pluripotency (Subramanyam et al. 2011). Induction rates of nearly 100%

pluripotency have been achieved by inhibiting Mbd3 in addition to production of the four transcription factors, reprogramming skin cells into iPSCs within seven days (Kaji et al. 2007, Rais et al. 2013).

iPSCs generated via one of the methods described above can also facilitate elastic matrix regeneration by differentiation (Table 7.1). Exosomes from MSCs derived from iPSCs were shown to accelerate wound closure in a rat model by increasing elastin expression in resident fibroblasts with increased time and concentration exposure to the exosomes (Zhang et al. 2015). In addition, these exosomes in culture showed increased fibroblast migration in culture (Zhang et al. 2015). In culture, iPSCs can also be differentiated into SMCs through supplementation of exogenous platelet-derived growth factor–two beta chains (PDGF-BB), and TGF-β1 to the media (Wanjare et al. 2013). Wanjare et al. (2013) found that iPSCs could be induced to differentiate into SMCs with a contractile phenotype by depriving them of PDGF and reducing the serum concentration while not altering TGF-β1 concentration.

iPSCs can also be used to generate ex vivo culture-based model systems to screen for prospective elastic matrix regenerative therapeutics, and investigate intrinsic defects of elastogenesis. For example, iPSCs from patients with an ELN mutation have been used to generate a culture model of SVAS, which has been used to assess defects of the elastic fiber assembly process and to investigate regenerative therapies (Ge et al. 2012).

It is important to note that although potentially any differentiated cell could be transformed into an iPSC, the most popular source of differentiated cells as a source of iPSCs are skin fibroblasts (Novosadova and Grivennikov 2014). Other cell types used to produce iPSCs are skin cells, lymphocytes, hepatocytes, epithelial cells of the stomach, and hair follicles (Novosadova and Grivennikov 2014). iPSCs overcome the major critique of ESCs by not using embryos, with the added benefit of allowing for the choice of an allogeneic or autologous donor source. However, major obstacles that remain include directed differentiation, similar to that of ESCs, as well as the potential for complications due to viral integration.

7.3.3 Hematopoietic Stem Cells

The two major types of HSCs are primitive and defined HSCs (Orkin and Zon 2008). Primitive HSCs are obtained from the blood island cells of embryos and give rise to erythrocytes, myeloid cells, and hemogenic endothelium (Orkin 2000). There has been a continuing debate on whether primitive HSCs contribute to adult hematopoiesis (Baron 2013). Defined HSCs are obtained from bone marrow, peripheral blood, and umbilical cord blood in adults (Chen et al. 2015). Defined HSCs can differentiate into red blood cells, white blood cells, lymphocytes, and platelets causing them to be referred to as bone marrow progenitor cells (Orkin 2000), as illustrated in Figure 7.1. Defined HSCs are primarily used in research and are normally cultured on a plate coated with fibronectin, with a medium containing an endothelial basal medium (Kishore et al. 2013).

Defined mice HSCs negatively express Lin and stain positive for c-kit surface proteins, whereas defined human HSCs stain negative for both Lin and c-kit (Ayach et al. 2006, Kim et al. 2014). HSCs are known to migrate to vascular tissues that express CXCL12 (SDF-1) (Kiel and Morrison 2006, Nervi et al. 2006). The age of the donor is an important factor in determining the biology of HSCs (Orkin and Zon 2008), because HSCs from older donor mice have different self-renewal properties and gene expression patterns than HSCs derived from younger mice (Rossi et al. 2005). Older HSCs are less effective at homing in response to CXCL12 expression and have a stronger tendency to differentiate into myeloid cells than other cell lines (Sudo et al. 2000, Orkin and Zon 2008). A couple of studies have demonstrated a number of genes to be downregulated in older HSCs; it is therefore reasonable to assume that this would be the case for genes of proteins involved in elastic fiber assembly and homeostasis, although this requires confirmation (Rossi et al. 2005, Nijnik et al. 2007).

The ability of HSCs to home to heart tissue in response to CXCL12 release after vascular injury has made them important for regeneration of vascular tissues (Ayach et al. 2006; Kim et al. 2014). Once HSCs home to injured vascular tissues, such as in myocardial infarction, they secrete HGF, IGF-1, and TGF-β1, all of which promote elastogenesis (Kim et al. 2014). Additionally, HSCs cultured under conditions optimized for endothelial cells and then delivered to an infarcted heart were found to generate IGF-1 and TGF-β1, factors known to promote elastogenesis, although elastic fiber formation itself was not assessed (Kim et al. 2014). HSCs can also differentiate into SMCs when cultured on fibrin-coated substrates (Sreerekha et al. 2006). Although these cells could potentially be used for matrix regeneration in proteolytically disrupted tissues, not much is known about their elastogenic potential.

The major limitation of HSCs is the difficulty of expanding them (Chen et al. 2015). Few HSCs can be harvested from bone marrow and other sources, which has led to the interest in using HSCs generated from iPSCs instead (Chen et al. 2015).

7.3.4 Mesenchymal Stem Cells

MSCs have also been referred to as stromal stem cells and pericytes, cells known to be associated with the capillaries. They are no longer referred to as stromal stem cells, because there are no major differences between MSCs and pericytes of different tissue types (Mills et al. 2013), although the two cell types have been shown to differ in their regenerative properties (Sundberg et al. 1993). MSCs have been harvested from multiple tissues, including bone marrow, muscle, adipose, and renal tissues in multiple species (Ding et al. 2011). Except for minor differences between species, the conditions necessary for MSC culture are rather similar (Peister et al. 2004, Barzilay et al. 2009). Culture of human MSCs is moving away from the medium containing animal proteins to a more defined media, often involving serum replacement for similar reasons as those for ESCs: to enable therapy without xenogeneic risks due to animal proteins in the culture media (Capelli et al. 2007).

MSCs were first defined by their ability to adhere to the culture flask after being harvested from bone marrow (Friedenstein et al. 1970), and are now defined by the presence or absence of multiple cell surface markers. Human MSCs are positive for CD73, CD90, CD105, and CD106 and negative for CD11b, CD14, CD31, CD34, and CD45 (Barzilay et al. 2009, Castro-Manrreza and Montesinos 2015). In contrast, mouse MSCs have been shown to stain positive for CD34 and negative for CD90 (Peister et al. 2004). In addition to cell surface markers, MSCs must also display an ability to differentiate into adipocytes, chondrocytes, and osteocytes *in vitro* (Castro-Manrreza and Montesinos 2015), as outlined in Figure 7.1. MSCs are prized for their immunoregulatory properties, which are an advantage for their application to allogeneic regenerative therapies. Studies have shown that MSCs can prevent activation of CD29 and CD69 in T-lymphocytes, preventing activation of the immune response (Castro-Manrreza and Montesinos 2015). Another feature of MSCs that makes them useful for *in situ* tissue repair is their ability to home to areas of injury following a CCL7 (MCP-3) gradient (Schenk et al. 2007). It is this ability that has led to investigation into their potential use for wound-healing applications

(Gnecchi et al. 2008, Deng et al. 2015). These studies suggest that the secretome of these cells facilitates matrix regeneration and tissue recovery, and regeneration rather than physical engraftment of the MSCs at the injury site and their subsequent differentiation (Caplan et al. 2006, Penn 2012, Tran and Damaser 2015). Modulating the culture conditions of these cells is one means of augmenting their paracrine secretions of elastogenic and antiproteolytic enzymes, *in vivo*. Alternatively, the conditioned medium collected from these cell cultures may be used for regenerative therapy, although there are likely to be issues related to quality control and patient-to-patient variability. For example, MSCs cultured in hypoxic conditions produce greater amounts of bFGF and HGF (Tsai et al. 2012). Similarly, when cultured in a 3D spheroid, MSCs increase production of bFGF, HGF, MMP2, MMP9, and TGF-β1, while culturing them in serum-free media increases TIMP1, TIMP2, IGF-1, and HGF production (Oskowitz et al. 2011, Santos et al. 2015), all of which are known to influence one of more aspects of elastic matrix neoassembly and regenerative repair.

Recent research has begun to elucidate the mechanisms underlying the proelastin regenerative effects of MSCs and MSC-based therapies (Swaminathan et al. 2014, Tian et al. 2014). In one study, rat aorta tissue from an abdominal aortic aneurysm model was harvested and cocultured with either adipose-derived MSCs or bone marrow-derived MSCs and demonstrated increased elastin fiber formation compared to control aorta tissue not cocultured with either MSC type (Tian et al. 2014). In another study, when bone marrow-derived MSCs were first differentiated into SMC-like cells, and then cocultured with aneurysmal SMCs from rats in noncontact mode, gene expression of elastin, fibulin 1, and fibulin 5 was increased (Swaminathan et al. 2014). Elastin deposition was also increased in this group, as seen in Figure 7.2, demonstrating that MSCs have the ability to regenerate elastin even when predifferentiated into SMCs.

MSCs injected into the infarcted heart have also been shown to decrease fibrosis (Mias et al. 2009). Gel zymography assays of the medium from cardiac fibroblasts cultured with the MSC-conditioned medium showed increased activity of both MMP2 and MMP9 compared to either the fibroblast-conditioned medium or the MSC-conditioned medium alone, suggesting that MSCs could have an effect on the local fibroblast population, causing them to change their expression of TIMP2 and MMP2 (Mias et al. 2009, Chen et al. 2014). This effect is likely via factors secreted by MSCs that act on the local fibroblasts to promote a more synthetic phenotype.

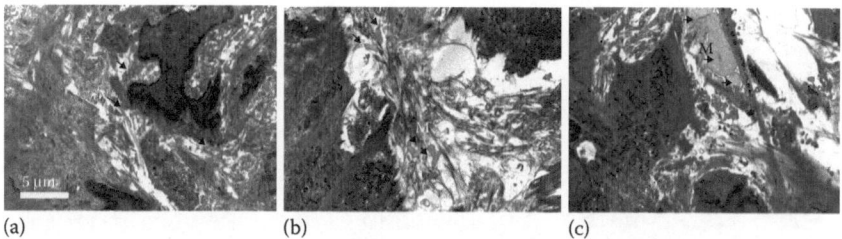

(a)   (b)   (c)

FIGURE 7.2   Representative TEM images illustrating the impact of culture with SMLC-conditioned medium on elastic matrix deposition by rat aneurysmal SMC (RASMCs). Cells were cultured for a total of 21 days. The arrows show amorphous elastin deposits and "M" shows microfibrillar structures in cultures corresponding to 0:1 (a), 0.5:1 (b), and 2:1 (c) ratios of seeding counts of SMLCs to RASMCs. While an increased number of amorphous elastin deposits were observed in test cultures relative to controls, few mature elastic fibers were seen. (Reprinted with permission from Swaminathan, G. et al., *J. Tissue Eng. Regen. Med.*, 2014. doi: 10.1002/term.1964.)

In similar studies, Deng et al. (2015) demonstrated that either MSCs or concentrated aliquots of CCM from MSCs could facilitate elastic fiber formation *in vivo* in a rat model of stress urinary incontinence. In this study, the MSCs were delivered via a tail vein injection and CCM was injected intraperitoneally in different animals with their own set of controls. Three weeks later, elastic fibers were increased in the urethra of both treatment groups compared to sham treatment, as seen in Figure 7.3, demonstrating that (a) physical engraftment at the site of tissue injury of MSCs is not necessary for tissue repair and that (b) nonlocal administration of MSC CCM can facilitate new elastin fiber formation. This study reinforced the idea that secretions of MSCs stimulate elastogenesis by fibroblasts and SMCs (Deng et al. 2015).

7.3.5 Fibroblasts

Fibroblasts are progenitor cells whose normal function is to maintain homeostasis of the ECM and facilitate in wound healing (Sivaraman et al. 2012, Chang et al. 2014). They are one of the most abundant cells in connective tissue and have been studied extensively (Chang et al. 2014). Fibroblasts originate from MSCs, as illustrated in Figure 8.1. They can also arise from other sources, including innate fibroblasts or from

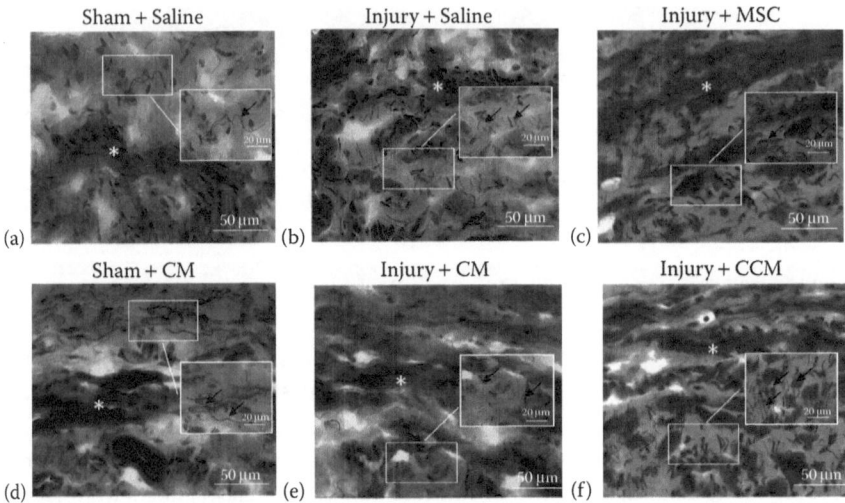

FIGURE 7.3 Representative images of urethras stained with elastin von Gieson stain. (a) and (d) received sham injury and sham treatment with either saline (a) or control media (d). (b) and (e) received the injury and sham treatment with either saline (b) or control media (e). (c) and (f) received the injury and the treatment with either MSC (c) or CCM (f). The white asterisk indicates the external urethral sphincter. Similar increases in elastin fibers were seen in both MSC and CCM treatments compared to injured sham-treated animals. (Reprinted with permission from Deng, K. et al., *Am. J. Physiol. Renal. Physiol.*, 308, F92, 2015.)

epithelial cells, through a process called epithelial–mesenchymal transition in which epithelial cells dedifferentiate into fibroblasts (Chang et al. 2014). Monocytes and HSCs can also differentiate into fibroblasts (Cossu and Bianco 2003, Chang et al. 2014).

Fibroblasts have been collected from multiple tissues, including heart, smooth muscle, and tendon from multiple species (Chang et al. 2014). Their nomenclature is generally based on their tissue of origin. For example, fibroblasts harvested from cardiac tissue are referred to as cardiac fibroblasts. Due to their diverse distribution, fibroblasts have been harvested from many different tissues. To properly identify them, a list of specific fibroblast markers has been defined (Chang et al. 2014), which include positive expression of vimentin, discoidin domain receptor (DDR2), CD90, alpha 8 beta 1 ($\alpha 8\beta 1$) integrin, fibroblast specific protein 1 (FSP1), smooth muscle α actin, and fibroblast-activation protein (Chang et al. 2014, Walmsley et al. 2015). There are also similarities in gene expression between stem cells and fibroblasts. Cultured fibroblasts express OCT4, a transcription factor also expressed by ESCs and iPSCs. Embryonic fibroblasts express CD70 and CD105, and stain negative for CD11b and CD45, similar to bone marrow derived MSCs (Chang et al. 2014). Embryonic fibroblasts can also differentiate into adipocytes and chondrocytes, similar to MSCs (Chang et al. 2014).

In the early 1990s, Fleischmajer et al. (1993) demonstrated that fibroblasts cocultured with keratinocytes stimulated ECM formation by keratinocytes. This was prior to identification of many of the previously mentioned elastogenic factors. Gogly et al. (2007) showed that fibroblasts decrease elastin fiber degradation in cultured aortic rings obtained from abdominal aortic aneurysm segments. Immunohistochemistry showed aneurysmal aorta rings cultured without fibroblasts generated higher levels of MMP9 compared to those cultured with fibroblasts (Gogly et al. 2007). Expression of TIMP1, an inhibitor of MMP9, was also increased in the aneurysmal aorta rings cultured with fibroblasts (Gogly et al. 2007). Conditioned media from the aorta culture were compared and indicated the TIMP1 levels to be much greater in the cocultured rings compared to either the stand-alone aorta ring or fibroblast cultures, with positive implications as to the integrity of neoassembled elastic fibers. This was confirmed to result from synergy in TIMP1 release between aorta SMCs and fibroblasts.

Additional benefits of cell-to-cell communication involving fibroblasts to alleviate fibrosis was demonstrated when fibroblasts were injected into an infarcted heart. While the injected fibroblasts reduced the size of the infarct and prevented fibrosis, when the fibroblasts were injected together with endothelial progenitor cells, scar formation was further reduced and functional recovery of the heart was promoted (Kobayashi et al. 2008). Cardiac fibroblasts have also been shown to differentiate into myofibroblast cell types capable of elastin synthesis in a hypoxic microenvironment, suggesting that these conditions could be useful for elastic matrix regeneration by fibroblasts (Watson et al. 2014). The involvement of fibroblasts in ECM homeostasis under both normal and pathologic conditions makes them an important option in cellular regeneration of elastin, as shown in Table 7.1.

7.4 CONCLUSIONS

There are many stem cells and progenitor cells used in research today, with different mechanisms of action, that is, via their directed differentiation along specific lineages, or via their secretions. While stem cell/progenitor engraftment and *in situ* differentiation was the method of action long presumed to account for the regenerative benefits of stem cells, it is known to not be the case for all cell types in all situations today. In light of the regenerative benefits of stem cell secretions, even when the source stem cells are not physically present, it is clear that they are sufficient for therapeutic action. However, there are issues related to (a) inherent difficulties in maintaining quality control over CCM, (b) significant patient-to-patient variability in CCM composition, (c) presence of other biological factors not involved in influencing or regulating elastogenesis but with potentially adverse or undesired effects, and (d) potentially adverse systemic effects associated with systemic CCM delivery. On this basis, ongoing research is focused on identifying key factors in the stem cell secretome that are necessary and sufficient for their proelastogenic and antiproteolytic effects, which can drive emerging stem cell-inspired small molecular therapeutic strategies based on delivery of these specific identified biological factors.

ACKNOWLEDGMENTS

Funding was received from NIH Grant 1R21HD078820 and RO1 HD059859 and the Cleveland Clinic and VA 101RX000228.

REFERENCES

All AH, Bazley FA, Gupta S et al. Human embryonic stem cell-derived oligodendrocyte progenitors aid in functional recovery of sensory pathways following contusive spinal cord injury. *PLoS One* 7(10) 2012: e47645.

Amantea CM, Kim WK, Meliton V, Tetradis S, Parhami F. Oxysterol-induced osteogenic differentiation of marrow stromal cells is regulated by Dkk-1 inhibitable and PI3-kinase mediated signaling. *J Cell Biochem* 105(2) 2008: 424–436.

Arikawa T, Matsukawa A, Watanabe K et al. Galectin-9 accelerates transforming growth factor beta3-induced differentiation of human mesenchymal stem cells to chondrocytes. *Bone* 44(5) 2009: 849–857.

Ayach BB, Yoshimitsu M, Dawood F et al. Stem cell factor receptor induces progenitor and natural killer cell-mediated cardiac survival and repair after myocardial infarction. *Proc Natl Acad Sci USA* 103(7) 2006: 2304–2309.

Ayatollahi M, Soleimani M, Tabei SZ, Kabir SM. Hepatogenic differentiation of mesenchymal stem cells induced by insulin like growth factor-I. *World J Stem Cells* 3(12) 2011: 113–121.

Balsam LB, Wagers AJ, Christensen JL, Kofidis T, Weissman IL, Robbins RC. Haematopoietic stem cells adopt mature haematopoietic fates in ischaemic myocardium. *Nature* 428(6983) 2004: 668–673.

Baron MH. Concise review: Early embryonic erythropoiesis: not so primitive after all. *Stem Cells* 31(5) 2013: 849–856.

Barzilay R, Sadan O, Melamed E, Offen D. Comparative characterization of bone marrow-derived mesenchymal stromal cells from four different rat strains. *Cytotherapy* 11(4) 2009: 435–442.

Baxter RC. Insulin-like growth factor (IGF)-binding proteins: Interactions with IGFs and intrinsic bioactivities. *Am J Physiol Endocrinol Metab* 278(6) 2000: E967–E976.

Bendall SC, Hughes C, Campbell JL et al. An enhanced mass spectrometry approach reveals human embryonic stem cell growth factors in culture. *Mol Cell Proteomics* 8(3) 2009: 421–432.

Benkerrou M. Indications for allogeneic hematopoietic stem cell transplantion in sickle cell disease. *Rev Prat* 64(8) 2014: 1130–1131.

Boiani M, Scholer HR. Regulatory networks in embryo-derived pluripotent stem cells. *Nat Rev Mol Cell Biol* 6(11) 2005: 872–884.

Boyd NL, Robbins KR, Dhara SK, West FD, Stice SL. Human embryonic stem cell-derived mesoderm-like epithelium transitions to mesenchymal progenitor cells. *Tissue Eng Part A* 15(8) 2009: 1897–1907.

Budatha M, Roshanravan S, Zheng Q et al. Extracellular matrix proteases contribute to progression of pelvic organ prolapse in mice and humans. *J Clin Invest* 121(5) 2011: 2048–2059.

Burdon T, Smith A, Savatier P. Signalling, cell cycle and pluripotency in embryonic stem cells. *Trends Cell Biol* 12(9) 2002: 432–438.

Capelli C, Domenghini M, Borleri G et al. Human platelet lysate allows expansion and clinical grade production of mesenchymal stromal cells from small samples of bone marrow aspirates or marrow filter washouts. *Bone Marrow Transplant* 40(8) 2007: 785–791.

Caplan AI, Dennis JE. Mesenchymal stem cells as trophic mediators. *J Cell Biochem* 98(5) 2006: 1076–1084.

Castro-Manrreza ME, Montesinos JJ. Immunoregulation by Mesenchymal Stem Cells: Biological Aspects and Clinical Applications. *J Immunol Res* 2015 2015: 394917.

Chang Y, Li H, Guo Z. Mesenchymal stem cell-like properties in fibroblasts. *Cell Physiol Biochem* 34(3) 2014: 703–714.

Chen HF, Chuang CY, Shieh YK, Chang HW, Ho HN, Kuo HC. Novel autogenic feeders derived from human embryonic stem cells (hESCs) support an undifferentiated status of hESCs in xeno-free culture conditions. *Hum Reprod* 24(5) 2009: 1114–1125.

Chen P, Wu R, Zhu W et al. Hypoxia preconditioned mesenchymal stem cells prevent cardiac fibroblast activation and collagen production via leptin. *PLoS One* 9(8) 2014: e103587.

Chen T, Wang F, Wu M, Wang ZZ. Development of hematopoietic stem and progenitor cells from human pluripotent stem cells. *J Cell Biochem* 116(7) 2015: 1179–1189.

Cheng L, Hammond H, Ye Z, Zhan X, Dravid G. Human adult marrow cells support prolonged expansion of human embryonic stem cells in culture. *Stem Cells* 21(2) 2003: 131–142.

Cheng L, Sung MT, Cossu-Rocca P et al. OCT4: Biological functions and clinical applications as a marker of germ cell neoplasia. *J Pathol* 211(1) 2007: 1–9.

Conley BJ, Young JC, Trounson AO, Mollard R. Derivation, propagation and differentiation of human embryonic stem cells. *Int J Biochem Cell Biol* 36(4) 2004: 555–567.

Cossu G, Bianco P. Mesoangioblasts – vascular progenitors for extravascular mesodermal tissues. *Curr Opin Genet Dev* 13(5) 2003: 537–542.

Dang CV, O'Donnell KA, Zeller KI, Nguyen T, Osthus RC, Li F. The c-Myc target gene network. *Semin Cancer Biol* 16(4) 2006: 253–264.

Dang DT, Pevsner J, Yang VW. The biology of the mammalian Kruppel-like family of transcription factors. *Int J Biochem Cell Biol* 32(11–12) 2000: 1103–1121.

Deng K, Lin DL, Hanzlicek B et al. Mesenchymal stem cells and their secretome partially restore nerve and urethral function in a dual muscle and nerve injury stress urinary incontinence model. *Am J Physiol Renal Physiol* 308(2) 2015: F92–F100.

Ding DC, Shyu WC, Lin SZ. Mesenchymal stem cells. *Cell Transplant* 20(1) 2011: 5–14.

Ferreira LS, Gerecht S, Shieh HF et al. Vascular progenitor cells isolated from human embryonic stem cells give rise to endothelial and smooth muscle like cells and form vascular networks in vivo. *Circ Res* 101(3) 2007: 286–294.

Fleischmajer R, MacDonald ED, Contard P, Perlish JS. Immunochemistry of a keratinocyte-fibroblast co-culture model for reconstruction of human skin. *J Histochem Cytochem* 41(9) 1993: 1359–1366.

Friedenstein AJ, Chailakhjan RK, Lalykina KS. The development of fibroblast colonies in monolayer cultures of guinea-pig bone marrow and spleen cells. *Cell Tissue Kinet* 3(4) 1970: 393–403.

Fulcher YG, Van Doren SR. Remote exosites of the catalytic domain of matrix metalloproteinase-12 enhance elastin degradation. *Biochemistry* 50(44) 2011: 9488–9499.

Fusaki N, Ban H, Nishiyama A, Saeki K, Hasegawa M. Efficient induction of transgene-free human pluripotent stem cells using a vector based on Sendai virus, an RNA virus that does not integrate into the host genome. *Proc Jpn Acad Ser B Phys Biol Sci* 85(8) 2009: 348–362.

Gacchina CE, Ramamurthi A. Impact of pre-existing elastic matrix on TGFbeta1 and HA oligomer-induced regenerative elastin repair by rat aortic smooth muscle cells. *J Tissue Eng Regen Med* 5(2) 2011: 85–96.

Ge X, Ren Y, Bartulos O et al. Modeling supravalvular aortic stenosis syndrome with human induced pluripotent stem cells. *Circulation* 126(14) 2012: 1695–1704.

Gilbert SF. The stem cell concept. In: *Developmental Biology.* Sunderland, MA: Sinauer Associates, 2010; 323–331.

Ginis I, Luo Y, Miura T et al. Differences between human and mouse embryonic stem cells. *Dev Biol* 269(2) 2004: 360–380.

Gnecchi M, Zhang Z, Ni A, Dzau VJ. Paracrine mechanisms in adult stem cell signaling and therapy. *Circ Res* 103(11) 2008: 1204–1219.

Gogly B, Naveau A, Fournier B et al. Preservation of rabbit aorta elastin from degradation by gingival fibroblasts in an ex vivo model. *Arterioscler Thromb Vasc Biol* 27(9) 2007: 1984–1990.

Guo X, Stice SL, Boyd NL, Chen SY. A novel in vitro model system for smooth muscle differentiation from human embryonic stem cell-derived mesenchymal cells. *Am J Physiol Cell Physiol* 304(4) 2013: C289–C298.

Halper J, Kjaer M. Basic components of connective tissues and extracellular matrix: Elastin, fibrillin, fibulins, fibrinogen, fibronectin, laminin, tenascins and thrombospondins. *Adv Exp Med Biol* 802, 2014: 31–47.

Harvey A, Yen TY, Aizman I, Tate C, Case C. Proteomic analysis of the extracellular matrix produced by mesenchymal stromal cells: implications for cell therapy mechanism. *PLoS One* 8(11) 2013: e79283.

Hashizume R, Yamawaki-Ogata A, Ueda Y, Wagner WR, Narita Y. Mesenchymal stem cells attenuate angiotensin II-induced aortic aneurysm growth in apolipoprotein E-deficient mice. *J Vasc Surg* 54(6) 2011: 1743–1752.

Hayashi K, Fong KS, Mercier F, Boyd CD, Csiszar K, Hayashi M. Comparative immunocytochemical localization of lysyl oxidase (LOX) and the lysyl oxidase-like (LOXL) proteins: Changes in the expression of LOXL during development and growth of mouse tissues. *J Mol Histol* 35(8–9) 2004: 845–855.

Hirano S, Bless D, Heisey D, Ford C. Roles of hepatocyte growth factor and transforming growth factor beta1 in production of extracellular matrix by canine vocal fold fibroblasts. *Laryngoscope* 113(1) 2003: 144–148.

Hung SP, Ho JH, Shih YR, Lo T, Lee OK. Hypoxia promotes proliferation and osteogenic differentiation potentials of human mesenchymal stem cells. *J Orthop Res* 30(2) 2012: 260–266.

Itskovitz-Eldor J, Schuldiner M, Karsenti D et al. Differentiation of human embryonic stem cells into embryoid bodies compromising the three embryonic germ layers. *Mol Med* 6(2) 2000: 88–95.

Kaji K, Nichols J, Hendrich B. Mbd3, a component of the NuRD co-repressor complex, is required for development of pluripotent cells. *Development* 134(6) 2007: 1123–1132.

Kaufman DS, Hanson ET, Lewis RL, Auerbach R, Thomson JA. Hematopoietic colony-forming cells derived from human embryonic stem cells. *Proc Natl Acad Sci USA* 98(19) 2001: 10716–10721.

Kiel MJ, Morrison SJ. Maintaining hematopoietic stem cells in the vascular niche. *Immunity* 25(6) 2006: 862–864.

Kielty CM, Sherratt MJ, Shuttleworth CA. Elastic fibres. *J Cell Sci* 115(Pt 14) 2002: 2817–2828.

Kim JH, Lee EH, Park HJ et al. The role of lysyl oxidase-like 2 in the odontogenic differentiation of human dental pulp stem cells. *Mol Cells* 35(6) 2013: 543–549.

Kim SW, Houge M, Brown M, Davis ME, Yoon YS. Cultured human bone marrow-derived CD31(+) cells are effective for cardiac and vascular repair through enhanced angiogenic, adhesion, and anti-inflammatory effects. *J Am Coll Cardiol* 64(16) 2014: 1681–1694.

Kishore R, Verma SK, Mackie AR et al. Bone marrow progenitor cell therapy-mediated paracrine regulation of cardiac miRNA-155 modulates fibrotic response in diabetic hearts. *PLoS One* 8(4) 2013: e60161.

Kobayashi H, Shimizu T, Yamato M et al. Fibroblast sheets co-cultured with endothelial progenitor cells improve cardiac function of infarcted hearts. *J Artif Organs* 11(3) 2008: 141–147.

Kothapalli CR, Ramamurthi A. Benefits of concurrent delivery of hyaluronan and IGF-1 cues to regeneration of crosslinked elastin matrices by adult rat vascular cells. *J Tissue Eng Regen Med* 2(2–3) 2008: 106–116.

Kothapalli CR, Taylor PM, Smolenski RT, Yacoub MH, Ramamurthi A. Transforming growth factor beta 1 and hyaluronan oligomers synergistically enhance elastin matrix regeneration by vascular smooth muscle cells. *Tissue Eng Part A* 15(3) 2009: 501–511.

Kubal C, Sheth K, Nadal-Ginard B, Galinanes M. Bone marrow cells have a potent anti-ischemic effect against myocardial cell death in humans. *J Thorac Cardiovasc Surg* 132(5) 2006: 1112–1118.

Lau AC, Duong TT, Ito S, Yeung RS. Matrix metalloproteinase 9 activity leads to elastin breakdown in an animal model of Kawasaki disease. *Arthritis Rheum* 58(3) 2008: 854–863.

Levenberg S, Golub JS, Amit M, Itskovitz-Eldor J, Langer R. Endothelial cells derived from human embryonic stem cells. *Proc Natl Acad Sci USA* 99(7) 2002: 4391–4396.

Loebel DA, Watson CM, De Young RA, Tam PP. Lineage choice and differentiation in mouse embryos and embryonic stem cells. *Dev Biol* 264(1) 2003: 1–14.

Losy F, Dai J, Pages C et al. Paracrine secretion of transforming growth factor-beta1 in aneurysm healing and stabilization with endovascular smooth muscle cell therapy. *J Vasc Surg* 37(6) 2003: 1301–1309.

Makridakis M, Roubelakis MG, Vlahou A. Stem cells: Insights into the secretome. *Biochim Biophys Acta* 1834(11) 2013: 2380–2384.

Mallanna SK, Rizzino A. Emerging roles of microRNAs in the control of embryonic stem cells and the generation of induced pluripotent stem cells. *Dev Biol* 344(1) 2010: 16–25.

Mias C, Lairez O, Trouche E et al. Mesenchymal stem cells promote matrix metalloproteinase secretion by cardiac fibroblasts and reduce cardiac ventricular fibrosis after myocardial infarction. *Stem Cells* 27(11) 2009: 2734–2743.

Milewicz DM, Urban Z, Boyd C. Genetic disorders of the elastic fiber system. *Matrix Biol* 19(6) 2000: 471–480.

Mills SJ, Cowin AJ, Kaur P. Pericytes, mesenchymal stem cells and the wound healing process. *Cells* 2(3) 2013: 621–634.

Murry CE, Soonpaa MH, Reinecke H et al. Haematopoietic stem cells do not transdifferentiate into cardiac myocytes in myocardial infarcts. *Nature* 428(6983) 2004: 664–668.

Nakagawa M, Koyanagi M, Tanabe K et al. Generation of induced pluripotent stem cells without Myc from mouse and human fibroblasts. *Nat Biotechnol* 26(1) 2008: 101–106.

Nervi B, Link DC, DiPersio JF. Cytokines and hematopoietic stem cell mobilization. *J Cell Biochem* 99(3) 2006: 690–705.

Nijnik A, Woodbine L, Marchetti C et al. DNA repair is limiting for haematopoietic stem cells during ageing. *Nature* 447(7145) 2007: 686–690.

Novosadova EV, Grivennikov IA. Induced pluripotent stem cells: From derivation to application in biochemical and biomedical research. *Biochemistry (Mosc)* 79(13) 2014: 1425–1441.

Okada Y, Morodomi T, Enghild JJ et al. Matrix metalloproteinase 2 from human rheumatoid synovial fibroblasts. Purification and activation of the precursor and enzymic properties. *Eur J Biochem* 194(3) 1990: 721–730.

Orkin SH. Diversification of haematopoietic stem cells to specific lineages. *Nat Rev Genet* 1(1) 2000: 57–64.

Orkin SH, Zon LI. Hematopoiesis: An evolving paradigm for stem cell biology. *Cell* 132(4) 2008: 631–644.

Orlic D, Kajstura J, Chimenti S, Bodine DM, Leri A, Anversa P. Bone marrow stem cells regenerate infarcted myocardium. *Pediatr Transplant* 7(Suppl 3) 2003: 86–88.

Oskowitz A, McFerrin H, Gutschow M, Carter ML, Pochampally R. Serum-deprived human multipotent mesenchymal stromal cells (MSCs) are highly angiogenic. *Stem Cell Res* 6(3) 2011: 215–225.

Peister A, Mellad JA, Larson BL, Hall BM, Gibson LF, Prockop DJ. Adult stem cells from bone marrow (MSCs) isolated from different strains of inbred mice vary in surface epitopes, rates of proliferation, and differentiation potential. *Blood* 103(5) 2004: 1662–1668.

Penn MS. Are stem cells the teacher or the student? *Curr Opin Organ Transplant* 17(6) 2012: 663–669.

Qa'aty N, Wang Y, Wang A et al. The antidiabetic hormone glucagon-like peptide-1 induces formation of new elastic fibers in human cardiac fibroblasts after cross-activation of IGF-IR. *Endocrinology* 156(1) 2015: 90–102.

Rais Y, Zviran A, Geula S et al. Deterministic direct reprogramming of somatic cells to pluripotency. *Nature* 502(7469) 2013: 65–70.

Reubinoff BE, Itsykson P, Turetsky T et al. Neural progenitors from human embryonic stem cells. *Nat Biotechnol* 19(12) 2001: 1134–1140.

Reubinoff BE, Pera MF, Fong CY, Trounson A, Bongso A. Embryonic stem cell lines from human blastocysts: Somatic differentiation in vitro. *Nat Biotechnol* 18(4) 2000: 399–404.

Rossi DJ, Bryder D, Zahn JM et al. Cell intrinsic alterations underlie hematopoietic stem cell aging. *Proc Natl Acad Sci USA* 102(26) 2005: 9194–9199.

Salmon M, Johnston WF, Woo A et al. KLF4 regulates abdominal aortic aneurysm morphology and deletion attenuates aneurysm formation. *Circulation* 128(11 Suppl 1) 2013: S163–S174.

Santos JM, Camoes SP, Filipe E et al. 3D spheroid cell culture of umbilical cord tissue-derived MSCs (UCX) leads to enhanced paracrine induction of wound healing. *Stem Cell Res Ther* 6(1) 2015: 90.

Schenk S, Mal N, Finan A et al. Monocyte chemotactic protein-3 is a myocardial mesenchymal stem cell homing factor. *Stem Cells* 25(1) 2007: 245–251.

Schuldiner M, Yanuka O, Itskovitz-Eldor J, Melton DA, Benvenisty N. Effects of eight growth factors on the differentiation of cells derived from human embryonic stem cells. *Proc Natl Acad Sci USA* 97(21) 2000: 11307–11312.

Sekiya N, Matsumiya G, Miyagawa S et al. Layered implantation of myoblast sheets attenuates adverse cardiac remodeling of the infarcted heart. *J Thorac Cardiovasc Surg* 138(4) 2009: 985–993.

Shabbir A, Zisa D, Suzuki G, Lee T. Heart failure therapy mediated by the trophic activities of bone marrow mesenchymal stem cells: a noninvasive therapeutic regimen. *Am J Physiol Heart Circ Physiol* 296(6) 2009: H1888–H1897.

Shen M, Lee J, Basu R et al. Divergent roles of matrix metalloproteinase 2 in pathogenesis of thoracic aortic aneurysm. *Arterioscler Thromb Vasc Biol* 35(4) 2015: 888–898.

Shynlova O, Bortolini MA, Alarab M. Genes responsible for vaginal extracellular matrix metabolism are modulated by women's reproductive cycle and menopause. *Int Braz J Urol* 39(2) 2013: 257–267.

Simionescu A, Philips K, Vyavahare N. Elastin-derived peptides and TGF-beta1 induce osteogenic responses in smooth muscle cells. *Biochem Biophys Res Commun* 334(2) 2005: 524–532.

Sivaraman B, Bashur CA, Ramamurthi A. Advances in biomimetic regeneration of elastic matrix structures. *Drug Deliv Transl Res* 2(5) 2012: 323–350.

Sreerekha PR, Divya P, Krishnan LK. Adult stem cell homing and differentiation in vitro on composite fibrin matrix. *Cell Prolif* 39(4) 2006: 301–312.

Srisuma S, Bhattacharya S, Simon DM et al. Fibroblast growth factor receptors control epithelial-mesenchymal interactions necessary for alveolar elastogenesis. *Am J Respir Crit Care Med* 181(8) 2010: 838–850.

Subramanyam D, Lamouille S, Judson RL et al. Multiple targets of miR-302 and miR-372 promote reprogramming of human fibroblasts to induced pluripotent stem cells. *Nat Biotechnol* 29(5) 2011: 443–448.

Sudo K, Ema H, Morita Y, Nakauchi H. Age-associated characteristics of murine hematopoietic stem cells. *J Exp Med* 192(9) 2000: 1273–1280.

Sundberg C, Ljungstrom M, Lindmark G, Gerdin B, Rubin K. Microvascular pericytes express platelet-derived growth factor-beta receptors in human healing wounds and colorectal adenocarcinoma. *Am J Pathol* 143(5) 1993: 1377–1388.

Swaminathan G, Gadepalli VS, Stoilov I, Mecham RP, Rao RR, Ramamurthi A. Pro-elastogenic effects of bone marrow mesenchymal stem cell-derived smooth muscle cells on cultured aneurysmal smooth muscle cells. *J Tissue Eng Regen Med* 2014. doi: 10.1002/term.1964.

Takahashi K, Yamanaka S. Induction of pluripotent stem cells from mouse embryonic and adult fibroblast cultures by defined factors. *Cell* 126(4) 2006: 663–676.

Tanabe K, Takahashi K, Yamanaka S. Induction of pluripotency by defined factors. *Proc Jpn Acad Ser B Phys Biol Sci* 90(3) 2014: 83–96.

Thomson JA, Itskovitz-Eldor J, Shapiro SS et al. Embryonic stem cell lines derived from human blastocysts. *Science* 282(5391) 1998: 1145–1147.

Thomson JA, Marshall V.S. Primate embryonic stem cells. *Curr Top Dev Biol* 38 1998: 133–165.

Tian X, Fan J, Yu M et al. Adipose stem cells promote smooth muscle cells to secrete elastin in rat abdominal aortic aneurysm. *PLoS One* 9(9) 2014: e108105.

Tran C, Damaser MS. Stem cells as drug delivery methods: Application of stem cell secretome for regeneration. *Adv Drug Deliv Rev* 82–83C 2015: 1–11.

Tsai CC, Yew TL, Yang DC, Huang WH, Hung SC. Benefits of hypoxic culture on bone marrow multipotent stromal cells. *Am J Blood Res* 2(3) 2012: 148–159.

Wagenseil JE, Mecham RP. New insights into elastic fiber assembly. *Birth Defects Res C Embryo Today* 81(4) 2007: 229–240.

Walmsley GG, Rinkevich Y, Hu MS et al. Live fibroblast harvest reveals surface marker shift in vitro. *Tissue Eng Part C Methods* 21(3) 2015: 314–321.

Wanjare M, Kuo F, Gerecht S. Derivation and maturation of synthetic and contractile vascular smooth muscle cells from human pluripotent stem cells. *Cardiovasc Res* 97(2) 2013: 321–330.

Watson CJ, Collier P, Tea I et al. Hypoxia-induced epigenetic modifications are associated with cardiac tissue fibrosis and the development of a myofibroblast-like phenotype. *Hum Mol Genet* 23(8) 2014: 2176–2188.

Wolfe BL, Rich CB, Goud HD et al. Insulin-like growth factor-I regulates transcription of the elastin gene. *J Biol Chem* 268(17) 1993: 12418–12426.

Xu C, Inokuma MS, Denham J et al. Feeder-free growth of undifferentiated human embryonic stem cells. *Nat Biotechnol* 19(10) 2001: 971–974.

Xu RH, Chen X, Li DS et al. BMP4 initiates human embryonic stem cell differentiation to trophoblast. *Nat Biotechnol* 20(12) 2002: 1261–1264.

Yamawaki-Ogata A, Fu X, Hashizume R et al. Therapeutic potential of bone marrow-derived mesenchymal stem cells in formed aortic aneurysms of a mouse model. *Eur J Cardiothorac Surg* 45(5) 2014: e156–e165.

Yanagisawa H, Davis EC. Unraveling the mechanism of elastic fiber assembly: the roles of short fibulins. *Int J Biochem Cell Biol* 42(7) 2010: 1084–1093.

Yang JR, Hsu CW, Liao SC, Lin YT, Chen LR, Yuan K. Transplantation of embryonic stem cells improves the regeneration of periodontal furcation defects in a porcine model. *J Clin Periodontol* 40(4) 2013: 364–371.

Yousef H, Conboy MJ, Li J et al. hESC-secreted proteins can be enriched for multiple regenerative therapies by heparin-binding. *Aging (Albany NY)* 5(5) 2013: 357–372.

Zhang J, Guan J, Niu X et al. Exosomes released from human induced pluripotent stem cells-derived MSCs facilitate cutaneous wound healing by promoting collagen synthesis and angiogenesis. *J Transl Med* 13(1) 2015: 49.

Zhang WG, He L, Shi XM et al. Regulation of transplanted mesenchymal stem cells by the lung progenitor niche in rats with chronic obstructive pulmonary disease. *Respir Res* 15 2014: 33.

Zhao P, Schulz TC, Sherrer ES, Weatherly DB, Robins AJ, Wells L. The human embryonic stem cell proteome revealed by multidimensional fractionation followed by tandem mass spectrometry. *Proteomics* 15(2–3) 2015: 554–566.

Zhuang W, Li L, Lin G, Deng Z. Autologous myoblasts transplantation improves heart function after myocardiac infarction. *Zhong Nan Da Xue Xue Bao Yi Xue Ban* 36(4) 2011: 286–293.

CHAPTER 8

Regulating Elastogenesis Using Proteoglycans

Mervyn J. Merrilees, Inkyung Kang,
Aleksander Hinek, and Thomas N. Wight

CONTENTS

8.1 INTRODUCTION

The formation of elastic fibers during development and repair takes place at cell surfaces and in the pericellular matrix compartment (Kozel et al. 2006, Wagenseil and Mecham 2007). This same space contains matrix proteoglycans (PGs), multifunctional and complex molecules that are emerging as key regulators in the assembly of elastic fibers. The large PGs whose glycosaminoglycan (GAG) side chains contain chondroitin sulfate (CS) are especially important as negative regulators of tropoelastin assembly, thus preventing formation of elastic fibers (Hinek et al. 1991, Wight and Merrilees 2004). In addition, PGs carrying heparan sulfate (HS) have been shown to positively influence events associated with elastogenesis (Buczek-Thomas et al. 2002, Kielty 2006, Tu and Weiss 2010). As a result, regulation of the synthesis of PGs and modulation of their type and levels in the extracellular matrix (ECM) may provide novel therapeutic strategies for the control of elastogenesis. Translational research is currently focused on restoring elastic fibers to organs, such as blood vessels, lung, and skin, which lose their elastic fibers with age and disease. This chapter discusses the inhibitory and stimulatory roles of the CS PGs and their potential use as a new class of therapeutic agent for replenishing elastic fibers destroyed by disease or creating elastic fibers for bioengineered constructs.

8.2 A MODEL FOR INHIBITORY EFFECTS OF MATRIX PGs ON ASSEMBLY OF ELASTIC FIBERS

Initial deposition of tropoelastin molecules onto the microfibrillar scaffold of elastic fibers takes place at the surface of elastogenic cells (Kielty et al. 2002, Merrilees et al. 2002, Kozel et al. 2006). The mechanism by which tropoelastin aggregates on the scaffold prior to cross-linking remains to be fully elucidated, but likely involves self-assembly of tropoelastin monomers that have been shown to coacervate through their hydrophobic domains (Muiznieks et al. 2010). Prior to self-assembly and cross-linking, delivery of monomers through the cell, to the surface, and then to the microfibrillar scaffold involves a molecular chaperone, an elastin-binding protein (EBP) whose affinity for tropoelastin is influenced by galactosugars (Hinek et al. 1991). EBP is an inactive variant of β-galactosidase and functions as a chaperone for tropoelastin rather than as an integral membrane receptor. It has two relevant binding sites, one for hydrophobic sequences of tropoelastin and one for galactosugars. Occupation of the latter binding pocket lowers the affinity for tropoelastin, resulting in its release from EBP. EBP is further complexed with neuraminidase that is proposed to remove terminal sialic acid sugars on the glycosylated microfibrils, exposing penultimate galactosugars for interaction with EBP, resulting in release of tropoelastin monomers immediately adjacent to the fibrillar framework (Hinek et al. 2006, Starcher et al. 2008). Aggregation and lysyl oxidase cross-linking then follow. Pericellular matrix containing a high level of CS disrupts this ordered sequence of events and results in the premature release of tropoelastin from EBP and diminished elastic fiber formation (Hinek et al. 1992). Conversely, low levels of pericellular CS favor enhanced fiber formation (Wight and Merrilees 2004). Accumulating evidence, discussed below, provides increasing support for this model of pericellular PG control over the assembly of elastic fibers.

8.3 PERICELLULAR MATRIX PGs

Versican and biglycan, two interstitial CS PGs found in the pericellular matrix, have been demonstrated to inhibit elastic fiber formation. Decorin, with its single galactosamine dermatan sulfate (DS) chain, can also inhibit elastogenesis (Hinek and Wilson 2000). Decorin is not usually found in significant amounts immediately adjacent to the cell surfaces; rather it is associated with collagen bundles in the interstitial matrix (Krusius and Ruoslahti 1986, Reed and Iozzo 2002, Iozzo 2011). Versican, which interacts with cell surface hyaluronan (Evanko et al. 2007), constitutes the bulk of cell-associated PGs and is present in most fibrous tissues including those of vessels, lung, and skin and is notably increased in many of the diseases that affect these organs (Wight et al. 2014). The versican gene and protein follow a domain template. The amino-terminal globular domain (G1) binds hyaluronan and the carboxy-terminal globular domain (G3) resembles the selectin family consisting of a C-type lectin adjacent to two epidermal growth factor repeats and a complement regulatory region. Interestingly, this region does possess the capacity to bind to proteins associated with the microfibrillar scaffold, such as fibulin-1 and -2 and fibrillin-1 (Aspberg et al. 1999, Olin et al. 2001, Isogai et al. 2002). This scaffold serves as a template for developing elastic fibers. Thus, two different parts of the versican molecule can have either positive or negative effects on elastogenesis and may explain some of the studies that show elastic fibers and versican colocalized in tissues such as in the skin (Zimmermann et al. 1994). The middle region of the versican core protein is encoded by two large exons that specify the CS attachment regions. Alternate splicing of these two exons gives rise to isoforms of different sizes. The CS attached to the core protein of versican is a galactosamine sugar and thus possesses the ability to bind to EBP.

Versican exists in at least four different isoforms (Figure 8.1): V0, the largest variant with two (α and β) GAG binding regions, V1 with the β GAG exon, V2 with the α GAG exon, and V3 the smallest formed from G1 and G3 and without either GAG exon, reviewed in Zimmermann (2000) and Wight (2002). Interactions of the variants with other cell surface molecules are numerous (Wu et al. 2005) and have an influence on cell phenotypes (Wight et al. 2014). The importance of versican in development is reflected by the early lethality of versican-null mice (Hatano et al. 2012). Synthesis and degradation is highly regulated, and there are several transcription factor binding sites in the versican promoter region (Wight and Merrilees 2004, Rahmani et al. 2006, 2012, Domenzain-Reyna et al. 2009, Wight 2012). In addition, versican synthesis is under *microRNA (miRNA) control* (Wang et al. 2010, Rutnam et al. 2013).

The V0 isoform of versican is more prominent during embryonic development (Perissinotto et al. 2000) and less abundant in adult tissues (Cattaruzza et al. 2002). V1 is most abundant in adult tissues and is the isoform most prominent in repair and remodeling associated with injury and disease, except for the nervous system where V2 is most abundant (Zimmermann and Dours-Zimmermann 2008). V3 is expressed

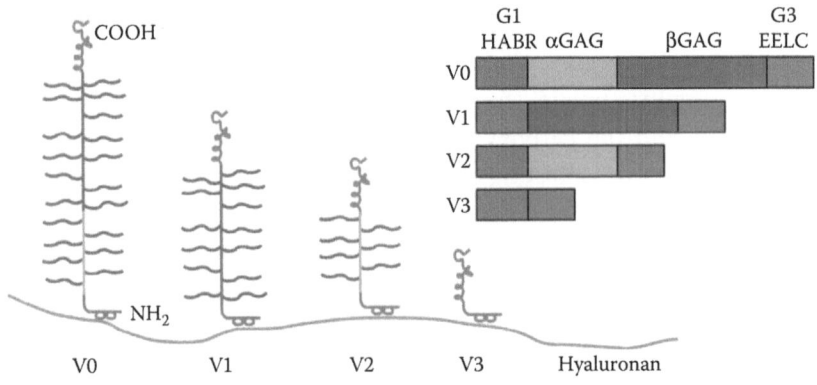

FIGURE 8.1 Schematic representation of the isoforms of versican generated by alternate splicing of mRNA transcript. All isoforms possess a hyaluronan binding region (HABR) in the G1 domain, and a common G3 domain with two epidermal growth factor repeats (EE), a lectin binding domain (L), and a complement regulatory region (C). The αGAG and βGAG regions, to which GAG chains attach, are alternately spliced to give rise to the four isoforms V0–V3. (Reproduced from *Curr. Opin. Cell Biol.*, 14, Wight T.N., Versican: A versatile extracellular matrix proteoglycan in cell biology, 617–623, Copyright 2002, with permission from Elsevier.)

in a variety of tissues (Cattaruzza et al. 2002, Zimmermann and Dours-Zimmermann 2008), but V3 protein is difficult to detect in tissues or cells. Recently, secretion of V3 protein by primary human skeletal muscle cells was detected by proteomic analysis (Hartwig et al. 2014). Some success has been achieved in localizing V3 in tissues, such as in developing heart in the myocardium proximal to the outflow track using tagged primer constructs in overexpression systems (Kern et al. 2007). Other studies demonstrated that forced expression of V3 can have marked effects on the proliferation and migration of different cell types such as chondrocytes (Kamiya et al. 2006), arterial smooth muscle cells (SMCs), fibroblasts (Lemire et al. 2002, Hinek et al. 2004), and melanoma cells (Serra et al. 2005, Miquel-Serra et al. 2006, Hernandez et al. 2011). One particularly impressive effect of expressing V3 in a variety of cells is its effects on ECM remodeling, including promoting the synthesis of tropoelastin and the assembly of elastic fibers (see Section 8.7).

Biglycan is a PG that exists also in the pericellular matrix and consists of a leucine-rich core protein and two galactosamine-containing GAG chains (either CS or DS; Zimmermann 2000). Biglycan interacts with numerous ECM components including collagens and elastin and is sequestered in the matrix of most organs. An osteoporosis-like phenotype and abnormalities in collagen fibrils in biglycan-deficient animals (Xu et al. 1998) supports a structural role, while its ability to bind growth factors and cytokines adds an additional role in the modulation of responses to damage and repair. Furthermore, biglycan expression is altered in human aortic aneurysms (Tamarina et al. 1998, Theocharis and Karamanos 2002) and biglycan knockout animals are characterized by both aortic dissections and aneurysms (Heegaard et al. 2007, Tang et al. 2014), suggesting a role in ECM remodeling possibly involving elastin.

8.4 DISTRIBUTION OF ELASTIC FIBERS IN TISSUES AND RELATIONSHIP TO PG PATTERNS

In developing organs, adult tissues, and wound repair tissues, there is a reciprocal relationship between elastin and versican and/or biglycan content in some phenotypes. This relationship is exemplified in the *elastic organs* that are dependent on elastin for proper physiological function and is seen in developing lung and the emphysematous lung diseases, in arteries with intimal hyperplasia and atherosclerosis, and in skin and scar tissue. In developing lung, the deposition of elastin is critical to secondary alveolar septa formation, defining the crests or rims of new alveoli that develop late during gestation. For example, in fetal sheep, from days 128 to 135 (term 147), there is a significant increase of elastin in the alveolar crest and in other regions, including the pleura (Willet et al. 1999), and this increase, along with increases in collagen deposition, occurs following a significant and progressive reduction in perisaccular and alveolar versican and hyaluronan levels from days 90 through 128, along with a concomitant reduction in tissue volume (Faggian et al. 2007). In diseases of the lung in adults, this reciprocal relationship between elastin and versican is also evident. In chronic obstructive pulmonary disease (COPD), elastin in the alveolar walls and alveolar rims is decreased and versican increased, as a function of the forced expiratory volume in 1 second (FEV1) (Figure 8.2) (Black et al. 2008, Merrilees et al. 2008). EBP also decreases with decreasing FEV1 and matches the decrease in elastin (Merrilees et al. 2008). Importantly, the failure of elastic fibers to repair in COPD is not

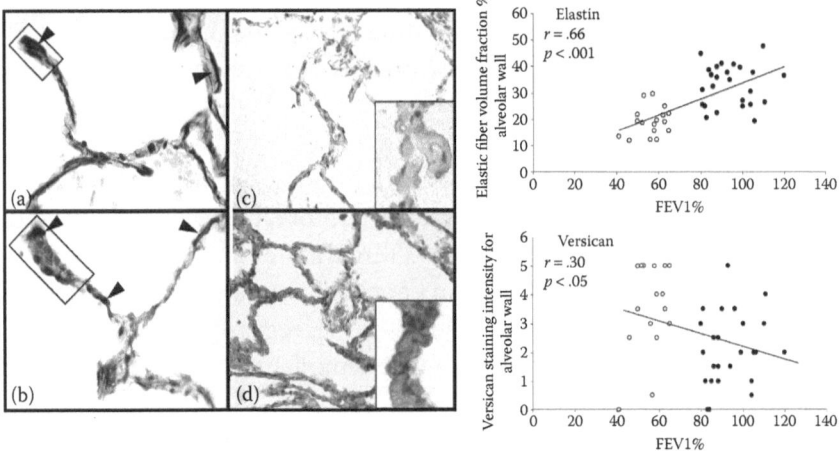

FIGURE 8.2 Elastin (arrow heads) in alveolar walls and rims (boxed regions) of normal (a) and COPD (b) lung showing loss of fibers with disease. Versican immunostaining of normal (c) and COPD (d) lung showing increased staining intensity in COPD lung. Graphs of elastin and versican content in alveolar walls of normal (filled circles) and COPD (open circles) patients, demonstrate the reciprocal relationship between elastin and versican, as a function of FEV1%. (Modified and reproduced from Merrilees, M. J. et al., *Respir. Res.*, 9, 41, 2008, under terms of the Creative Commons Attribution License, http://creativecommons.org/licenses/by/2.0.)

due to impaired tropoelastin synthesis. Several early studies, on emphysematous lungs in humans (Belton et al. 1977, Fukuda et al. 1989) and in animal models (Morris et al. 1981, Osman et al. 1985), have shown that tropoelastin as well as insoluble elastin is produced, but with disordered patterns of deposition, often in the alveolar rims where remodeling is most pronounced (Lucey et al. 1998). Repair of functional fibers does not occur. Of interest, sections of aorta from elastin knockout mice show elevated levels of versican staining in the aortas along with increased versican transcript levels when compared with age-matched wild-type animals (Wight, Mecham, and Davis unpublished observations, 2008). Similarly, in the rare lung disease lymphangioleiomyomatosis (LAM) the extensive remodeling to the parenchyma associated with LAM cell invasion results in disordered patterns of elastin, with elastic fibers absent in expanded parenchymal areas that stain strongly for versican, and also for biglycan (Merrilees et al. 2004). In regions with comparatively normal parenchyma, free of LAM cell invasion, alveoli appear similar to control lung, but versican is increased and elastin decreased, indicating early remodeling.

A similar relationship has been observed in blood vessels. Thickened intima of human atherosclerotic-susceptible vessels (Merrilees et al. 2001) and neointima formed in rabbit vessels in response to balloon catheter injury (Merrilees et al. 2011) are characterized by high versican and low elastic fiber content. This relationship is most apparent in the subendothelial zone of thickened intima and neointima, which has been formally described as the *PG layer* to distinguish it from the deeper *musculoelastic layer* in which PG levels are lower and elastin deposits are present, although not in an organized network of fibers (Figure 8.3) (Stary et al. 1992). The PGs in vessels are predominately the versican variants V0 and V1 (Theocharis et al. 2001) that, along with biglycan, also play a role in trapping lipoproteins, thereby initiating atherosclerosis (Williams and Tabas 1995). Similar to fibroblasts in alveolar wall, the intimal SMCs in the PG-rich zone actively synthesize tropoelastin (Nikkari et al. 1994), but these monomers are not assembled into functional elastic fibers (Stary et al. 1992).

In human skin, the reticular layer of the dermis contains prominent elastic fibers, organized in networks aligned with collagen fiber bundles (Starcher et al. 2005) and with the lines of skin tension (Flint 1976). In the papillary layer immediately adjacent to the epidermis, the elastin content is lower with fine elastic fibers extending through the hydrated matrix,

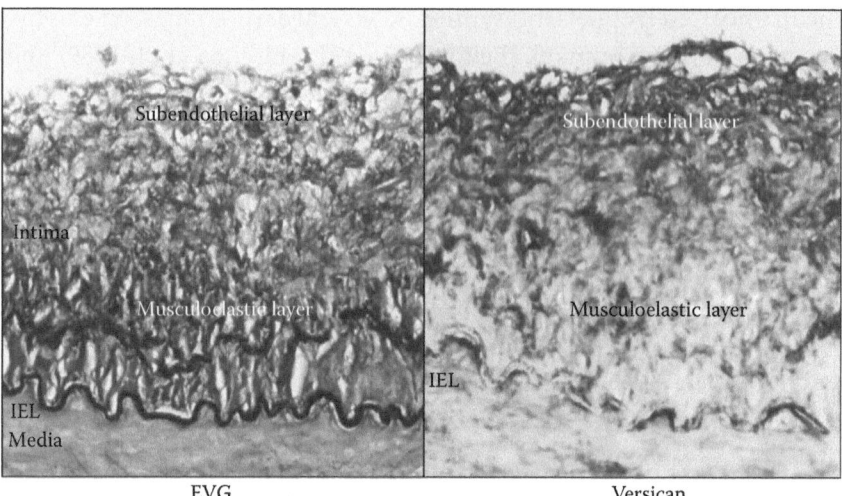

EVG   Versican

FIGURE 8.3 Thickened intima from human coronary artery stained with Verhoeff's van Gieson (EVG) for elastin, and for versican by immunostaining. Versican staining is most intense in the subendothelial (proteoglycan) layer that does not contain elastic fibers. Conversely the deeper musculoelastic layer, and notably the intimal tissue close to the internal elastic lamina (IEL), stains weakly for versican and contains elastic fibers.

often from the reticular layer to the epidermal junction (Zimmermann et al. 1994). Versican is present in this region, often colocated with the fine fibers, and hyaluronan levels are elevated (Bertheim and Hellstrom 1994). In healed dermal wounds and in hypertrophic scars, elastic fibers are generally absent. During the early phases of wound healing, in nodules and bands of scars, and in contractures such as Dupuytren's, CS levels are elevated compared with normal skin (Flint 1990, McFarlane and McGrouther 1991). The inverse relationship between elastin and PGs in the dermis is also evident in Costello syndrome and Hurler disease patients in whom low levels of dermal elastin are associated with excess production of CS and DS PGs, respectively (discussed in Section 8.5).

Collectively, these observations in lung, vessels, and skin demonstrate a common pattern of exclusion of elastic fibers from matrices rich in CS-containing PGs. Experimental studies, *in vitro* and *in vivo*, support a direct inhibitory role for CS in preventing the assembly of tropoelastin monomers onto microfibrillar scaffolds, thereby inhibiting the deposition of insoluble elastic fibers (Hinek et al. 1991, Merrilees et al. 2011).

8.5 STIMULATION OF ELASTIC FIBER FORMATION BY CHONDROITINASES AND VERSICAN ANTISENSE

Evidence that the formation of elastic fibers is inhibited by CS comes from several studies, including investigations on cultured skin fibroblasts from normal and Costello syndrome patients (Hinek et al. 2000). Costello syndrome, a rare genetic disorder involving mutations in the HRAS gene, manifests as poor postnatal growth, neural deficits, flexible joints, loose skin, cardiovascular abnormalities, and uncontrolled growth leading to papillomas and soft tissue rhabdomyosarcomas, among other abnormalities. Histological analyses have shown impaired elastin deposition in skin and other organs, including lung and vessels. Elastin deposition is also impaired in cultured dermal fibroblasts from Costello syndrome patients compared with fibroblasts from normal patients. Costello fibroblasts also show enhanced proliferation and increased production of CS-containing versican as well as biglycan. The phenotype of normal fibroblasts can be changed to mimic the Costello phenotype by the addition of CS that inhibits elastin deposition and reduces cell layer EBP. Correspondingly, the Costello fibroblast phenotype, of high CS production and deficiency of elastin, can be reverted to normal, with deposition of a network of elastic fibers and reduced proliferation, by treatment of cultures with chondroitinase ABC. Importantly, tropoelastin and fibrillin production by both normal and Costello syndrome fibroblasts are similar, as are the initial levels of EBP, indicating that the early events of elastogenesis are not affected. Costello fibroblasts, however, show increased shedding of EBP over time into the culture media in the presence of excess CS.

Hurler disease, in which DS and HS GAGs accumulate due to a primary deficiency in lysosomal α-L-iduronidase, results in widespread connective tissue lesions and sparse thin elastin fibers in numerous organs. Similar to Costello syndrome, the elastin-deficient and proliferative phenotype of dermal fibroblasts can be restored to normal by chondroitinase ABC treatment (Hinek and Wilson 2000). Normally DS, as a component of decorin, is not abundant in tissues; however, in those tissues in which it is the dominant PG, such as tendon, the levels are much lower than in tissues containing the CS PGs (Gillard et al. 1977). Similar to the increase in CS in Costello syndrome, the accumulation of DS on the surface of Hurler disease fibroblasts interferes with EBP-mediated assembly of elastic fibers. As predicted by this model, the addition of DS, but not HS, to normal dermal fibroblasts inhibits elastogenesis *in vitro* (Hinek and Wilson 2000).

Collectively, these findings in Hurler disease and Costello syndrome elegantly demonstrate a central role for matrix galactosugars in modulating elastogenesis in skin fibroblasts.

CS is similarly central to the modulation of elastogenesis by SMCs in blood vessels, both in culture and *in vivo*. Transduction of Fischer rat aortic SMCs with a full-length versican antisense strand of variant V3, resulting in efficient knockdown of all versican variants, significantly increases tropoelastin expression and elastin deposited in cultures (Figure 8.4) (Huang et al. 2006). Proliferation, migration, and pericellular CS are also decreased. The increase in insoluble elastin by versican antisense-expressing cultures is blocked by CS add-back. Correspondingly, levels of EBP (the 67 kDa inactive β-galactosidase enzyme) increase in antisense-expressing cells, and decrease following CS add-back. Both control and antisense-expressing cells, however, contain similar levels of the 88 kDa β-galactosidase precursor and the smaller 64 kDa mature active form of the enzyme, and both control and antisense-expressing cells treated with CS show reduced levels of the 67 kDa variant or EBP, indicating that reduced elastin deposition is associated with a functional deficiency in EBP, not an effect on synthesis of its precursor.

Seeding of the versican antisense-expressing cells into balloon-injured rat carotid arteries demonstrates that versican impacts elastogenesis *in vivo* as well (Huang et al. 2006). Following balloon catheter injury and removal

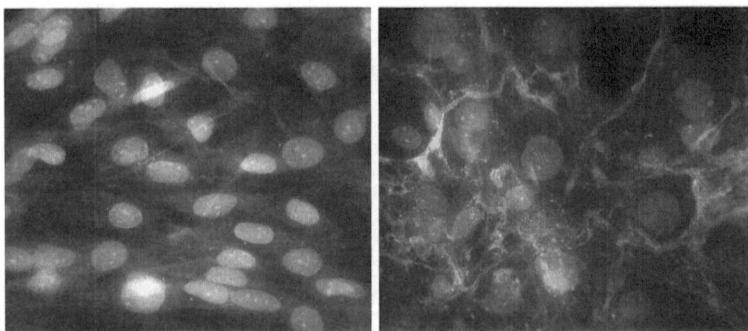

FIGURE 8.4 Cultures of rat aortic smooth muscle cells transduced with empty retroviral vector (left panel) and with vector containing versican antisense sequence (right panel) and immunostained for elastin. Knockdown of versican (all variants) markedly increases elastin deposition in the matrix around cells. (Modified and reproduced with permission from Huang, R. et al., *Circ. Res.* 98, 370, 2006. *Circulation Research* is published by the American Heart Association.)

of the enothelium, the intima responds over a period of several weeks by producing a thickened neointima. SMCs seeded onto the injured surface immediately after ballooning adhere and proliferate along with host cells to produce a neointima that is markedly different from that formed by seeding of empty vector cells. Control neointima is characterized by a myxoid morphology of rounded or stellate cells embedded in a matrix that stains strongly for PGs in general and specifically for versican. That matrix also contains little elastin, mostly in the form of small scattered deposits. In contrast, neointima containing versican antisense-expressing cells shows reduced staining for PGs and versican, increased staining for EBP, and a marked increase in elastin deposition. More importantly, the elastin is organized into circumferentially arranged fibers and lamellae, present throughout the full thickness of the neointima (Figure 8.5). The neointima is also compact and highly structured with elongated SMCs arranged parallel to the elastic lamellae and collagen bundles. This regular organization, not as evident in culture, is interpreted as attributable to the mechanical forces associated with systole and diastole, in association with an appropriate balance of ECM components. In this regard, it is notable that significantly reduced elastin, achieved by elastin gene

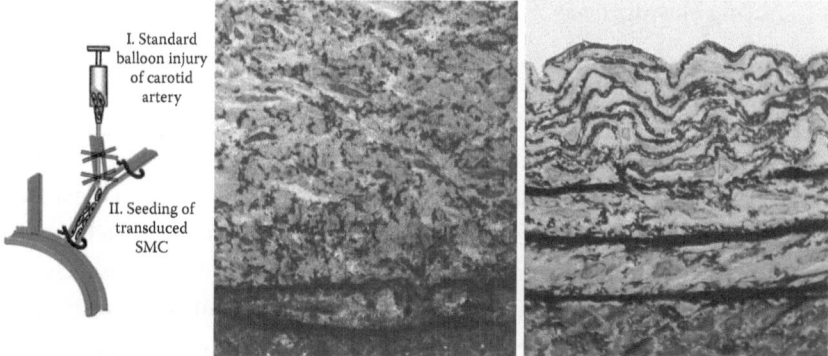

FIGURE 8.5   Forced expression of versican antisense by rat aortic smooth muscle cells seeded into balloon-injured common carotid artery induces a compact, layered, and elastin-rich neointima, in contrast to vector control in which the resulting thick neointima contains small scattered deposits of elastin and a proteoglycan-rich metachromatic matrix. (Images in right panels are reproduced with permission from: Huang, R. et al., *Circ. Res.* 98, 370, 2006. *Circulation Research* is published by the American Heart Association; Diagram in left panel is reused with permission from: Wight, T. N. et al., *Matrix Biol.* 35, 152, 2014.)

knockout, induces intimal SMC proliferation to the extent that the lumen is obstructed (Li et al. 1998).

Using the same experimental approaches, elastin production has also been investigated *in vitro* and *in vivo* in Fischer rat SMCs overexpressing normal biglycan and a GAG-deficient form of biglycan in which the serines of the two GAG attachment sites of the core protein have been replaced by alanine residues (Hwang et al. 2008). Overexpression of the GAG-deficient biglycan results in marked upregulation of tropoelastin message and insoluble elastin deposition, a decrease in collagen, and an increase in fibulin-5, but no change in fibrillin-1. Conversely, overexpression of normal biglycan reduces tropoelastin message and insoluble elastin compared with control cells expressing normal levels of biglycan. In the balloon injury model, elastin increases in neointima containing cells expressing GAG-deficient biglycan, with elastin deposits aggregated into bands, although not into continuous fibers or lamellae as occur with overexpression of versican antisense. While the mechanism(s) responsible for the elastogenic inhibitory activity of the mutated biglycan is not known, it is important to emphasize that the mutated biglycan carries no galactosamine moieties because no GAGs are present. As proposed a number of years ago (Hinek et al. 1991), it may be the lack of the galactosamine sugars that allows proper binding of EBP to its surface protein receptors promoting elastogenesis.

8.6 ROLE OF CS/DS SULFOTRANSFERASES IN ELASTOGENESIS

A significant amount of data indicates that it is the GAG-containing components of the PGs that influence events associated with elastogenesis. The biosynthesis of GAGs is a multistep process that includes the attachment of sulfate groups to specific positions of the polysaccharide chains by sulfotransferases. While HS and HS-sulfotransferases have been appreciated as important regulators of growth factor signaling and animal development, the biological importance of chondroitin sulfation during mammalian development and growth factor signaling is poorly understood. Kluppel et al. (2005) demonstrated that a trap mutation induced in chondroitin-4-sulfotransferase 1 (C4ST1) gene (also called carbohydrate sulfotransferase 11 – ChST11), which encodes an enzyme specific for the transfer of sulfate groups to the 4-O-position in chondroitin, causes severe chondrodysplasia characterized by a disorganized cartilage growth plate. A detailed investigation of cells derived from skin, arteries, and hearts of Costello syndrome patients revealed that this mutation also impacts elastic fiber formation in these tissues (Kluppel et al. 2012). Indeed, it has been established that Costello syndrome tissues display an excessive accumulation of chondroitin-6-sulfate-bearing PGs, associated with both impaired formation of elastic fibers and an unusually high rate of cellular proliferation. In contrast, deposition of chondroitin-4-sulfate is below the level detected in normal tissues. Thus, it has been proposed that an imbalance in sulfation of CS molecules and subsequent compensatory accumulation of chondroitin-6-sulfate in pericellular space may contribute to the development of the Costello syndrome phenotype including defective elastogenesis. Of interest is the observation that accumulation of chondroitin-6-sulfate causes shedding of EBP from cell surfaces, thereby disrupting the process of tropoelastin secretion and preventing its extracellular assembly into elastic fibers (Hinek et al. 2000, 2005). Notably, forced expression of C4ST1 in Costello fibroblasts rescues the abnormal phenotype, promoting elastic fiber formation (Kluppel et al. 2012). It has also been demonstrated that C4ST1 is regulated by transforming growth factor β (TGFβ) signaling, and that treatment of Costello cells with TGFβ normalizes elastic fiber production and proliferation (Hinek et al. 1991, Hinek and Wilson 2000, Kluppel et al. 2005).

Further investigations indicate that a mutation in the CHST14 gene, which codes for dermatan 4-O-sulfotransferase, may contribute to the impaired elastogenesis seen in fibroblasts from Ehlers Danlos syndrome (variant EDS CHST14) (Girirajan et al. 2007), through lower than normal production of fibrillin-1-containing microfibrils and increased chondroitin-6 sulfate. These findings reinforce the concept that imbalance of GAG content can interfere with deposition of elastic fibers.

As discussed, the inhibition of tropoelastin assembly by pericelluar galactosugars occurs at the cell surface through premature shedding of EBP, of which the major component is the spliced variant of β-galactosidase, S-Gal. Inhibition of assembly can also occur where S-Gal is deficient, as occurs in patients with Morquio B disease and Infantile GM1-gangliosidosis (Hinek et al. 2000). Similar to the restoration of elastin assembly by modulating pericellular galactosugar levels, S-Gal-deficient cells can have their elastin production restored by coculture with cells transduced with S-Gal cDNA. Collectively, these data on the effects of CS and DS on EBP and on the assembly of elastic fibers indicate functional deficiencies of elastogenesis, not primary defects in tropoelastin or microfibrillar synthesis.

8.7 STIMULATION OF ELASTOGENESIS BY FORCED EXPRESSION OF VERSICAN VARIANT V3

In contrast to PGs containing CS and DS GAG chains, V3, the smallest variant of versican and without GAG chains, is elastogenic. V3 is also anti-proliferative and anti-inflammatory, and promotes tissue differentiation. V3 is not present to any significant extent in tissues, but V3 transcript has been detected in fetal and adult cells in mouse, rat, and human (Zako et al. 1995, Paulus et al. 1996, Perissinotto et al. 2000, Cattaruzza et al. 2002, Koga et al. 2005) and more recently it has been identified as part of the secretome of primary skeletal muscle cells by proteomic profiling (Hartwig et al. 2014). Findings on its effects on elastin, inflammation and differentiation have all come from investigations involving forced expression of V3, and its roles *in vivo* have yet to be fully elucidated.

Initial investigations on expression of V3, by cultured rat aortic SMCs, demonstrated several changes consistent with induction of a differentiated phenotype; increased cell adhesion to the culture substrate through an increase in focal contacts, flattening and spreading of cells, a reduction in the extent of the pericellular (hyaluronan and versican) coat, and decreases in migration and proliferation (Lemire et al. 2002). Notably, the latter findings differ from G1 and G3 domain effects, both of which stimulate proliferation while G1 promotes migration (Zhang et al. 1998, Ang et al. 1999, Yang et al. 1999). Furthermore, long-term (~3-week) culture of these V3-expressing aortic SMCs led to the unexpected discovery that V3 stimulates tropoelastin message and results in the deposition of extensive elastic fiber networks beneath the cells, on the substrate, and in the matrix between the multilayered cells (Merrilees et al. 2002). This elastin was closely associated with the cell surfaces (Figure 8.6).

The same V3-expressing cells seeded into balloon-injured rat carotid arteries, as done for cells expressing versican antisense, retained their elastogenic phenotype (Figure 8.7) (Merrilees et al. 2002). Neointima, formed over four weeks from both donor and host SMCs, contains a significantly increased volume fraction of elastin in the ECM. Importantly, V3 neointima is highly structured with elongated and circumferentially oriented SMCs embedded in a compact ECM of collagen and elastin, a structure more similar to the media than to normal neointima. These layers are characterized by rounded or stellate cells in a hydrated myxoid matrix containing increased levels of CS, a matrix that inhibits the deposition of elastic fibers.

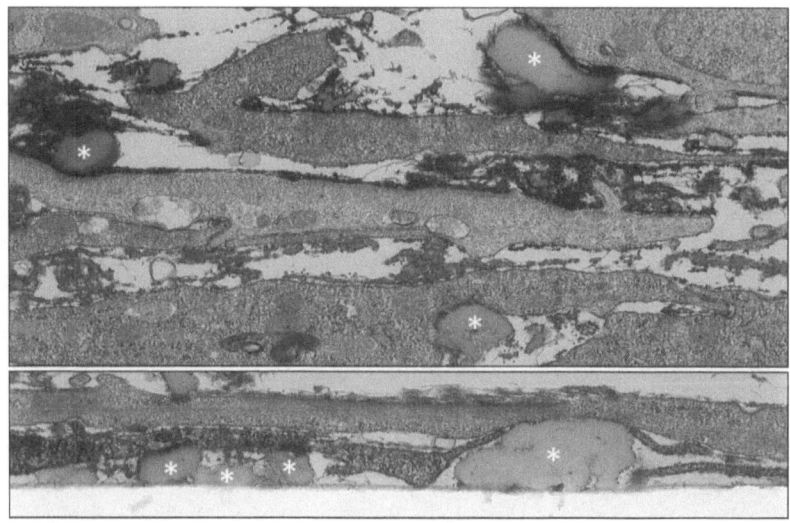

FIGURE 8.6 Electron micrographs of cultured rat aortic smooth muscle cells expressing versican variant V3 showing elastin deposits (*) at cell surfaces (upper panel) and on the culture dish substrate (lower panel). (Modified and reproduced with permission from Merrilees, M.J. et al., *Circ. Res.* 90, 481, 2002. *Circulation Research* is published by the American Heart Association.)

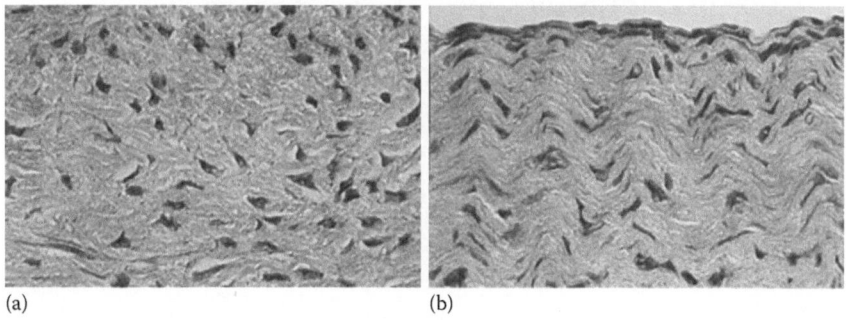

(a)   (b)

FIGURE 8.7 Masson trichrome stained neointima of rat carotid artery, formed from vector alone (a) and V3-expressing (b) smooth muscle cells. Forced expression of V3 induces a highly structured neointima with elongated cells sandwiched between an organized extracellular matrix of collagen and elastin, in contrast to the control neointima of stellate cells embedded in a myxoid matrix of woven collagen fibers. (Modified and reproduced with permission from Merrilees, M.J. et al., *Circ. Res.* 90, 481, 2002. *Circulation Research* is published by the American Heart Association.)

V3 similarly promotes elastogenesis by dermal fibroblasts. Demonstration of the potential usefulness of V3 comes from several studies, including those of Costello syndrome and Hurler disease patients who, as discussed above, have sparse, thin, and poorly formed elastic fibers in the dermis due to accumulation of CS and DS, respectively. Retroviral transduction of patient fibroblasts with V3 reverses the impaired elastogenesis, as well as the characteristic heightened proliferation, to match normal skin fibroblasts (Figure 8.8)

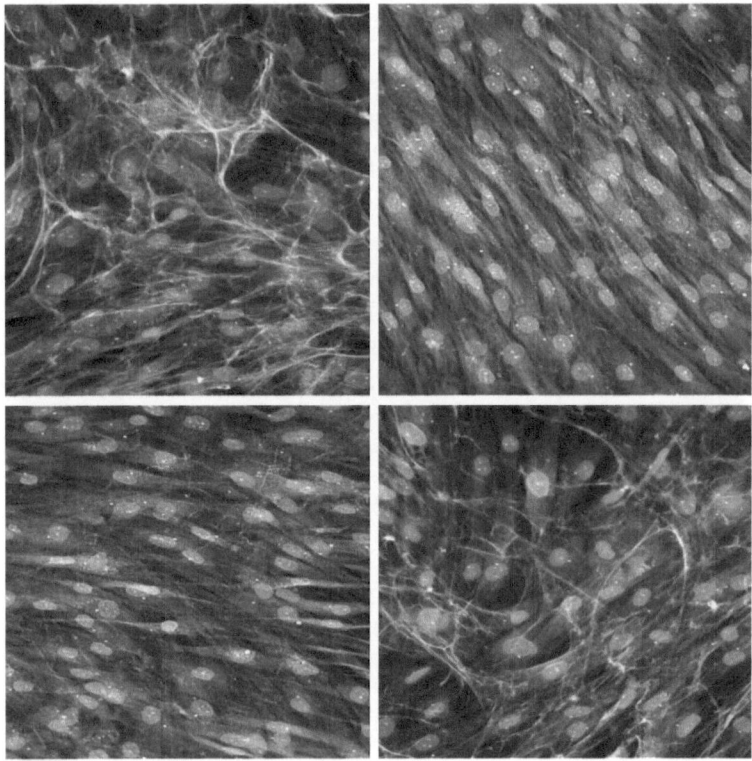

FIGURE 8.8 *Upper panels:* Cultured human dermal fibroblasts immunostained for elastin under normal culture conditions (left panel) and following treatment with chondroitin sulfate (right panel) showing inhibition of elastin network deposition. *Lower panels:* Cultured human dermal fibroblasts from a Costello Syndrome patient immunostained for elastin showing characteristic elastin deficiency (left panel), and the restoration of elastin deposition in cultures of Costello fibroblasts expressing versican variant V3 (right panel). (Modified and reprinted from *Am. J. Pathol.*, 164, Hinek A. et al., Retrovirally mediated overexpression of versican V3 reverses impaired elastogenesis and heightened proliferation exhibited by fibroblasts from Costello syndrome and Hurler disease patients, 119–132, Copyright 2004, with permission from Elsevier.)

(Hinek et al. 2004). The restoration of elastogenesis is accompanied by the loss of CS and DS from the cell surfaces and increases in EBP levels. V3 transduction of skin fibroblasts from GM1-gangliosidosis patients which lack EBP fails to restore impaired elastogenesis, indicating that tropoelastin needs to be delivered to cell surfaces before V3 affects the assembly of tropoelastin onto the microfibrillar scaffold.

8.8 V3 PROMOTES DIFFERENTIATION AND IS ANTI-INFLAMMATORY

In the rabbit-ballooned artery model (Merrilees et al. 2011), the reduced ingress of macrophages supports an anti-inflammatory role for V3. In that study, it was found that matrix generated by V3-expressing SMCs is significantly less adherent for monocytes than matrices generated by control SMCs (Merrilees et al. 2011). V3-expressing SMCs resist monocyte adhesion due to the generation of an ECM enriched in elastin and depleted in hyaluronan, as well as a decrease in vascular cell adhesion molecule 1 (VCAM-1), a key monocyte-binding cell surface molecule, via differentially regulating TGFβ-, epidermal growth factor receptor (EGFR)-, and nuclear factor κB (NFκB)-dependent signaling pathways (Kang et al. 2014). V3 expression induces enhanced expression of tropoelastin and fibulin-5 that is mediated by TGFβ-dependent signaling pathways (Kang et al. 2014). Furthermore, in addition to the effects on elastic fiber accumulation, expression of V3 also reduces hyaluronan accumulation in the ECM through EGFR- and NFκB-dependent activation and negatively impacts monocyte adhesion to the ECM (Kang et al. 2014). V3 expression also induces significant remodeling of the ECM, indicated by changes observed by microarray analysis of differentially expressed genes in ECM molecules, growth factors, cytokines, components of the complement cascades, proteases and protease inhibitors, as well as molecules involved in cell–cell adhesion (Kang et al. 2015). Moreover, V3 expression increases a number of contractile SMC markers such as SMA, calponin 1, and myocardin, the latter a key transcription factor promoting muscle differentiation. Myocardin has been shown to repress versican through induction of miRNA 143 (Wang et al. 2010, Rangrez et al. 2011), consistent with the decrease in total versican transcript induced by V3 expression, suggesting that V3 may promote SMC differentiation by decreasing the GAG-containing isoforms of versican. V3 expression also reduces other inflammatory chemokines, such as lipopolysaccharide-binding protein, Cxcl1, Ccl20, Ccl2, Cxcl6, Cxcl12, and macrophage migration inhibitory factor, accompanied by downregulation of the proinflammatory transcription factors, C/EBPβ and NFκB1. V3 expression significantly increases expression of endogenous inhibitor of focal adhesion kinase (FAK) known as Frnk that has been shown to be selectively expressed by SMCs and large conduit blood vessels and negatively regulates proliferative and migratory phenotypes (Taylor et al. 2001) while reinforcing expression of differentiated SMC markers (Sayers et al. 2008). FAK mediates key signaling pathways elicited by extracellular stimuli activating integrins or growth factors, and further regulates cell proliferation, survival, and migration via PI3K, MAP kinase, and/or NFκB (Morla and Mogford 2000, Mitra et al. 2005, Urbinati et al. 2005, Huang et al. 2007, Petzold et al. 2009). The effect of V3 on reprogramming SMC phenotype may be due to altered FAK signaling pathways leading to increases in differentiated SMC marker expression and decreases in activation of PI3K and NFκB. Our findings that V3 expression induces increases in the differentiated SMC markers as well as in components of basement membrane and elastic fibers suggest that SMCs can be reprogrammed to actively synthesize the ECM components present in healthy arteries while maintaining a differentiated and contractile phenotype. Our earlier work showed that forced expression of V3 results in a dramatic cell shape change creating a more flattened, highly spread cell with large areas of close contacts potentially altering cell adhesion through FAK signaling (Lemire et al. 2002). Such shape changes most likely come about as a result of the dramatic changes in the composition of the ECM, for example, a decrease in the loose pericellular coat enriched in GAG and CS PGs deposited by the cells (Lemire et al. 2002, Merrilees et al. 2002, Hinek et al. 2004). There is extensive evidence that compositional changes in the ECM can lead to changes in cell shape and micromechanical properties that in turn will alter gene expression and associated cell phenotypes (Iwasaki et al. 2000, Wipff et al. 2007, DuFort et al. 2011, Paszek et al. 2014). These findings suggest that altering the ECM microenvironment around the cells by regulating PGs associated with the cell surface can reprogram cell phenotypes including elastogenesis.

8.9 THE USE OF PGs TO ENGINEER ELASTIC FIBER-CONTAINING TISSUES

Extended culture of V3-transduced dermal fibroblasts has also been used to engineer human bilayered skin composed of an epidermis and dermis. This dermis is characterized by an increased content of insoluble elastin, reduced synthesis of versican V1, and reduced deposition of CS in the cell layer (Merrilees et al. 2014). The V3-expressing dermal layer is also more compact and exhibits increased stiffness and an increased elastic modulus compared with controls. Similar, although less marked, effects are seen with forced expression of versican antisense. These results emphasize the potential therapeutic value of modulating PGs to favor an elastogenic phenotype. There is a large body of literature reporting on the use of autologous cultured keratinocytes and dermal fibroblasts, often in combination with acellular scaffolds, to produce skin substitutes. Despite recent improvements, however, none provide a covering that matches normal skin. The long-term result is often formation of scar tissue with a high collagen content and a deficiency of elastic fibers. While the V3-induced elastin-enriched skin sheets have yet to be tested *in vivo*, the use of V3 provides a new approach in this field.

V3 expression has also been used to engineer vascular constructs made from aortic SMCs cultured for extended periods, initially for 12 weeks in culture flasks to create tissue sheets, followed by rolling of the sheets around Teflon™-coated stainless steel mandrels followed by further culture for 18 weeks (Keire et al. 2010). The tissue tubes formed from V3-expressing cells, in addition to containing increased elastin arranged in the form of lamellae and a reduced PG content, demonstrate favorable mechanical properties compared with control constructs. V3 constructs are more elastic at low strains (0%–12%) and have significantly higher burst pressures than control constructs, features enhanced if ascorbate, which reduces tropoelastin, fibulin-5, and lysyl oxidase expression, is removed from the medium. These vessel constructs are also responsive to vasoconstriction and vasodilation agents.

As discussed above, the benefit of V3 *in vivo* for remodeling injured artery wall is clearly demonstrated in the rat using the balloon catheter model followed by cell seeding. The benefit of increasing elastin in the neointimal repair tissue, and lowering PG content, has been demonstrated in a rabbit model in which cholesterol feeding results in lipid deposition and associated inflammatory changes (Merrilees et al. 2011). Balloon injury of rabbit carotid artery, followed by seeding of V3-transduced rabbit SMCs, results in a significant increase in insoluble elastin, organized into multiple layers of fibers and lamellae throughout the neointima, and a decrease in CS (Figure 8.9). Cells and other matrix components, mainly collagen, are similarly highly organized, producing a compact differentiated tissue. Importantly, in the face of a cholesterol challenge lasting for four weeks

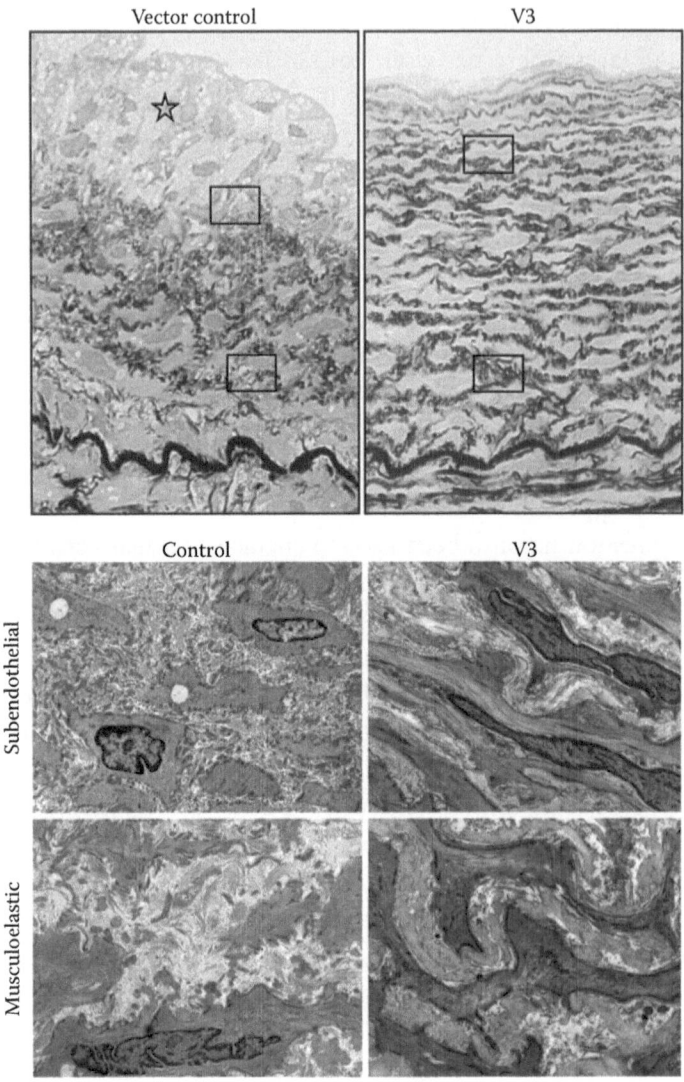

FIGURE 8.9 *Upper panels*: Toluidine Blue stained neointima in rabbit carotid arteries formed from vector alone and V3-expressing SMCs seeded in ballooned vessels. Forced expression of V3 results in multiple elastic laminae throughout the neointima, in contrast to vector control neointima in which fragmented fibers are confined to the deeper layers. Cholesterol feeding results in foam cell formation (star) in control, but not in V3-expressing neointima. *Lower panels*: Electron micrograph images of boxed areas in upper panels. V3 induces highly structured neointima more similar to medial organization than normal neo-imtima. (Modified and reproduced with permission from Merrilees, M.J. et al., *Arterioscler. Thromb. Vasc. Biol.* 31, 1309, 2011.)

and in which plasma cholesterol levels increased to a very high level (>20 mmol/L), V3 neointima is resistant to cholesterol deposition and to macrophage accumulation and foam cell formation. Control neointima, containing vector-alone SMCs, displays typical myxoid morphology, with rounded or stellate cells, a matrix rich in PGs, and in the subendothelial zone, accumulation of lipid-rich macrophages and SMCs (foam cells). Effectively, V3 expression not only increases elastin but also inhibits the initiation of atherosclerotic changes in this model (Figure 8.9).

8.10 CONCLUDING REMARKS

The pericellular matrix PGs play a central role in controlling the assembly of elastic fibers. Matrices with high levels of CS-containing PGs, as found in early development, and in repair and inflamed tissues, prevent or disrupt the ordered delivery of tropoelastin to the microfibrillar scaffold at cell surfaces. As a result, new fibers either do not form or the elastin is deposited in irregular patterns. Importantly, this inhibitory process has been shown to be reversible by modulating the composition of the pericellular matrix. Thus, a reciprocal relationship can exist between some PGs, such as versican, and elastic fibers, suggesting that versican accumulation can interfere with elastic fiber formation and assembly, creating an unstable tissue architecture and promoting inflammation, while the opposite occurs when versican content is low, facilitating elastic fiber formation and assembly (Figure 8.10). During development, this happens naturally when PG-rich tissues of early organogenic phases are remodeled during differentiation to create environments with lower concentrations of PGs in which organized elastin and collagen fibers are deposited. PG content and form can also be modulated exogenously, for example, by enzymatic digestion of the GAG chains, or endogenously, by expression of antisense or siRNA directed at core protein synthesis, with both approaches able to restore elastic fiber formation. Conversely, the exogenous addition of CS PGs or just CS, or enhanced production of the CS PGs through vector-mediated forced expression will decrease elastic fiber formation by elastogenic cells.

The discovery that the spliced variant of versican, V3, which does not have GAG chains, is strongly elastogenic supports the model by which CS is a major endogenous inhibitor of elastic fiber assembly. But it is also evident that the effects of V3 are much broader, with expression affecting large numbers of genes that promote differentiation and formation of highly organized ECMs. The ECMs of these V3-expressing tissues are additionally resistant to inflammatory changes.

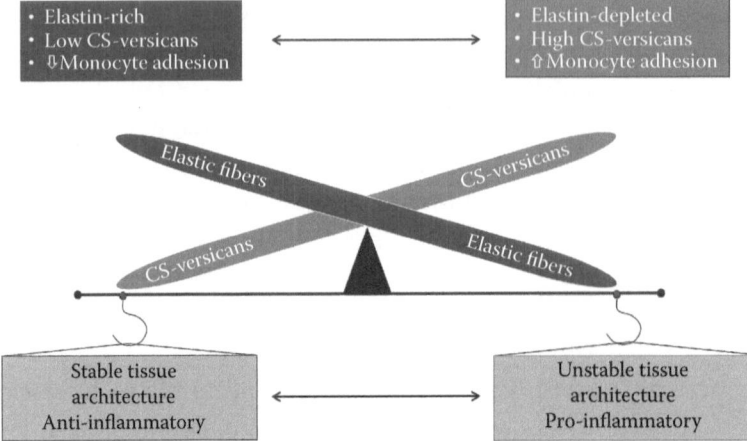

FIGURE 8.10 Schematic depiction of the inverse relationship between the chondroitin sulfate-containing versicans and elastic fibers. The glycososaminoglycan-containing forms of versican interfere with elastogenesis, creating an unstable and pro-inflammatory tissue architecture. A stable and anti-inflammatory tissue architecture occurs when CS-containing versicans are low and elastic fiber content is high. (From Wight, T. N. et al., *Matrix Biol.* 35, 152, 2014, with permission.)

The point at which PGs inhibit or promote elastogenesis, is at the time of release and transfer of tropoelastin monomers from accompanying chaperone EBP to the microfibrillar scaffold for aggregation and cross-linking, seems to be ideally suited for therapeutic interventions designed to modulate elastin in tissues. Synthesis and passage of tropoelastin to the cell surface is not generally affected, and in tissues in which elastin deposition is compromised, the cells continue to synthesize and secrete tropoelastin. Targeting the composition of the pericellular matrix, by changing the content and balance of the PGs, provides for a focused approach at a key step in the sequence of events that make up the elastogenic process. The discovery that this target also affects differentiation and susceptibility to inflammation will likely broaden therapeutic applications to numerous conditions beyond deficiency in elastic fibers.

ACKNOWLEDGMENTS

This study was supported by grants from the National Institutes of Health R01 HL064387, P01 HL18645, R41 HL106967, P01 HL098067, R01 EB012558 (to TNW); the Health Research Council of New Zealand, National Heart Foundation of New Zealand, Auckland Medical Research Foundation, Marsden Fund of the Royal Society of New Zealand, Lottery Health

Research, New Zealand LAM Trust, Maurice and Phyllis Paykel Trust, William and Lois Manchester Trust, The University of Auckland (to MJM); and American Heart Association Predoctoral Fellowship 0310062Z to Paul A. Keire. The authors thank Dr. Michael G. Kinsella for helpful discussions and Dr. Virginia M. Green for preparation and editing of the manuscript.

REFERENCES

Ang, L. C., Y. Zhang, L. Cao, B. L. Yang, B. Young, C. Kiani, V. Lee, K. Allan, and B. B. Yang. 1999. Versican enhances locomotion of astrocytoma cells and reduces cell adhesion through its G1 domain. *J Neuropathol Exp Neurol* 58(6): 597–605.

Aspberg, A., S. Adam, G. Kostka, R. Timpl, and D. Heinegard. 1999. Fibulin-1 is a ligand for the C-type lectin domains of aggrecan and versican. *J Biol Chem* 274 (29): 20444–20449.

Belton, J. C., N. Crise, R. F. McLaughlin, Jr., and E. E. Tueller. 1977. Ultrastructural alterations in collagen associated with microscopic foci of human emphysema. *Hum Pathol* 8(6): 669–677.

Bertheim, U. and S. Hellstrom. 1994. The distribution of hyaluronan in human skin and mature, hypertrophic and keloid scars. *Br J Plast Surg* 47(7): 483–489.

Black, P. N., P. S. Ching, B. Beaumont, S. Ranasinghe, G. Taylor, and M. J. Merrilees. 2008. Changes in elastic fibres in the small airways and alveoli in COPD. *Eur Respir J* 31(5): 998–1004.

Buczek-Thomas, J. A., C. L. Chu, C. B. Rich, P. J. Stone, J. A. Foster, and M. A. Nugent. 2002. Heparan sulfate depletion within pulmonary fibroblasts: Implications for elastogenesis and repair. *J Cell Physiol* 192(3): 294–303.

Cattaruzza, S., M. Schiappacassi, A. Ljungberg-Rose, P. Spessotto, D. Perissinotto, M. Morgelin, M. T. Mucignat, A. Colombatti, and R. Perris. 2002. Distribution of PG-M/versican variants in human tissues and de novo expression of isoform V3 upon endothelial cell activation, migration, and neoangiogenesis in vitro. *J Biol Chem* 277(49): 47626–47635.

Domenzain-Reyna, C., D. Hernandez, L. Miquel-Serra, M. J. Docampo, C. Badenas, A. Fabra, and A. Bassols. 2009. Structure and regulation of the versican promoter: The versican promoter is regulated by AP-1 and TCF transcription factors in invasive human melanoma cells. *J Biol Chem* 284(18): 12306–12317.

DuFort, C. C., M. J. Paszek, and V. M. Weaver. 2011. Balancing forces: Architectural control of mechanotransduction. *Nat Rev Mol Cell Biol* 12(5): 308–319.

Evanko, S. P., M. I. Tammi, R. H. Tammi, and T. N. Wight. 2007. Hyaluronan-dependent pericellular matrix. *Adv Drug Deliv Rev* 59(13): 1351–1365.

Faggian, J., A. J. Fosang, M. Zieba, M. J. Wallace, and S. B. Hooper. 2007. Changes in versican and chondroitin sulphate proteoglycans during structural development of the lung. *Am J Physiol Regul Integr Comp Physiol* 293(2): R784–R792.

Flint, M. H. 1990. Connective tissue biology. In *Dupuytren's Disease Biology and Treatment.*, edited by R. M. McFarlane, D. H. McGrouther and M. H. Flint, pp. 13–24. Edinburgh, Scotland: Churchill Livingstone.

Flint, M. H. 1976. The biological basis of Langer's lines. In *The Ultrastructure of Collagen*, edited by J. J. Longacre, pp. 132–140. Springfield, IL: Charles C. Thomas.

Fukuda, Y., Y. Masuda, M. Ishizaki, Y. Masugi, and V. J. Ferrans. 1989. Morphogenesis of abnormal elastic fibers in lungs of patients with panacinar and centriacinar emphysema. *Hum Pathol* 20(7): 652–659.

Gillard, G. C., M. J. Merrilees, P. G. Bell-Booth, H. C. Reilly, and M. H. Flint. 1977. The proteoglycan content and the axial periodicity of collagen in tendon. *Biochem J* 163(1): 145–151.

Girirajan, S., R. Mendoza-Londono, C. N. Vlangos, L. Dupuis, N. J. Nowak, D. J. Bunyan, E. Hatchwell, and S. H. Elsea. 2007. Smith-Magenis syndrome and Moyamoya disease in a patient with del(17)(p11.2p13.1). *Am J Med Genet A* 143A (9): 999–1008.

Hartwig, S., S. Raschke, B. Knebel, M. Scheler, M. Irmler, W. Passlack, S. Muller et al. 2014. Secretome profiling of primary human skeletal muscle cells. *Biochim Biophys Acta* 1844(5): 1011–1017.

Hatano, S., K. Kimata, N. Hiraiwa, M. Kusakabe, Z. Isogai, E. Adachi, T. Shinomura, and H. Watanabe. 2012. Versican/PG-M is essential for ventricular septal formation subsequent to cardiac atrioventricular cushion development. *Glycobiology* 22(9): 1268–1277.

Heegaard, A. M., A. Corsi, C. C. Danielsen, K. L. Nielsen, H. L. Jorgensen, M. Riminucci, M. F. Young, and P. Bianco. 2007. Biglycan deficiency causes spontaneous aortic dissection and rupture in mice. *Circulation* 115(21): 2731–2738.

Hernandez, D., L. Miquel-Serra, M. J. Docampo, A. Marco-Ramell, J. Cabrera, A. Fabra, and A. Bassols. 2011. V3 versican isoform alters the behavior of human melanoma cells by interfering with CD44/ErbB-dependent signaling. *J Biol Chem* 286(2): 1475–1485.

Hinek, A., J. Boyle, and M. Rabinovitch. 1992. Vascular smooth muscle cell detachment from elastin and migration through elastic laminae is promoted by chondroitin sulfate-induced "shedding" of the 67-kDa cell surface elastin binding protein. *Exp Cell Res* 203: 344–353.

Hinek, A., K. R. Braun, K. Liu, Y. Wang, and T. N. Wight. 2004. Retrovirally mediated overexpression of versican v3 reverses impaired elastogenesis and heightened proliferation exhibited by fibroblasts from Costello syndrome and Hurler disease patients. *Am J Pathol* 164(1): 119–131.

Hinek, A., R. P. Mecham, F. Keeley, and M. Rabinovitch. 1991. Impaired elastin fiber assembly related to reduced 67-kD elastin-binding protein in fetal lamb ductus arteriosus and in cultured aortic smooth muscle cells treated with chondroitin sulfate. *J Clin Invest* 88: 2083–2094.

Hinek, A., A. V. Pshezhetsky, M. von Itzstein, and B. Starcher. 2006. Lysosomal sialidase (neuraminidase-1) is targeted to the cell surface in a multiprotein complex that facilitates elastic fiber assembly. *J Biol Chem* 281(6): 3698–3710.

Hinek, A., A. C. Smith, E. M. Cutiongco, J. W. Callahan, K. W. Gripp, and R. Weksberg. 2000. Decreased elastin deposition and high proliferation of fibroblasts from Costello syndrome are related to functional deficiency in the 67-kD elastin-binding protein. *Am J Hum Genet* 66(3): 859–872.

Hinek, A., M. A. Teitell, L. Schoyer, W. Allen, K. W. Gripp, R. Hamilton, R. Weksberg, M. Kluppel, and A. E. Lin. 2005. Myocardial storage of chondroitin sulfate-containing moieties in Costello syndrome patients with severe hypertrophic cardiomyopathy. *Am J Med Genet A* 133A(1): 1–12.

Hinek, A. and S. E. Wilson. 2000. Impaired elastogenesis in Hurler disease: Dermatan sulfate accumulation linked to deficiency in elastin-binding protein and elastic fiber assembly. *Am J Pathol* 156(3): 925–938.

Huang, D., M. Khoe, M. Befekadu, S. Chung, Y. Takata, D. Ilic, and M. Bryer-Ash. 2007. Focal adhesion kinase mediates cell survival via NF-kappaB and ERK signaling pathways. *Am J Physiol Cell Physiol* 292(4): C1339–C1352.

Huang, R., M. J. Merrilees, K. Braun, B. Beaumont, J. Lemire, A. W. Clowes, A. Hinek, and T. N. Wight. 2006. Inhibition of versican synthesis by antisense alters smooth muscle cell phenotype and induces elastic fiber formation in vitro and in neointima after vessel injury. *Circ Res* 98(3): 370–377.

Hwang, J. Y., P. Y. Johnson, K. R. Braun, A. Hinek, J. W. Fischer, K. D. O'Brien, B. Starcher, A. W. Clowes, M. J. Merrilees, and T. N. Wight. 2008. Retrovirally mediated overexpression of glycosaminoglycan-deficient biglycan in arterial smooth muscle cells induces tropoelastin synthesis and elastic fiber formation in vitro and in neointimae after vascular injury. *Am J Pathol* 173(6): 1919–1928.

Iozzo, R. 2011. Small leucine-rich proteoglycans. In *The Extracellular Matrix: An Overview*, edited by Mecham R. P., Heidelberg, Germany: Springer.

Isogai, Z., A. Aspberg, D. R. Keene, R. N. Ono, D. P. Reinhardt, and L. Y. Sakai. 2002. Versican interacts with fibrillin-1 and links extracellular microfibrils to other connective tissue networks. *J Biol Chem* 277(6): 4565–4572.

Iwasaki, H., S. Eguchi, H. Ueno, F. Marumo, and Y. Hirata. 2000. Mechanical stretch stimulates growth of vascular smooth muscle cells via epidermal growth factor receptor. *Am J Physiol Heart Circ Physiol* 278(2):H521H529.

Kamiya, N., H. Watanabe, H. Habuchi, H. Takagi, T. Shinomura, K. Shimizu, and K. Kimata. 2006. Versican/PG-M regulates chondrogenesis as an extracellular matrix molecule crucial for mesenchymal condensation. *J Biol Chem* 281(4): 2390–2400.

Kang, I., J. L. Barth, E. P. Sproul, D. W. Yoon, G. A. Workman, K. R. Braun, W. S. Argraves et al. 2015. Expression of V3 versican by rat arterial smooth muscle cells promotes differentiated and anti-inflammatory phenotypes. *J Biol Chem* 290: 21629–21641.

Kang, I., D. W. Yoon, K. R. Braun, and T. N. Wight. 2014. Expression of versican V3 by arterial smooth muscle cells alters TGFβ-, EGF-, and NFkB-dependent signaling pathways, creating a microenvironment that resists monocyte adhesion. *J Biol Chem* 289(22): 15393–15404.

Keire, P. A., N. L'Heureux, R. B. Vernon, M. J. Merrilees, B. Starcher, E. Okon, N. Dusserre, T. N. McAllister, and T. Wight. 2010. Expression of versican isoform V3 in the absence of ascorbate improves elastogenesis in engineered vascular constructs. *Tissue Eng Part A* 15: 501–512.

Kern, C. B., R. A. Norris, R. P. Thompson, W. S. Argraves, S. E. Fairey, L. Reyes, S. Hoffman, R. R. Markwald, and C. H. Mjaatvedt. 2007. Versican proteolysis mediates myocardial regression during outflow tract development. *Dev Dyn* 236(3): 671–683.

Kielty, C. M. 2006. Elastic fibres in health and disease. *Expert Rev Mol Med* 8(19): 1–23.

Kielty, C. M., M. J. Sherratt, and C. A. Shuttleworth. 2002. Elastic fibres. *J Cell Sci* 115(Pt 14): 2817–2828.

Kluppel, M., P. Samavarchi-Tehrani, K. Liu, J. L. Wrana, and A. Hinek. 2012. C4ST-1/CHST11-controlled chondroitin sulfation interferes with oncogenic HRAS signaling in Costello syndrome. *Eur J Hum Genet* 20(8): 870–877.

Kluppel, M., T. N. Wight, C. Chan, A. Hinek, and J. L. Wrana. 2005. Maintenance of chondroitin sulfation balance by chondroitin-4-sulfotransferase 1 is required for chondrocyte development and growth factor signaling during cartilage morphogenesis. *Development* 132(17): 3989–4003.

Koga, T., M. Inatani, A. Hirata, Y. Inomata, M. Zako, K. Kimata, A. Oohira, T. Gotoh, M. Mori, and H. Tanihara. 2005. Expression of a chondroitin sulfate proteoglycan, versican (PG-M), during development of rat cornea. *Curr Eye Res* 30(6): 455–463.

Kozel, B. A., B. J. Rongish, A. Czirok, J. Zach, C. D. Little, E. C. Davis, R. H. Knutsen, J. E. Wagenseil, M. A. Levy, and R. P. Mecham. 2006. Elastic fiber formation: A dynamic view of extracellular matrix assembly using timer reporters. *J Cell Physiol* 207(1): 87–96.

Krusius, T. and E. Ruoslahti. 1986. Primary structure of an extracellular matrix proteoglycan core protein deduced from cloned cDNA. *Proc Natl Acad Sci USA* 83: 7683–7687.

Lemire, J. M., M. J. Merrilees, K. R. Braun, and T. N. Wight. 2002. Overexpression of the V3 variant of versican alters arterial smooth muscle cell adhesion, migration, and proliferation in vitro. *J Cell Physiol* 190(1): 38–45.

Li, D. Y., B. Brooke, E. C. Davis, R. P. Mecham, L. K. Sorensen, B. B. Boak, E. Eichwald, and M. T. Keating. 1998. Elastin is an essential determinant of arterial morphogenesis. *Nature* 393(6682): 276–280.

Lucey, E. C., R. H. Goldstein, P. J. Stone, and G. L. Snider. 1998. Remodeling of alveolar walls after elastase treatment of hamsters. Results of elastin and collagen mRNA in situ hybridization. *Am J Respir Crit Care Med* 158(2): 555–564.

McFarlane, R. M. and D. A. McGrouther. 1991. *Dupuytren's Disease: Biology and Treatment*. New York: Elsevier Health Sciences.

Merrilees, M, P. S. T Ching, B. Beaumont, A. Hinek, T. N. Wight, and P. N. Black. 2008. Changes in elastin, elastin binding protein and versican in alveoli in chronic obstructive pulmonary disease. *Respir Res* 18(9): 41–50.

Merrilees, M. J., B. Beaumont, and L. J. Scott. 2001. Comparison of deposits of versican, biglycan and decorin in saphenous vein and internal thoracic, radial and coronary arteries: Correlation to patency. *Coron Artery Dis* 12(1): 7–16.

Merrilees, M. J., B. W. Beaumont, K. R. Braun, A. C. Thomas, I. Kang, A. Hinek, A. Passi, and T. N. Wight. 2011. Neointima formed by arterial smooth muscle cells expressing versican variant v3 is resistant to lipid and macrophage accumulation. *Arterioscler Thromb Vasc Biol* 31(6): 1309–1316.

Merrilees, M. J., E. J. Hankin, J. L. Black, and B. Beaumont. 2004. Matrix proteoglycans and remodelling of interstitial lung tissue in lymphangioleiomyomatosis. *J Pathol* 203(2): 653–660.

Merrilees, M. J., J. M. Lemire, J. W. Fischer, M. G. Kinsella, K. R. Braun, A. W. Clowes, and T. N. Wight. 2002. Retrovirally mediated overexpression of versican v3 by arterial smooth muscle cells induces tropoelastin synthesis and elastic fiber formation in vitro and in neointima after vascular injury. *Circ Res* 90(4): 481–487.

Merrilees, M. J., B. A. Falk, N. Zuo, M. E. Dickinson, B. C. H. May, and T. N. Wight. 2014. Use of versican variant V3 and versican antisense expression to engineer cultured human skin containing increased content of insoluble elastin. *J Tiss Eng Regen Med*. doi: 10.1002/term.1913.

Miquel-Serra, L., M. Serra, D. Hernández, C. Domenzain, M. J. Docampo, R. M. Rabanal, I de Torres, T. N. Wight, A. Fabra, and A. Bassols. 2006. V3 versican isoform expression has a dual role in human melanoma tumor growth and metastasis. *Lab Invest* 86(9): 889–901.

Mitra, S. K., D. A. Hanson, and D. D. Schlaepfer. 2005. Focal adhesion kinase: In command and control of cell motility. *Nat Rev Mol Cell Biol* 6(1): 56–68.

Morla, A. O. and J. E. Mogford. 2000. Control of smooth muscle cell proliferation and phenotype by integrin signaling through focal adhesion kinase. *Biochem Biophys Res Commun* 272(1): 298–302.

Morris, S. M., P. J. Stone, G. L. Snider, J. T. Albright, and C. Franzblau. 1981. Ultrastructural changes in hamster lung four hours to twenty-four days after exposure to elastase. *Anat Rec* 201(3): 523–535.

Muiznieks, L. D., A. S. Weiss, and F. W. Keeley. 2010. Structural disorder and dynamics of elastin. *Biochem Cell Biol* 88(2): 239–250.

Nikkari, S. T., H. T. Järveläinen, T. N. Wight, M. Ferguson, and A. W. Clowes. 1994. Smooth muscle cell expression of extracellular matrix genes after arterial injury. *Am J Pathol* 144: 1348–1356.

Olin, A. I., M. Morgelin, T. Sasaki, R. Timpl, D. Heinegard, and A. Aspberg. 2001. The proteoglycans aggrecan and Versican form networks with fibulin-2 through their lectin domain binding. *J Biol Chem* 276(2): 1253–1261.

Osman, M., J. O. Cantor, S. Roffman, S. Keller, G. M. Turino, and I. Mandl. 1985. Cigarette smoke impairs elastin resynthesis in lungs of hamsters with elastase-induced emphysema. *Am Rev Respir Dis* 132(3): 640–643.

Paszek, M. J., C. C. DuFort, O. Rossier, R. Bainer, J. K. Mouw, K. Godula, J. E. Hudak, J. N. Lakins, A. C. Wijekoon, L. Cassereau, M. G. Rubashkin, M. J. Magbanua, K. S. Thorn, M. W. Davidson, H. S. Rugo, J. W. Park, D. A. Hammer, G. Giannone, C. R. Bertozzi, and V. M. Weaver. 2014. The cancer glycocalyx mechanically primes integrin-mediated growth and survival. *Nature* 511(7509): 319–325.

Paulus, W., I. Baur, M. T. Dours-Zimmerman, and D. R. Zimmermann. 1996. Differential expression of versican isoforms in brain tumors. *J Neuropathol Exp Neurol* 55: 528–533.

Perissinotto, D., P. Iacopetti, I. Bellina, R. Doliana, A. Colombatti, Z. Pettway, M. Bronner-Fraser et al. 2000. Avian neural crest cell migration is diversely regulated by the two major hyaluronan-binding proteoglycans PG-M/versican and aggrecan. *Development* 127(13): 2823–2842.

Petzold, T., A. W. Orr, C. Hahn, K. A. Jhaveri, J. T. Parsons, and M. A. Schwartz. 2009. Focal adhesion kinase modulates activation of NF-kappaB by flow in endothelial cells. *Am J Physiol Cell Physiol* 297(4): C814–C822.

Rahmani, M., J. M. Carthy, and B. M. McManus. 2012. Mapping of the Wnt/beta-catenin/TCF response elements in the human versican promoter. *Methods Mol Biol* 836: 35–52.

Rahmani, M., B. W. Wong, L. Ang, C. C. Cheung, J. M. Carthy, H. Walinski, and B. M. McManus. 2006. Versican: Signaling to transcriptional control pathways. *Can J Physiol Pharmacol* 84(1): 77–92.

Rangrez, A. Y., Z. A. Massy, V. Metzinger-Le Meuth, and L. Metzinger. 2011. miR-143 and miR-145: Molecular keys to switch the phenotype of vascular smooth muscle cells. *Circ Cardiovasc Genet* 4(2): 197–205.

Reed, C. C. and R. V. Iozzo. 2002. The role of decorin in collagen fibrillogenesis and skin homeostasis. *Glycoconj J* 19(4–5): 249–255.

Rutnam, Z. J., T. N. Wight, and B. B. Yang. 2013. miRNAs regulate expression and function of extracellular matrix molecules. *Matrix Biol* 32(2): 74–85.

Sayers, R. L., L. J. Sundberg-Smith, M. Rojas, H. Hayasaka, J. T. Parsons, C. P. Mack, and J. M. Taylor. 2008. FRNK expression promotes smooth muscle cell maturation during vascular development and after vascular injury. *Arterioscler Thromb Vasc Biol* 28(12): 2115–2122.

Serra, M., L. Miquel, C. Domenzain, M. J. Docampo, A. Fabra, T. N. Wight, and A. Bassols. 2005. V3 versican isoform expression alters the phenotype of melanoma cells and their tumorigenic potential. *Int J Cancer* 114(6): 879–886.

Starcher, B., R. L. Aycock, and C. H. Hill. 2005. Multiple roles for elastic fibers in the skin. *J Histochem Cytochem* 53(4): 431–443.

Starcher, B., A. d'Azzo, P. W. Keller, G. K. Rao, D. Nadarajah, and A. Hinek. 2008. Neuraminidase-1 is required for the normal assembly of elastic fibers. *Am J Physiol Lung Cell Mol Physiol* 295(4): L637–L647.

Stary, H. C., D. H. Blankenhorn, A. B. Chandler, S. Glagov, W. Insull, Jr., M. Richardson, M. E. Rosenfeld et al. 1992. A definition of the intima of human arteries and of its atherosclerosis-prone regions. A report from the Committee on Vascular Lesions of the Council on Arteriosclerosis, American Heart Association. *Circulation* 85(1): 391–405.

Tamarina, N. A., M. A. Grassi, D. A. Johnson, and W. H. Pearce. 1998. Proteoglycan gene expression is decreased in abdominal aortic aneurysms. *J Surg Res* 74(1): 76–80.

Tang, T., J. C. Thompson, P. G. Wilson, M. H. Yoder, J. Mueller, J. W. Fischer, K. J. Williams, and L. R. Tannock. 2014. Biglycan deficiency: Increased aortic aneurysm formation and lack of atheroprotection. *J Mol Cell Cardiol* 75: 174–180.

Taylor, J. M., C. P. Mack, K. Nolan, C. P. Regan, G. K. Owens, and J. T. Parsons. 2001. Selective expression of an endogenous inhibitor of FAK regulates proliferation and migration of vascular smooth muscle cells. *Mol Cell Biol* 21(5): 1565–1572.

Theocharis, A. D. and N. K. Karamanos. 2002. Decreased biglycan expression and differential decorin localization in human abdominal aortic aneurysms. *Atherosclerosis* 165(2): 221–230.

Theocharis, A. D., I. Tsolakis, A. Hjerpe, and N. K. Karamanos. 2001. Human abdominal aortic aneurysm is characterized by decreased versican concentration and specific downregulation of versican isoform V(0). *Atherosclerosis* 154(2): 367–376.

Tu, Y. and A. S. Weiss. 2010. Transient tropoelastin nanoparticles are early-stage intermediates in the coacervation of human tropoelastin whose aggregation is facilitated by heparan sulfate and heparin decasaccharides. *Matrix Biol* 29(2): 152159.

Urbinati, C., A. Bugatti, M. Giacca, D. Schlaepfer, M. Presta, and M. Rusnati. 2005. alpha(v)beta3-integrin-dependent activation of focal adhesion kinase mediates NF-kappaB activation and motogenic activity by HIV-1 Tat in endothelial cells. *J Cell Sci* 118(Pt 17): 3949–3958.

Wagenseil, J. E. and R. P. Mecham. 2007. New insights into elastic fiber assembly. *Birth Defects Res C Embryo Today* 81(4): 229–240.

Wang, X., G. Hu, and J. Zhou. 2010. Repression of versican expression by microRNA-143. *J Biol Chem* 285(30): 23241–23250.

Wight, T. N. 2002. Versican: A versatile extracellular matrix proteoglycan in cell biology. *Curr Opin Cell Biol* 14(5): 617–623.

Wight, T. N., I. Kang, M. J. Merrilees. 2014. Versican and the control of inflammation. *Matrix Biol.* 35: 152–161.

Wight, T. N., M. G. Kinsella, S. P. Evanko, S. Potter-Perigo, and M. J. Merrilees. 2014. Versican and the regulation of cell phenotype in disease. *Biochim Biophys Acta* 1840(8): 2441–2451.

Wight, T. N. and M. J. Merrilees. 2004. Proteoglycans in atherosclerosis and restenosis: Key roles for versican. *Circ Res* 94(9): 1158–1167.

Wight, T. N. 2012. The pathobiology of versican. In *Extracellular Matrix: Pathobiology and Signaling*, edited by N. Karamanos, 154–170 Berlin, Germany: Walter De Gruyter GMBH & Co., KG.

Willet, K. E., P. McMenamin, K. E. Pinkerton, M. Ikegami, A. H. Jobe, L. Gurrin, and P. D. Sly. 1999. Lung morphometry and collagen and elastin content: Changes during normal development and after prenatal hormone exposure in sheep. *Pediatr Res* 45(5 Pt 1): 615–625.

Williams, K. J. and I. Tabas. 1995. The response-to-retention hypothesis of early atherogenesis. *Arterioscler Thromb Vasc Biol* 15: 551–561.

Wipff, P. J., D. B. Rifkin, J. J. Meister, and B. Hinz. 2007. Myofibroblast contraction activates latent TGF-beta1 from the extracellular matrix. *J Cell Biol* 179(6): 1311–1323.

Wu, Y. J., D. P. La Pierre, J. Wu, A. J. Yee, and B. B. Yang. 2005. The interaction of versican with its binding partners. *Cell Res* 15(7): 483–494.

Xu, T., P. Bianco, L. W. Fisher, G. Longenecker, E. Smith, S. Goldstein, J. Bonadio, A. Boskey, A. M. Heegaard, B. Sommer, K. Satomura, P. Dominguez, C. Zhao, A. B. Kulkarni, P. G. Robey, and M. F. Young. 1998. Targeted disruption of the biglycan gene leads to an osteoporosis-like phenotype in mice. *Nat Genet* 20(1): 78–82.

Yang, B. L., Y. Zhang, L. Cao, and B. B. Yang. 1999. Cell adhesion and proliferation mediated through the G1 domain of versican. *J Cell Biochem* 72(2): 210–20.

Zako, M., T. Shinomura, M. Ujita, K. Ito, and K. Kimata. 1995. Expression of PG-M (V3), an alternatively spliced form of PG-M without a chondroitin sulfate attachment region in mouse and human tissues. *J Biol Chem* 270: 3914–3918.

Zhang, S., M. C. Y. Chang, D. Zylka, S. Turley, R. Harrison, and E. A. Turley. 1998. The hyaluronan receptor RHAMM regulates extracellular-regulated kinase. *J Biol Chem* 273: 11342–11348.

Zimmermann, D. R. 2000. Versican. In *Proteoglycans: Structure, Biology and Molecular Interactions*, edited by RV Iozzo, pp. 327–341. New York: Marcel Dekker.

Zimmermann, D. R. and M. T. Dours-Zimmermann. 2008. Extracellular matrix of the central nervous system: From neglect to challenge. *Histochem Cell Biol* 130(4): 635–653.

Zimmermann, D. R., M. T. Dours-Zimmermann, M. Schubert, and L. Bruckner-Tuderman. 1994. Versican is expressed in the proliferating zone in the epidermis and in association with the elastic network in the dermis. *J Cell Biol* 124: 817–825.

CHAPTER 9

Recent Approaches and Future Perspectives on Elastin Regeneration and Repair

Jyotsna Joshi and Chandrasekhar Kothapalli

CONTENTS

9.1 INTRODUCTION

Elastin is found in a wide range of soft tissues such as arteries, tracheo-bronchial tree, heart valves, urinary bladder, pelvic floor tissues, vocal folds, and dermis, with detailed orientations and arrangements to meet the tissue-specific functionality (e.g., strength and direction of applied forces) (Culav et al. 1999, Sivaraman et al. 2012). The primary functions of elastin are mechanical and biological: elastin provides tissue elasticity and it also mediates cell proliferation, morphology, migration, and chemotaxis for a diverse range of cells, including smooth muscle cells (SMCs), endothelial cells, fibroblasts, and mesenchymal cells (Lisa and Anthony 2011).

As detailed in Chapters 1, 2, and 8, elastin biosynthesis is a highly controlled and coordinated, multicomponent, and multistep hierarchical process, which includes the intracellular synthesis of soluble tropoelastin monomers, their extracellular release, aggregation via coacervation, and deposition onto microfibrillar scaffold, which facilitates tropoelastin cross-linking and mature fiber formation (Kielty et al. 2002, Lisa and Anthony 2011). Thus, numerous factors play defined roles in elastin matrix maturation process, including but not limited to, the genetic expression of elastin and microfibril proteins with optimal posttranscriptional and posttranslational modifications, microfibril organization by calcium ions, stabilization of elastin and microfibrils via cross-links that are mediated by enzymes such as lysyl oxidase (LOX) and transglutaminase, respectively, and high-affinity association between fibrillin-1 and tropoelastin (Kielty et al. 2002, Rock et al. 2004). Such highly cross-linked elastin fibers generally remain stable throughout the lifetime in humans, with minimal turnover. However, various biological and environmental factors, such as aging, injuries, genetic defects, inflammation, UV exposure, and cigarette smoking, negatively impact the cross-linked elastin matrix and associated proteins, resulting in degradation and loss of elastic fibers in tissues (Tassabehji et al. 1997, Kozel et al. 2011, Rossetti et al. 2011, Chen et al. 2013, Vučević et al. 2014). On the other hand, unlike their elastin-producing neonatal counterparts, most adult cells have a very limited ability to synthesize and deposit new elastin precursors and to assemble them into mature matrix structures (Sivaraman et al. 2012).

Owing to the wide distribution of elastin matrix in the body and its susceptibility to various harmful chemical and biological factors under injury and diseased conditions, numerous approaches to repair, replace, and regenerate elastin are currently being investigated. As thoroughly detailed in Chapters 3 through 9, these approaches aim to identify the scope of various adult cells and stem cells, genes and oligonucleotides, pharmaceutical compounds, mechanical stimuli, chemical and biological signaling cues, and delivery platforms (e.g., tissue-engineered scaffolds, nanoparticles [NPs], microspheres), to promote elastin repair and/or regeneration. Some of these strategies are evolving with the advent of technologies such as sophisticated bioreactors, modular microfluidic platforms, and controllable drug delivery devices, and the availability of appropriate knockout cell lines and animal models. This final chapter summarizes some of the most recent developments in the field of elastin repair, replacement, and regeneration and highlights the grand challenges that still need to be overcome for successful clinical outcomes. A list of recent intellectual property filings and start-up companies working toward this goal are also tabled.

9.2 RECENT APPROACHES AND CHALLENGES FOR ELASTIN REGENERATION

Recent approaches for elastin repair and regeneration are exploring how to (a) stimulate the biosynthesis of tropoelastin monomers from adult elastin-producing cells (SMCs and fibroblasts); (b) induce stem cell differentiation into elastin-producing cells such as SMCs; (c) increase cross-linking and maturation of elastin synthesized and released into extracellular matrix (ECM); (d) upregulate the expressions of elastin-associated proteins (fibrillin, fibulin, etc.); (e) prevent inflammation within ECM microenvironment and suppress elastolysis of the existing cross-linked elastin matrix; (f) specifically target elastin fibers *in vivo* using custom-designed NPs for imaging, diagnostic, and therapeutic purposes; (g) block expression of certain biological molecules that are proven to be detrimental to elastic fiber formation (e.g., versican); and (h) develop scaffolds made of elastin-like peptides (ELPs), or derivatives of natural/synthetic polymers, to replace the lost elastic tissues. In the following sections, we will highlight the recent attempts and successes in elastin regeneration and repair within specific tissues and regions of the body, with a commentary on future perspectives in the field.

9.2.1 Elastin Repair within Abdominal Aortic Aneurysms

Abdominal aortic aneurysms (AAAs) involve a detrimental matrix remodeling of the abdominal aorta, such as matrix calcification and degradation of elastic lamellae, mediated by infiltration of the immune and inflammatory cells, and their secretion of matrix metalloproteinases (MMPs) and inflammatory cytokines (e.g., TNF-α, IL-1-β) (Wills et al. 1996). Numerous studies suggest that this process could be initiated by defective genetic and environmental signals, such as mutations of fibrillin-1 gene (Marfan syndrome), heterozygous disruption of elastin gene (supravalvular aortic stenosis), lipid deposition, bacterial infections, and reactive oxygen species (ROS), which lead to alterations in SMC phenotype and negatively impact vascular matrix remodeling (Kothapalli and Ramamurthi 2010, Dong and Majesky 2012, Merk et al. 2012, Zhang et al. 2012, Bashur et al. 2013). The result of such processes leads to elastic matrix degradation (including collagen) and thinning, generation of soluble peptides that signal elastin–laminin receptors of the vascular cells for further secretion of elastases, tissue weakening, and an ultimate rupture of the abdominal aortic wall (Kothapalli and Ramamurthi 2010, Bashur et al. 2013).

Thus, anti-inflammatory agents and gene and drug targeting for inhibiting MMP activities (e.g., TIMPs) have been proposed as potential therapeutics for treatment of AAAs in animal models (Isenburg et al. 2007). However, current clinical options for AAA are limited to either open surgery, minimally invasive surgical procedures (deployment of stent graft), or drug therapy, which are selected on the basis of the patient age and the growth rate of the aneurysm (Bashur et al. 2013). These clinical approaches have considerably helped to prevent from the catastrophic failures and have aided to slow or arrest the pathological progression of disease; however, there is an unmet demand for a regenerative procedure that can entail enhanced elastogenesis at the site of aneurysm while simultaneously suppressing elastolysis for aneurysm therapy (Bashur et al. 2013).

Current pharmaceutical/biomolecular approaches to elastin repair and regeneration within aortic aneurysms are focused on investigating the following:

1. Utility of hyaluronic acid (HA) oligomers (<1 kDa size) and transforming growth factor-beta (TGF-β1) (Dai et al. 2005) to enhance tropoelastin production, suppress elastase and SMC activation, and promote the elastin matrix yield and cross-linking by chronically activated adult SMCs (Kothapalli and Ramamurthi 2010).

2. Benefits of endovascular delivery of adenovirus encoding TGF-β, in experimental AAA rat models, to preserve the medial elastin, stabilize the aorta diameter, and decrease the infiltration of inflammatory cells (Dai et al. 2005).

3. Advantages of treating adult SMCs with LOX peptides or copper NPs to enhance elastin matrix synthesis and cross-linking efficiency (Kothapalli and Ramamurthi 2009a,b).

4. Impact of activated extracellular signal-regulated kinases 1/2 on elastin gene, and the utility of inhibitors for such activated kinases to increase elastin gene transcription (Lannoy et al. 2014).

5. Promising role of K-channel openers on the elastin synthesis by vascular SMCs (Lannoy et al. 2014).

6. Efficacy of elastin-binding phenolic tannins, such as pentagalloyl glucose, which stabilizes aortic elastin and retards their degradation during inflammatory conditions of AAA (Isenburg et al. 2007).

7. Benefits of antisense oligonucleotides in blocking miR-29b, a microRNA increased in ascending aorta of Marfan mice and are known to regulate apoptosis and matrix deposition, for preventing matrix deterioration and aneurysm development (Merk et al. 2012).

Further details on these approaches have been elaborated in Chapters 4 and 6 through 9. The following subsections elaborate on the recent approaches to elastin regeneration for aortic aneurysms and relevant vascular pathologies.

9.2.1.1 Theranostic NPs for Elastin Fiber Targeting and Repair

Despite recent progress, numerous challenges still persist in the development of clinically successful theranostic (*thera*peutic + dia*gnostic*) platforms. Ideally, these platforms (e.g., NPs) should mimic the mythological "trojan horse," that is, they should (a) be easily deliverable; (b) remain intact till they reach their intended target; (c) be able to precisely and accurately identify their designated target (e.g., cancer cells, tumors, tissues) using surface moieties; (d) have enough space to hold cargo (e.g., drug) either by physical or chemical bonding; (e) have minimal side effects; (f) be scalable to yield large quantities for on-demand applications; (g) be traceable on delivery *in vivo* using conventional imaging modalities such as MRI and CT scan; (h) deliver the drug or biomolecular cues in a sustainable fashion over longer distances and durations; and (i) successfully carry out the intended goal without being recognized by immune cells in the body. The same principles and expectations apply when developing NPs for targeted delivery of the drugs and regenerative cues for elastin repair, or as imaging moieties to specifically identify and associate with the diseased vasculature. It is worth mentioning that a high shear flow of blood in arteries necessitates delivery of high doses of drugs and therapeutic molecules, which might contribute to higher systemic and local toxicities (Sinha et al. 2014). Similarly, a rapid cellular uptake of NPs could reduce their retention in the ECM, which is not desirable for stimulating elastin synthesis and stabilization. On the other hand, there is continual shedding off of constitutively expressed endothelial markers as a result of negative feedback mechanism for leukocyte adhesion; hence, those common disease targets are also rendered transient and inconsistent (Sinha et al. 2014). Needless to mention, systemic delivery of MMP-inhibiting drugs could negatively impact the matrix remodeling process of tissues elsewhere in the body (Sivaraman and Ramamurthi 2013).

Thus, there is a critical need for a targeted therapeutic platform that can entail a precise spatiotemporal release of the drugs or regenerative cues with minimal local/systemic toxicity while simultaneously enabling tracking and imaging *in vivo*. The need for such therapy is more pronounced in conditions such as AAAs where the current treatment in human and animal models has been limited to oral routes. Although doxycycline (DOX), a tetracycline-based antibiotic, has been shown to retard AAA growth in both clinical and animal models and inhibit MMPs nonspecifically via direct coordination with their catalytic sites and inhibition of MMP mRNA transcription, higher doses in the blood negatively impact elastin deposition by vascular cells (Hanemaaijer et al. 1998, Pyo et al. 2000, Baxter et al. 2002, Prall et al. 2002, Liu et al. 2003, Bartoli et al. 2006, Franco et al. 2006). Thus, recent studies are investigating the utility of multifunctional NPs, such as NPs loaded with cues for elastin regeneration, magnetic particles for enhancing retention in aorta, fluorescent dyes for improved imaging, and physical and/or biochemical surface modification for specific disease targeting (Sivaraman et al. 2012, Sinha et al. 2014).

In a recent study, Vyavahare and coworkers developed a poly(D, L-lactide) (PLA) NP system decorated with an elastin antibody and loaded with DIR dye (Sinha et al. 2014). The rationale was that increased MMP activity erodes the elastin-associated proteins and exposes the elastin core in diseased vasculature, and the elastin antibody-decorated PLA NPs would specifically target and bind to such degraded elastic fibers and not their healthy counterparts (Figures 6.4 and 9.1).

Outcomes of their study showed (a) an increased NP attachment in explanted rat aortae, previously treated with elastase, with an increased surface concentration of elastin antibody; (b) no acute cytotoxicity of the NPs within rat aortic SMC cultures; (c) negatively charged NPs with ~200 nm size were retained in the extracellular space after 24 h of incubation, but those with ~100 nm size and negative charge were engulfed by the cells; (d) cellular uptake was furthered in smaller and positively charged NPs (Figures 9.1 and 6.4); (e) elastin antibody-decorated NPs exhibited a fivefold higher targeting efficacy to the injured abdominal

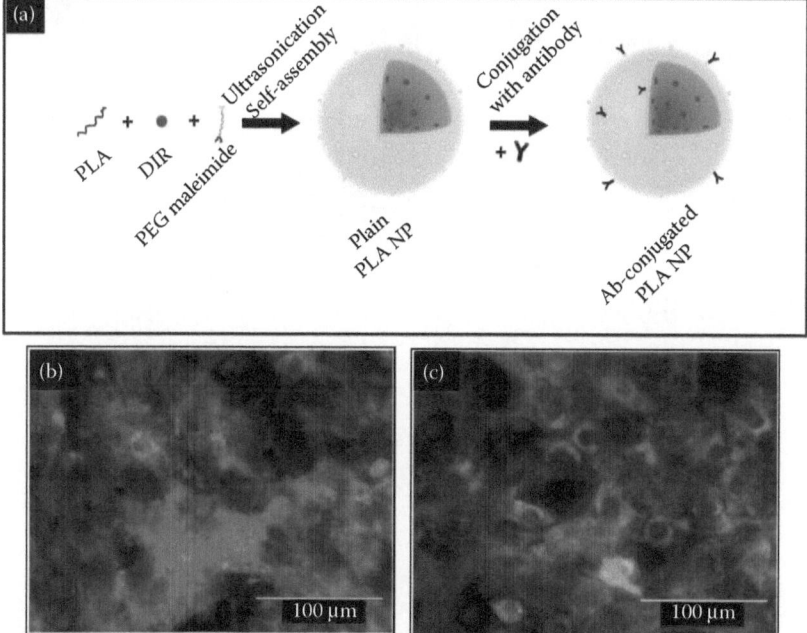

FIGURE 9.1 (a) Illustration of the PLA NP decoration with the functional groups specific to particle tracking (DIR), and antibody attachment. (b) Schematic depiction of the changes in elastic lamina fibers *in vivo* under healthy and diseased conditions, leading to elastin degradation. The decorated NPs would bind to such degraded elastic fibers in the diseased arteries, while they lack such binding capability in healthy arteries where elastin core is intact. (c) Smaller-sized PLA NPs (<100 μm) with a negative surface charge were taken up by rat aortic SMCs *in vitro*, and such uptake was more pronounced when the NP surface was modified with poly-L-lysine to create a positive charge. (Reprinted with permission from Sinha, A. et al., *Nanomed. Nanotech. Biol. Med.*, 10, 1003–12, 2014.)

aorta, compared to IgG antibody-decorated NPs; and (f) higher fluorescence from only elastin antibody-decorated NPs in the diseased but not in the healthy aortae (Figure 9.2).

In a separate recent study, which is discussed in greater detail in Chapter 4, the Ramamurthi group examined the utility of multifunctional NPs to inhibit proteolysis and simultaneously provide a conducive

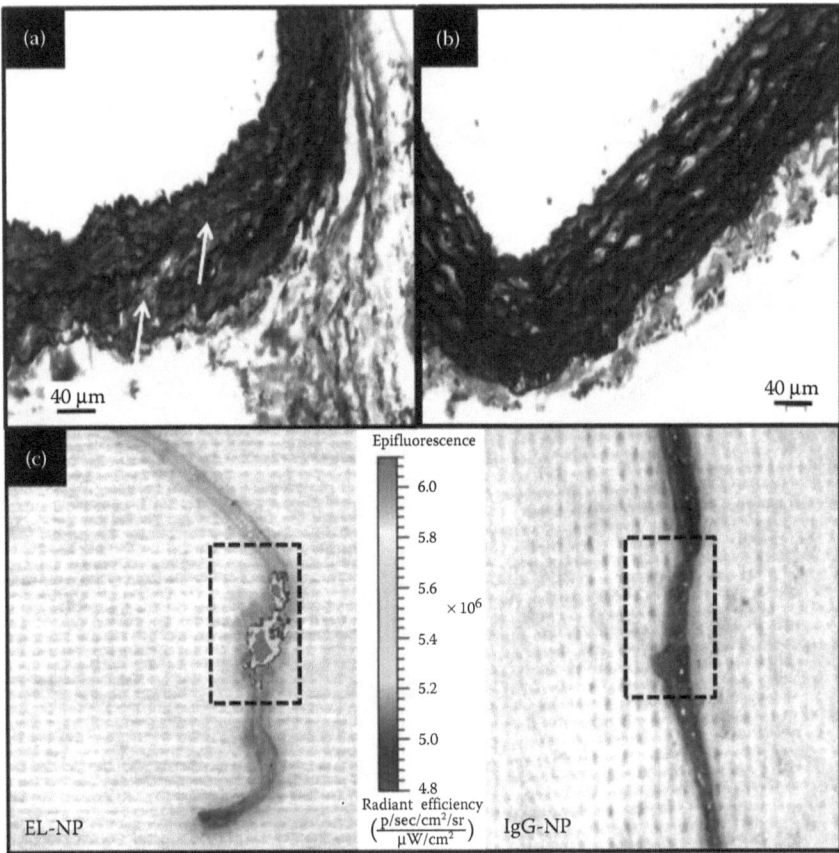

FIGURE 9.2 (a) Outcomes from *in vivo* studies show that the decorated PLA NPs specifically targeted exposed elastin core within degraded elastic fibers within the rat aortic aneurysmal blood vessels, while no such targeting was evident in the healthy rat aorta. (b) Quantification of these images suggested that the targeting of elastin antibody-decorated NPs was almost fivefold higher in the aneurysmal vessels compared to that in controls. (c) These results were verified by whole aorta imaging of aneurysmal vessels, 24 h postintravenous delivery of elastin antibody NPs or control NPs. (Reprinted with permission from Sinha, A. et al., *Nanomed. Nanotech. Biol. Med.*, 10, 1003, 2014.)

microenvironment for elastin stabilization (Sivaraman and Ramamurthi 2013). They fabricated DOX-loaded poly (lactic-*co*-glycolic acid) NPs (PLGA-NPs) using double emulsion-solvent evaporation technique. PLGA-NPs were surface modified with cationic amphiphiles such as dodecyl trimethyl ammonium bromide (DTAB), dodecyl amine hydrochloride, or didodecyl dimethyl ammonium bromide (DMAB). Such NPs were loaded with fluorescent dyes to enable their fluorometric detection. Preliminary results of their NP-based system on cellular retention, cytotoxicity studies, and drug release profile showed that (a) larger PLGA-NPs (size greater than 200 nm) were excluded by aneurysmal rat aortic SMCs, but smaller ones were rapidly engulfed by cells (Figure 9.3); (b) DOX-loaded PLGA-NPs did not impart cellular cytotoxicity at the tested concentrations and the loaded drug exhibited a characteristic biphasic release pattern, with an initial burst profile followed by a slower release pattern; and (c) the cumulative release of 2% DOX-loaded NPs over 21 days was lower than 5 μg/mL, a threshold that could limit the viability of aneurysmal SMCs.

Results of their study in terms of cellular proliferation, MMP activity, and elastin secretion suggested that (a) 2% DOX-loaded NPs caused a significant increment in cell proliferation irrespective of the NP concentration; (b) DOX release caused no significant difference to tropoelastin synthesis; (c) total elastin deposition was significantly higher in 2% DOX loaded within 0.2 mg/mL NPs; and (d) tropoelastin levels were inhibited on increasing the concentration of DOX-loaded PLGA NP, compared to

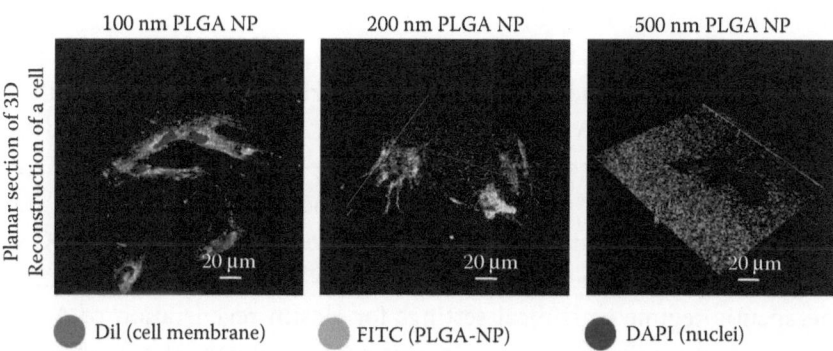

FIGURE 9.3 FITC-labeled PLGA NPs with particle sizes ranging between 100 and 500 nm were exposed to aneurysmal rat aortic SMC cultures, and their uptake patterns suggest that particles beyond 200 nm size were not taken up by these cells. (Reproduced with permission from Dr. Anand Ramamurthi, Cleveland Clinic Foundation, private communication.)

treatment controls and untreated controls. The authors anticipated that the decreased tropoelastin levels were due to increased DOX concentrations and/or due to "macromolecular crowding effect," a phenomenon supposed to inhibit the release of immature tropoelastin into the culture media. In addition, they speculated that the significant improvement in the total elastin matrix synthesis by the PLGA-NP, even in the absence of DOX, may be due to "macromolecular crowding effect" of NPs that would have potentiated the elastin stabilization and maturation process rather than the tropoelastin secretion. Similarly, results from DMAB- and DTAB-modified PLGA-NPs showed that these NPs exhibit a significantly higher binding affinity to elastin, higher interactions with SMCs, significant increment in LOX activity in the cell layers, and a significant inhibition of MMP-2 synthesis, when compared to PVA-modified NPs.

These studies suggest that the elastin matrix assembly and maturation process can be enhanced by (a) shielding the negatively charged cell membrane of SMCs with positively charged NPs, thereby preventing the interaction of pericellular matrix (e.g., negatively charged chondroitin sulfate of proteoglycans) with the elastin-binding proteins (EBPs) and reducing the immature release of tropoelastin-bound EBP; (b) providing positive charge on the NPs to enable their strong interaction with elastin and negatively charged LOX, which will enhance the recruitment of LOX at the elastogenic sites; (c) inhibiting MMP activity by charge repulsion between their active positive centers with cationic NPs; and (d) providing stearic hindrances to the active sites of MMPs due to larger surface moieties in the NP system (e.g., DMAB).

In a follow-up study, the same group investigated the utility of incorporating super paramagnetic iron oxide NPs (SPIONs) in DMAB-modified and DOX-loaded PLGA-NPs (Sivaraman et al. 2014). The rationale for the selection of SPION-based NPs was to enhance their localization in AAA wall using an external magnetic field. Incorporation of SPIONs did not significantly alter cell viability, NP size and the surface charge, and DOX-loading efficiency of the NPs. Thus, such an NP system offers a potential therapeutic regime in clinical settings for elastin regeneration of AAA. However, future research needs to elucidate the potential advantage of such NP systems over the conventional systems in terms of elastin secretion, matrix assembly, and maturation process.

Although their long-term *in vivo* efficiency is yet to be demonstrated with regard to their theranostic effects, these recent studies suggest that multifunctional NPs can specifically target elastic fibers *in vivo*, promote elastin synthesis, maturation, and stabilization, while simultaneously acting to prevent potential elastolytic events. From the above studies, we note that these NPs can inhibit the immature escape of tropoelastin from EBP–tropoelastin complex, interact with elastin and LOX molecules, suppress elastase and inhibit MMPs, and deliver the cargo with precise spatiotemporal release at the site of inflammation. In this context, Ramamurthi's group also examined the scope of hyaluronan-loaded PLGA NPs to achieve the targeted and controlled delivery of the hyaluronan oligomers, which are known to be elastogenic cues, for their possible *in vivo* applications (Sylvester et al. 2013). Within rat aortic SMC cultures, such NPs were able to (a) provide elastogenic doses of hyaluronan oligomers over 30 days, (b) provide a dose-dependent enhancement of elastin matrix synthesis, and (c) recruit and activate LOX. In conclusion, NP-mediated theranostic approaches offer a promising approach for AAA treatment, by not only identifying the extent and location of elastin fiber degradation in the vasculature, but also by enabling localized delivery of therapeutic and regenerative compounds for elastin repair and regeneration.

9.2.1.2 Nitric Oxide Cues for Elastogenesis within Adult Human SMC-EC Cocultures

Nitric oxide (NO) is a signaling molecule that helps to regulate vascular tone and is constantly released by the endothelial NO synthase (eNOS) of the vascular endothelium under healthy conditions (Ignarro et al. 1987, Palmer et al. 1987). Studies have shown that due to an injury or a pathological disorder in the endothelium, NO release is compromised. This activates SMC phenotype leading to their proliferation and migration, stimulates release of degradative enzymes that causes elastin matrix deterioration, and ultimately results in blocking of innate elastin-SMC signaling (Lüscher and Noll 1994, Alonso and Radomski 2003). Based on the hypothesis that restoring the native NO levels to SMCs might curtail their inflammatory phenotype and promote elastin synthesis and maturation by adult human SMCs, our group recently tested the utility of exogenously delivered NO cues within human SMC-EC cocultures in a microfluidic platform *in vitro* (Figure 9.4) (Simmers et al. 2015). Healthy adult human aortic SMCs (HA-SMC) were cocultured with HA endothelial cells (HA-ECs) in the presence or absence of S-nitrosoglutathione (GNSO, an NO donor; 0–100 nM) within 3D type I collagen scaffolds. This platform enables paracrine signaling between the two cell types via diffusion between their designated chambers, and the NO concentrations tested were within the physiological ranges.

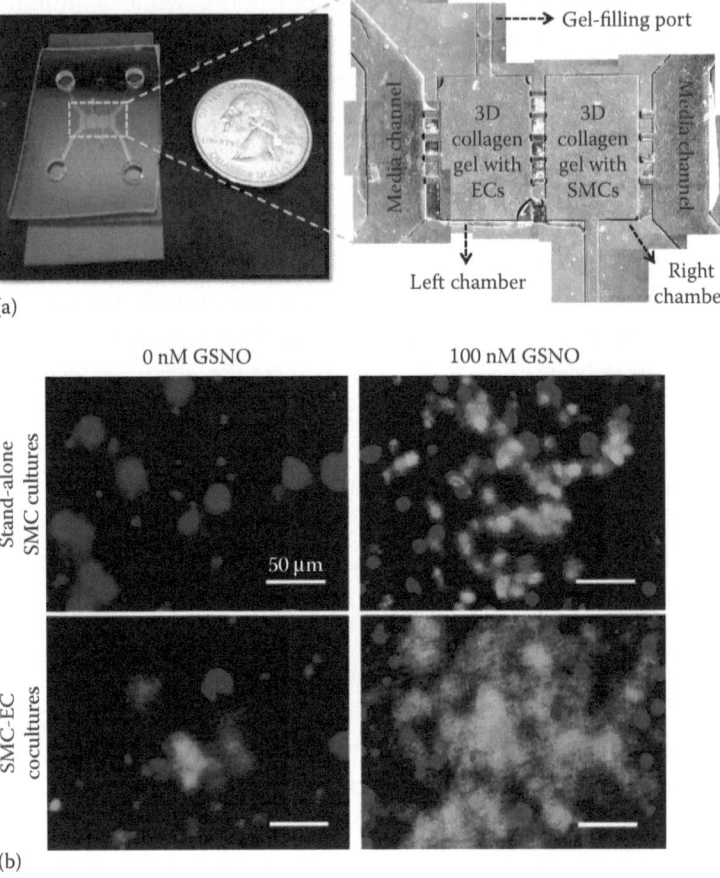

FIGURE 9.4 (a) A digital micrograph of the microfluidic platform designed for biomimetic cocultures. The platform was fabricated using soft-lithography and replica-molding techniques. Separate cell chambers with respective gel-filling ports and media channels are shown for clarity. In one of the configuration of this platform, HA-SMCs would be cultured within 3D collagen gels in the right chamber, while HA-ECs in the left chamber. (b) Cross-linked elastin matrix deposition within HA-SMC cultures, in the presence (100 nM) or absence of GSNO, and cocultures with human ECs.

Outcomes of their study suggested that (a) with increasing GSNO dosage, SMC proliferation was inhibited, either in the presence or absence of HA-EC cocultures; (b) multifold increases in the synthesis and deposition of elastin (Figure 9.4), HA, glycosaminoglycans (GAGs), TIMP-1, and LOX were noted at higher GNSO dosages and more so within HA-EC cocultures; (c) MMP-2 but not MMP-9 levels remain attenuated with increasing GSNO levels, and EC cocultures promoted these trends; and (d) a positive correlation between NO-induced matrix synthesis and an increase in the expression of eNOS and inducible NO synthase (iNOS) in adult EC and SMC cultures, respectively. Such elevation in iNOS might be beneficial to increase local NO levels via their interaction with L-arginine, which could potentially benefit in regulating blood vessel pathology and matrix remodeling. Although further studies are needed to identify the paracrine signaling between these cell types, optimize the NO concentration, and validate these outcomes *in vivo* within adult healthy and diseased animal models, these results point to the benefits of exogenously delivering physiologically relevant biological compounds to elastin synthesis and deposition. The microfluidic platform developed here for cocultures could easily be extended to culture other elastin-producing cell types such as dermal fibroblasts and lung epithelial cells, and investigate their response to exogenously delivered drugs and pharmacological compounds.

9.2.2 Elastogenesis within Elastin Haploinsufficient Diseases

Elastin replacement via protein or complementary DNA (cDNA)-based approach is not feasible because elastin gene encodes multiple splice variants and produces complex intracellular and extracellular proteins (Zhang et al. 2012). On the other hand, growth factors such as TGF-β1, IGF-1, bFGF, and so on may not be favorable for systemic delivery purposes because of their wider biological implications. Thus, there is a greater demand for an endogenous and a precise regulation of elastin gene for clinical purpose (Zhang et al. 2012).

Zhang et al. (2012) developed a mechanistic approach for targeted transcriptional activation of endogenous and intact wild-type allele in elastin haploinsufficiency, while simultaneously rescuing the generation of mutant elastin protein. They engineered transcription factors that would specifically bind to the elastin promoter sequence and enhance elastin expression from the normal intact allele of haploinsufficient cells (Zhang et al. 2012). In brief, three zinc-finger protein (ZFP) transcription factors were screened for specific binding to elastin promoter. These ZFPs were inserted to pcDNA 3.1 plasmid having cytomegalovirus promoter, nuclear translocation signal (SV40), and transactivation domain (VP16). Plasmids without VP16 were treated as controls. Human dermal fibroblasts (HDFs) and human embryonic kidney (HEK) cells were electroporated and transiently transfected with elastin-ZFP plasmids. Similarly, retroviral and lentiviral constructs of elastin-ZFPs were also constructed, and target cells were incubated with a retrovirus-conditioned and lentivirus-containing medium.

Results evinced greater than sixfold increment in elastin mRNA expression in HEK cells after treatment with all three elastin-ZFPs, with ZFP-3 being the most pronounced compared to controls. Similarly, a 12- to 32-fold increment in elastin mRNA expression in HDF cells was noted with elastin-ZFP1 and elastin-ZFP3, with enhanced secretion of tropoelastin by elastin-ZFP. The basal expression levels of vascular SMC elastin mRNA were enhanced by more than eightfold with lentiviral transduction; however, collagen mRNA expression remained unaltered implicating the specific role of ZFP on elastin gene alone. The potential of elastin-ZFP3 in inducing compensatory expression from the intact wild-type allele of dermal fibroblast cells, isolated from a patient with the Williams–Beuren syndrome, was also investigated. These cells exhibit a heterozygous microdeletion of elastin gene and express only 26%–36% of elastin mRNA. The effect of elastin-ZFP3 was very pronounced on elastin mRNA of these cells and caused almost a sevenfold increase. Next, the effect of elastin-ZFP on the isolated pulmonary vascular SMC from a patient with supravalvular aortic stenosis was examined. These cells had 4 bp inserted in exon 9 of elastin gene and a frameshift and a premature termination of codon in exon 10, which targets the mutant transcript to nonsense-mediated decay and caused elastin haploinsufficiency. Such cells were transduced with lentivirus encoding elastin-ZFP, which resulted in a ~fivefold increment in elastin mRNA, with no significant changes in collagen.

In addition, the authors investigated whether elastin-ZFP will increase the mutant elastin transcripts and potentially lead to their inefficacious clearance from nonsense-mediated decay mechanisms. They transduced haploinsufficient pulmonary vascular SMC with elastin-ZFP3 or control lentivirus, and with or without emetine (a translation inhibitor) posttransduction. They found that mutant mRNA was negligibly present, with no significant differences between cells transduced with elastin-ZFP and control virus at 72 h of posttransduction. However, on addition of emetine, there was an incremental change of mutant elastin mRNA levels in cells transduced with elastin-ZFP and control virus, with a greater increment in cells transduced with the former. Thus, it could be inferred that although the transduction of elastin-ZFP might cause an increment in the transcription of mutant elastin genes with haploinsufficient cells, it did not affect the functioning of the nonsense-mediated decay mechanism, and hence accumulation of mutant elastin protein via ZFP transduction is unlikely to happen.

However, adequate preclinical testing is necessary to ensure the efficacy of the engineered ZFP on the nonsense-mediated decay mechanism in other cell lines, before such transcriptional activation enters clinical trials (Zhang et al. 2012). Besides, the challenges associated with (a) delivery of elastin-ZFP to specific diseased cells during developmental stages, (b) ZFP as a cell permeable protein, and (c) systemic delivery for treating multiple vascular lesions need to be overcome. In this regard, it has been suggested that approaches based on catheter-based local elastin-ZFP gene delivery for site-specific lesions, prenatal or early postnatal gene delivery for early genomic integration, transduction of fetal/early postnatal cells (e.g., pluripotent cells, cord blood stem cells) with elastin-ZFP, and back delivery into the host could be areas of clinical relevance that merit further investigation.

9.2.3 Elastin Repair Mechanisms in Pelvic Floor Disorders

Disease, disorder, or trauma to the pelvic floor and associated structures and organs will result in a variety of medical conditions such as stress urinary incontinence (SUI), flatal incontinence, fecal incontinence, or pelvic organ prolapse (POP). The potential risk factors for these conditions, identified thus far, include genetic factors, pregnancy, vaginal delivery (VD), trauma, abnormal connective tissue metabolism, aging, constipation, and obesity (Couri et al. 2012, Pathi et al. 2012, Jiang et al. 2013). As multiple tissues, ligaments, muscles, and organs are involved in these disorders, recent reparative approaches are geared toward restoring the neural, mechanical, and other biological components of the damaged tissues and organs (Salcedo et al. 2012, Jiang et al. 2013, Dissaranan et al. 2014). This section highlights the recent cellular engineering approaches that are focused on elastin regeneration and repair.

Ramamurthi et al. (2012) investigated the utility of HA oligomers and TGF-β1 (termed as elastogenic factors, EFs) in improving the elastin fiber synthesis and deposition by adult vaginal SMCs isolated from prolapsed vagina (stage 3 and multiparous) of LOX-like 1 (LOXL1) knockout mouse, a well-characterized animal model to mimic clinical POP. LOXL1 is a member of the LOX family and is involved in oxidative deamination of lysine residues on tropoelastin monomers, causing cross-linking between monomers and forming elastin polymer. They treated the isolated cells with EFs for 21 days of culture and examined the cell layers and spent medium for elastin. The cell proliferation of the treatment and the control groups were similar; however, the treatment groups exhibited higher elastin mRNA expression and deposited higher total elastin, mainly as alkali-soluble elastin matrix, compared to the controls. Tropoelastin synthesis was higher, but not significantly different, in treatment group compared to the controls. In addition, transmission electron microscopy imaging depicted mature and abundant elastin fibers in the treatment groups, but intermittent and irregular fibers in the controls. Hence, it was hypothesized that EFs would have contributed to the matrix assembly process, posttropoelastin synthesis. The inability to significantly raise the alkali-insoluble cross-linked elastin would reflect the prime role of LOXL-1 in the elastin fiber cross-linking and mature fiber formation processes. Because LOX gene was upregulated in the treatment group compared to controls, although statistically insignificantly, future investigations need to examine the dose-dependent effect of EFs on LOX-mediated monomer cross-linking and elastin deposition. Overall, the study shows a promising approach for the development of a therapeutic approach for elastin matrix regeneration in pelvic floor tissues.

On the other hand, Dissaranan et al. (2014) examined the potential of delivering mesenchymal stem cells (MSCs) as a noninvasive therapeutic approach for recovering SUI following childbirth. In their studies, rat SUI models were used for simulating childbirth conditions. VD was achieved by inserting urethral dilators of increasing sizes sequentially, followed by inserting a Foley catheter and inflating the balloon for several hours. Sham VD was accomplished by catheter insertion, without balloon inflation, for the same time period as in VD. This study explored whether intravenously delivered MSCs will home in the injured tissues, influence tissue regeneration, or support the tissue functionality. One week posttreatment with MSCs, urethra, vagina, and spleen of rats receiving cells showed significantly higher homing to the injured organs compared to sham VD cases. Similar positive attributes were noted compared to sham VD cases, when MSCs were delivered intravenously to rats, or when rats received periurethral concentrated conditioned media of MSCs. These studies attest to the role of MSCs and its trophic factors in mediating the urethral recovery. Interestingly, delivering MSC and MSC-conditioned medium also provided contiguous SMC layers in the urethral tissues, where lining of smooth and striated urethral muscles was breached following VD. In addition, a week after MSC delivery, significant amounts of elastin fibers were found in the urethra, compared to sham controls (Figure 9.5).

Taken together, these results suggest that exogenously delivered MSCs influence the phenotype of urethral SMCs and fibroblasts under injury conditions, and mediate elastin recovery mostly via paracrine-signaling mechanisms. However, such studies should be conducted over longer durations to enable sufficient time frame for full elastin recovery, maturation, and organization. Besides there is a critical need to identify the specific signaling molecules (growth factors, cytokines, and chemokines) responsible for the elastin recovery.

In similar studies, Zou et al. (2010) investigated the utility of MSC-knitted silk slings in the treatment of SUI. They found that rats receiving MSC-knitted slings exhibited a higher collagen content and failure force compared to the bare sling implanted groups. Although this study did not investigate the effect of these implants on elastin matrix repair and regeneration, it demonstrated the potential benefits of cell-laden tissue-engineered slings over the conventional synthetic slings. Therefore, future studies could examine their utility for the functional recovery of the ECM, including elastin, before full-fledged clinical trials. Such slings could also

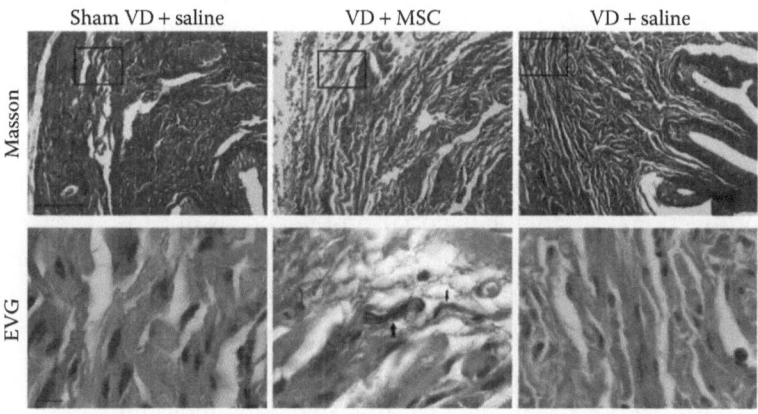

FIGURE 9.5 Histological staining of urethral tissues following MSC or saline treatment for VD or sham rats. Inset in the upper panel denotes area of magnification for elastin von Giesson stain (EVG) in the lower panel. Note: black arrows denote deposition of disorganized elastin fibers in the lower panel. Scale bars: 100 μM (Masson's trichrome) and 10 μm (EVG). (Reprinted with permission from Dissaranan, C. et al., *Cell Transplant.*, 11, 1395, 2014.)

be used for controlled release of drugs, cells, and other regenerative cues as described in Table 9.3.

A deeper understanding of the pathophysiology of pelvic floor disorders, such as POP, necessitates the application of suitable animal model because of longer durations involved in disorder progression, ethical concerns over human studies, and multifactorial causations for the disorders (Couri et al. 2012). Animal models need to mimic anatomical, histological, hormonal, and pathological characteristics of humans; however, not all parameters might be available simultaneously (Couri et al. 2012). Thus, both small and large animal models may provide answers to several factors contributing to the disorder, including (a) LOX knockout mice models on how an imbalance in elastin homeostasis can cause the development of POP, and restoration might alleviate the disorder; (b) sheep models on the role of hormones and biomechanics on the causation of POP; and (c) nonhuman primates in mimicking the human pathophysiology and providing useful clues on the efficacy of novel innovations/implants (Couri et al. 2012). Introduction of such animal models for the study purpose is by itself also a significant challenge; hence, studies should also take into account such needs.

9.2.4 Elastin Regeneration within Skin Disorders

Elastic fibers form ~2%–4% of the total dry weight of the dermis and confer elasticity and resilience (Uitto et al. 2013). However, adverse conditions, such as disease, age, trauma, and burns, can result in the abnormal matrix regulation of the skin, including that of elastin. For instance, elastin fiber degradation can be caused by the increased release of human neutrophils and macrophage elastases with age, or the continual buildup of nonfunctional elastolytic materials in the dermis due to UV exposure (Rossetti et al. 2011). Although a body of research has concentrated on the regeneration of skin tissue, with specific focus on collagen (Sheng et al. 2013, Bonvallet et al. 2015), studies aiming on elastin fiber regeneration are very limited.

Recently, various cell sources and signaling molecules have been examined to address elastin restoration in different skin disorders. For instance, dermal multipotent stem cells are being investigated as an alternative strategy to overcome skin photoaging, which involves reduction of fibroblasts and blockade of TGF-β/Smad and p38 MAPK signaling pathways (Zhong et al. 2011). These stem cells are hypothesized to possess the ability to differentiate into fibroblast lineage or activate existing fibroblasts and contribute to wound healing by releasing TGF-β, and therefore might induce elastin regeneration in photoaged skin (Zhong et al. 2011). Similarly, retinol treatment has been explored to aid in anti-aging by enhancing both elastin and collagen matrix formation (Rossetti et al. 2011). In particular, topical treatment with retinol has shown enhancements in mRNA and protein expression levels of tropoelastin and fibrillin-1 in cultured human skin (Rossetti et al. 2011). Likewise, a trifunctional peptide consisting of Val-Gly-Val-Ala-Pro-Gly motif (which increases matrix expression through the stimulation of EBP receptor), Gly-Ile-Leu tripeptide (which will occupy MMP-1 subsites and causes its inhibition), and Arg-Val-Arg-Leu linker (a competitive substrate for uro-kinase) was found to inhibit MMP-1 and activate elastin and collagen expression (Attia-Vigneau et al. 2014).

Young et al. reported that natural extracts such as that of the mycelium of *Tricholoma matsutake* (*T. matsutake*), which is an edible mushroom rich in polysaccharides such as β-glucan, can be a potential ingredient for antiaging treatments (Kim et al. 2014). They reported that such an extract exerts a significant reduction in gene and protein expressions of MMP-1 and MMP-3, and contributes to an increase in the levels of TIMP-1 and tropoelastin expressions of human fibroblasts, in a dose-dependent manner.

In addition to the role of these elastogenic molecules in rejuvenating burned or diseased skin, there is also an increasing attention toward the role of intracellular machinery, such as the Golgi apparatus and mitochondrial enzymes, in the transportation and release of tropoelastin monomers in skin disorders such as Cutis laxa (CL, Urban 2012). CL is a skin disorder characterized by a prematurely wrinkled skin with fragmented and disorganized dermal elastic fibers caused by acquired or inherited mutations in genes, affecting not only elastin or microfibrillar proteins but also the mitochondrial enzymes and Golgi secretory pathway (Urban 2012). Further research on mitochondrial enzymes involved in tropoelastin sorting and vesicular elastin preassembly, such as those implicated in proline (an important amino acid of elastin and collagen molecules) biosynthesis and in the Golgi trafficking machinery, will open new avenues for elastin repair and regeneration approaches.

In addition to the recent advances in elastin regeneration within tissues and organs highlighted earlier, other researchers have investigated elastin regeneration approaches in the heart, vocal cords, and urinary bladder, which are detailed in Table 9.1.

TABLE 9.1   Approaches Targeted for Elastin Regeneration in Different Organs/Tissues

Organ/Tissue	Study	Results	References
Myocardium	1. Transplantation of myoblast sheets, modified to secrete elastin, in the myocardial infarction (MI) region of rats	a. Significant improvement of cardiac function and the left ventricular end-diastolic volume b. Attenuation of left ventricular remodeling with concurrent formation of elastic fibers in the epicardial area	Uchinaka et al. (2012), Li et al. (2012)
	2. Transplantation of rat bone marrow stromal cells (BMSCs), transduced with elastin cDNA, in infarcted myocardium of rats	a. Elastin deposition in the infarcted tissue was correlated with the improved tissue integrity and functions b. For over 9 weeks, rats receiving transduced BMSCs maintained tissue organization via elastin overexpression, showed highest functional improvement, and reduced scar expansion	
Vocal folds	1. Treatment of human vocal fold fibroblasts (hVFFs) with granulocyte-macrophage colony-stimulating factor (GM-CSF)	Inhibited TGF-β1-induced collagen synthesis, enhanced HA production, and significant tropoelastin expression by hVFFs	Lim et al. (2013), Hughes et al. (2014)
	2. Culture of hVFFs on the aligned elastin-like peptide (ELP)-coated Tecoflex scaffold	a. ELP-coated aligned scaffolds provided highest elastin transcription level compared to unaligned or aligned fibronectin-coated scaffolds b. ELP-coated scaffolds did not elicit simultaneous upregulation of collagen synthesis	
Urinary bladder	1. An *ex vivo* organ culture of urinary bladder wall under strain-based mechanical stimuli and exogenous supplements of TGF-β	A 0.5 Hz strain frequency (at 15% strain) showed a significant increment in elastin production compared to static cultures. However, the cell phenotype was altered on addition of TGF-β, which caused higher collagen production	Heise et al. (2012)

9.3 DEVELOPMENT OF BIOENGINEERED ELASTIC CONSTRUCTS

There has been an increasing interest in expanding the utility of elasto-genic biomaterials to reconstruct and repair the elastic tissues, such as blood vessels, dermal grafts, and vocal folds. These elastogenic biomaterials are often combined with appropriate cells and signaling molecules and are provided with appropriate mechanical cues for the development of elastomeric constructs. The role of each of these components in the context of growing elastic tissue constructs *in vitro* and *in vivo* is discussed in Chapters 4, 5, and 7. The following subsections will however broadly highlight the recent developments in the applications of elastomeric constructs in conjunction with signaling cues for elastin regeneration.

9.3.1 Vascular Grafts

Combination of a variety of cell types (e.g., stem cells, vascular progenitor, or mature vascular cells) and scaffolds (decellularized animal tissues and various degradable or nondegradable scaffolds) can provide substitute materials for vascular constructs (Babczyk et al. 2014). However, being the major extracellular component of the arteries and contributing up to 50% of its dry weight (Patel et al. 2006), the quality and the quantity of the deposited elastic fibers influence the success of the vascular constructs. Numerous scaffolds based on collagen, HA, fibrin, polyglycolic acid (PGA), and its copolymers, silk fibroin, PCL, to name a few, have been recently investigated for their ability to induce elastogenesis within vascular constructs (Bashur et al. 2012).

Allen et al. (2014) examined neoarteriogenesis in rats 1 year post-implantation of a biodegradable arterial graft, made of microporous poly(glycerol sebacate) (PGS) and reinforced with nanofibrous PCL. Results suggested that the fast resorption of the scaffold facilitated formation of collagen and elastin fiber-sheathed new arteries, minimized tissue inflammation, and eliminated consequences of late graft failures. Such neoarteries responded to the vasoactive molecules and were found to be encapsulated by new nerves, although the elastin fiber organizations in them were not comparable to that of native tissue. Future studies should examine the feasibility of delivering vascular cells in such scaffolds to provide integrated functions of both neural and vascular circuitry at the transplanted site.

Zhang et al. (2012) utilized the elastogenic potential of ZFP (described in Section 9.2) on the engineered arteries, which were ~1 mm in diameter and had human vascular SMCs seeded onto a PGA scaffold strengthened with silicone tubes (Zhang et al. 2012). Such constructs were cultured for 6 weeks in a bioreactor in the presence of bFGF, PDGF-bb, and copper sulfate, and a pulsatile pump was used to provide pulsation to the arteries through the silicone tubes. Human vascular SMCs were transduced with lentivirus encoding elastin-ZFP3, seeded on engineered vessels, and cultured for 8 weeks under similar bioreactor conditions as control cells. The elastin-ZFP transduced vessels showed greater fibronectin, fibrillin-1, elastin, and desmosine (a marker of cross-linked elastin) amounts than controls. Elastin-ZFP did not cause any increment in the amount of hydroxyproline nor were there any differences in the cell number from controls. However, surprisingly, elastin-ZFP transduced vessels did not exhibit any mature elastin lamellae.

Lee et al. (2011) examined the synergistic effects of scaffold pore size and pulsatile flow on elastin synthesis and release by adult baboon primary SMCs. SMCs were seeded in the lumen of a porous and tubular PGS scaffolds and the whole constructs were strained under pulsatile flow for 3 weeks. Results suggest that SMCs deposit circumferentially organized elastin proteins, as seen in native tissue, with mature elastin equivalent to ~19% of the native tissue. In addition, the constructs exhibited higher mechanical properties, with compliance comparable to native tissue. The constructs with smaller pore sizes (25–32 μm) were found to support higher cellular organization, ECM protein deposition, including that of elastin fibers and microfibrillar proteins, compared to those with larger pores. However, lower mechanical properties of the construct and insufficient collagen matrix production suggest the need for a more appropriate coculture model of SMCs with fibroblasts, to enhance elastin and collagen deposition and boost the mechanical properties of the vascular constructs.

9.3.2 Dermal Grafts

Although split- or full-thickness autologous grafts are the gold standard for skin replacements in cases of burns and wounds, the limited availability of the donor sites in massive burns and wounds has led to the developments of alternative scaffolding materials for dermal applications, of which cultured epithelial autografts (CEA) is one example (Almine et al. 2010). CEA allows rapid wound closure; however, it is often associated with a few adverse events such as wound contraction, blistering, and scarring. In addition, elastin expression occurs only 4–5 years after the treatment of burn wounds with CEA, and presents with functional and spatial disorganization in scar tissues (Almine et al. 2010).

While elastin forms a crucial component of healthy skin dermis and plays a crucial role in dermal regeneration, it fails to adequately regenerate after severe wound healing. Elastin-based grafts are generally overlooked in the development of dermal grafts, as opposed to the readily obtained collagen-based grafts (Almine et al. 2010, Rnjak et al. 2011). However, the inherent problems associated with conventional collagen-based grafts on wound contractures often lead to severe scar formation and delayed wound healing. Recent progress on elastin isolation from animal tissues and the development of elastin-based constructs have accelerated interests in the design of elastin-based dermal grafts. Examples of clinically available, elastin-containing, dermal substituents include Alloderm®, a decellularized human cadaver skin, and Matriderm®, which consists of native bovine collagen and soluble α-elastin derived from bovine ligamentum nuchae (Rnjak et al. 2011).

Min et al. (2014) performed a retrospective study of 31 patients who underwent dermal replacements by autologous split-thickness skin grafts with Matriderm®. After ~12 months postsurgery, the graft success rate was reported to be ~96.7%, and the average elasticity on the skin portion where Matriderm was applied was 0.765 (range 0.635–0.800). In addition, other skin properties such as transepidermal water loss, humidification value, and erythema and melanin levels were within the normal limits in the grafted portions of the skin. More importantly, no significant differences were reported in the elasticity and transepidermal water loss between the nearby skin and the skin treated with Matriderm®. Similar outcomes were reported by Choi et al. (2014) on a total of 34 patients who had previously received skin graft along with Matriderm®. However, it is also important to note that while these grafts are clinically available for treating skin burns, there are risks of graft rejection, infection, failure, and batch-to-batch variability associated with these grafts (Rnjak et al. 2011). Hence, recent investigations are examining the utility of recombinant and synthetic elastin molecules for such applications.

9.4 ELASTOMERS FOR 3D CONSTRUCTS

The heavy cross-linking and insoluble nature of purified elastin has posed significant problems to incorporate these molecules as a scaffold for tissue engineering (Moore and Thibeault 2012). This, in addition to the problems associated with graft rejection and failures from tissue-derived elastin-based constructs, has led to the development of biodegradable elastomers for 3D construct applications. In this regard, recombinant tropoelastin, solubilized elastin (e.g., animal-derived soluble elastin such as α-elastin and κ-elastin), and elastin-based peptides are being investigated to construct electrospun fibers or hydrogels, and mimic the properties of the native tissue (Moore and Thibeault 2012, Annabi et al. 2013). These biomolecules have the ability to self-assemble under physiological conditions, as native tropoelastin monomers, and therefore have been evaluated as biomimetic scaffolds for elastin regeneration (Annabi et al. 2013). In particular, because elastin derived from animal sources has partial cross-links that will provide inadequate sites for cellular binding, synthetically or biosynthetically derived ELP and recombinant tropoelastin are being developed. Moreover, recombinant tropoelastin is known to produce long protein sequences with defined chain compositions by using *Escherichia coli*, yeast, or plants for protein expression (Annabi et al. 2013).

For the development of elastomeric constructs using these elastomeric biopolymers, other biomaterials are also utilized to provide adequate mechanical properties to the intended tissue of application (e.g., hydrogels for vocal fold constructs) (Moore and Thibeault 2012). Similarly, these biosynthetically derived elastins have also been utilized to develop elastin-coated vascular constructs; for instance, electrospun recombinant tropoelastin with PCL (Wise et al. 2011). Such tubular constructs have shown reduced thrombogenicity and optimal mechanical properties (permeability, elastic modulus, compliance, etc.) and provide a smooth elastic lamina in the luminal surface under circulating blood flow, and exhibited durability *in vivo* (Wise et al. 2011). These developments have provided useful insights for the incorporation of biosynthetic or synthetic elastin monomers for tissue engineering applications. However, further studies are required to investigate the cellular and physiological roles of such elastin monomers at the transplantation site, for example, the induction of the ECM, including the elastin fibers and their incorporation into the constructs.

9.5 RECENT PATENTS AND PRODUCTS ON ELASTIN

Tables 9.2 and 9.3 list some of the recent technologies and approaches pertinent to elastin regeneration and repair that have been patented since 2008. This is not a comprehensive listing as there could be numerous other technologies that are still in the provisional patenting or IP disclosure stages.

9.6 CONCLUSIONS AND FUTURE DIRECTIONS

At present, bulk of the elastin repair and regeneration strategies have been focused on investigating the benefits of delivering signaling cues, ECM and synthetic biomaterials, tissue grafts isolated from animals, and cellular gene transfection to elastin biosynthesis, maturation, or stabilization within

TABLE 9.2 List of Selected Companies and their Products for Elastin Repair and Regeneration in Humans

Company Name	Product Name	Elastin-Related Function	References
Elastagen	Elastatherapy®	Use of clinical-grade recombinant human elastin for dermal applications	http://www.elastagen.com/, http://www.ausbiotech.org/userfiles/file/ElastagenCaseStudy.pdf
Protein Genomics	Elastatropin®	Human tropoelastin produced by biotechnology methods in microorganisms and plants for wound healing and skin care products	http://www.proteingenomics.com/index-2.html
Life Cell	Alloderm®	Intended to home the circulating stem cells, differentiate into tissue-specific lineage, regenerate the matrix (including collagen and elastin), and vascularize the tissue	http://www.lifecell.com/health-care-professionals/lifecell-products/allodermr-regenerative-tissue-matrix/allodermr-tissue-matrix-defined/tissue-regeneration/
Medskin Solutions Dr. Suwelack AG	Matriderm®	The blend of collagen and elastin dermal substitute promotes cell migration, proliferation, matrix including elastin synthesis, and angiogenesis	http://www.medskin-suwelack.com/en/matriderm.html

TABLE 9.3 Patented Methods and Technologies Filed and Issued since 2008, in the Field of Elastin Regeneration and Repair

Patent Identifier	Patent Title	Elastin-Related Signaling Cues or Available Technologies
US 8618084 B2	Aldosterone induced vascular elastin production	Mineralocorticoid, such as aldosterone, can induce elastogenesis but downregulate collagen synthesis if provided in conjunction with mineralocorticoid receptor (MR) antagonists.
US 20140155335 A1	Elastin protective polyphenolics and methods of using the same	Polyphenols (ellagic acid and/or tannic acid) have inherent ability to scavenge ROS and reactive nitrogen species (RNS) and thereby protect the tropoelastin mRNA from its deterioration. In addition, their ability to bind with the elastin molecules further retards the degradation process of elastic fibers.
US 20110081322 A1	Elastin-producing fibroblast formulations and methods of using the same	Enzymatic digestion of bovine *ligamentum nuchae* (ProK-60), containing soluble elastin and microfibrillar peptides, can stimulate deposition of elastin fibers from dermal fibroblasts, also attested from organ cultures and animal models.
US 20150037382 A1	Microsphere skin treatment	Use of microspheres to bring controlled delivery and release of growth factors (connective tissue growth factor and basic fibroblast growth factor) for enhancing the extracellular matrix regeneration in skin.
US 20110091398 A1	Oleanoyl peptide composition and a method of treating skin aging	Peptide SEQ ID No. 1 when linked to oleanolic acid, and with or without plant derivatives (coconut liquid endosperm, amla, etc.), inhibits aging due to oxidation and high activity of elastase and collagenase, and so on.
US 20140161850 A1	Cosmetic compositions with near infrared (NIR) light-emitting material and methods thereof	Infrared or NIR light, generated from low-level laser therapy, can reactivate the mitochondrion functioning of the injured or damaged cells, stimulate collagen and elastin production, and can improve the skin texture by reducing wrinkles.
US 20150064268 A1	Nanoparticles for stimulating elastogenesis	Nanoparticles delivering elastogenic cues, MMP-inhibitory drugs (DOX), imaging agents, and surface functionalization with cationic amphiphiles will improve LOX recruitment but simultaneously reduce MMP activity. Such nanoparticle-based designs can be utilized for different elastic tissues. *(Continued)*

TABLE 9.3 (*Continued*) Patented Methods and Technologies Filed and Issued since 2008, in the Field of Elastin Regeneration and Repair

Patent Identifier	Patent Title	Elastin-Related Signaling Cues or Available Technologies
US 8529951 B1	Elastogenic cues and methods for using same	Elastogenic cues including hyaluronan fragments and oligomers, optionally in conjunction with growth factors and/or a source of copper ions, to encourage growth and development of elastin-containing cellular constructs.
WO 2014163178 A1	Elastin synthesis/regeneration promoting agent	8-[2-(2-Pentyl-cyclopropylmethyl)-cyclopropyl]-octanoic acid (DCP-LA) promotes elastin regeneration and synthesis. Hence, it is beneficial to prevent wrinkles and can be utilized as antiaging medicine.
WO 2012156641 A1	Use of kappa-elastin for the reconstruction and/ or regeneration of periodontal tissues	Kappa-elastin enhances tissue repair and healing and also regenerates the lost gum tissue during periodontal disease, as evidenced by increased expression of tropoelastin, collagen I, and fibrillin-I by human gingival fibroblasts.
EP 2412795 A1	Cross-linked material comprising elastin and collagen, and use thereof	Collagen/elastin cross-linked materials are obtained by cross-linking collagen and elastin, both derived from fish, and resembles the application as artificial dermis and cellular scaffold materials.
US 8940868 B2	Elastin-based growth factor delivery platform for wound healing and regeneration	The growth factor delivery system consists of a fusion polypeptide of keratinocyte growth factor (KGF) and ELP, where the bioactivity of KGF and inverse phase transition behavior of ELP are retained. At higher temperatures (>30°C), ELP will enhance the aggregation of particles, thereby will improve cellular growth, wound healing, and the subsequent internalization of the aggregates by keratinocytes.
WO 2011039728 A1	Home use electric machine and system with micro needles for stimulation of collagen and elastin-producing cells	Collagen and elastin fibers are induced to form due to mechanical action because as the skin is stimulated the body defends against the procedure, causing self-regulation. The machine will provide a precise action with no slippage but uniformity in the penetration of micro needles into the skin and will cause lesser trauma during the procedure.

(Continued)

TABLE 9.3 (*Continued*) Patented Methods and Technologies Filed and Issued since 2008, in the Field of Elastin Regeneration and Repair

Patent Identifier	Patent Title	Elastin-Related Signaling Cues or Available Technologies
US 20120010146 A1	Composite containing collagen and elastin as a dermal expander and tissue filler	The composite can be retained at the injection site for extended period of time and eliminate wrinkles and other skin. This is achieved via the natural resistance of elastin against degradation and the space filling ability due to collagen. Other proteins such as glycosaminoglycan and hyaluronic acid can also comprise the filler.
EP 1797899 A1	Preventive and remedy for collagen or elastin metabolic disorder	A therapeutic agent composed of an active ingredient possessing JNK inhibitory activity for preventing collagen and elastin metabolic disorders, particularly for aneurysms. JNK inhibitors inhibit MMPs that are involved in collagen and elastin degradation.
WO 2010135527 A2	Elastin for soft tissue augmentation	Compositions of isolated elastin and a pharmaceutical carrier, with growth factors, cells, and drugs, can improve folds, wrinkles, cleft lips, vocal fold defects, breast deformities, cheek and nose deformities, and so on.
WO 2009017646 A3	Compositions comprising human collagen and human elastin and methods for soft tissue augmentation	The invention presents the compositions of isolated human collagen and elastin (molecular weight greater than 100 kDa; insoluble in water) and a pharmaceutical carrier. It also provides methods and kits for soft tissue augmentation.
US 20130123364 A1	N6-(1-Iminoethyl)-L-lysine for regeneration of alveoli in lungs	Animal studies exhibited N6-(1-iminoethyl)-L-lysine treatment provided a complete regeneration of alveolar structure and lung functionality, including regeneration of elastic fibers, after tissue deterioration due to tobacco exposure.

(*Continued*)

TABLE 9.3 (*Continued*) Patented Methods and Technologies Filed and Issued since 2008, in the Field of Elastin Regeneration and Repair

Patent Identifier	Patent Title	Elastin-Related Signaling Cues or Available Technologies
US 20120100185 A1	Regeneration of tissue without cell transplantation	Articular cartilage regeneration include combination of biomolecules (needed for stem cell homing) with cell-free biodegradable scaffolds (e.g., collagen, PCL, elastin, etc.), where the temporal release of the biomolecules is determined by the scaffold degradation kinetics or their type (e.g., GAG holds cytokines and growth factors enable their retention or concentration following cell recruitment).
WO 2014110177 A2	Small molecules that promote skin regeneration	The method includes administration of an effective amount of small molecule (SL 327, ABT 702, fenobam, SX 011, EGF, prostaglandin E2, etc.) that will induce fibroblast proliferation and skin regeneration, including the production of collagen and elastin.
WO 2011044367 A1	Methods and compositions for skin regeneration	The methods and compositions include pharmaceutical or biological agents such as insulin-like growth factor-1 (IGF-1), NP-based systems for the release of such agents, and matrix components (e.g., hyaluronan) for skin regeneration.
US 8568761 B2	Compositions for regenerating defective or absent myocardium	Emulsified or injectable matrix components (e.g., urinary bladder submucosa and liver basement membrane) added with appropriate cells, proteins, or polypeptide (e.g., collagen, elastin, VEGF, EGF, etc.) can regenerate structure and function (e.g., contractility, conductivity, etc.) of the defective or diseased heart muscle. The matrix components will provide a conducive microenvironment needed for optimal cell–matrix, cell–cell, or protein–protein interactions required for the tissue regeneration.

(*Continued*)

TABLE 9.3 (*Continued*) Patented Methods and Technologies Filed and Issued since 2008, in the Field of Elastin Regeneration and Repair

Patent Identifier	Patent Title	Elastin-Related Signaling Cues or Available Technologies
EP 1860182 B1	Method of regenerating elastic fiber with the use of DANCE or factor enhancing the expression thereof	Secretory protein known as DANCE (developmental arteries and neural crest epidermal growth factor (EGF)-like, also known as fibulin-5) was cloned from developing cardiovascular tissues by the inventors. DANCE and/or fibulin-4 cause the efficient formation of elastic fibers in serum-free cultures of elastogenic cells, highlighting its essential role for elastic fiber regeneration *in vivo*.
US 20100316614 A1	Compositions and methods for urinary bladder regeneration	This method examines the utility of MSC and endothelial progenitor cells (EPC) for bladder regeneration, where elastin expression was increased that is required for the SMC development and functional requirement of the bladder.
EP 2740498 A2	Compositions and methods for tissue filling and regeneration	Compositions for immediate and long-term tissue filling include cellular components, filler components (e.g., HA-based fillers) optimal for cellular growth, and integrin binding components (e.g., laminin, fibronectin, elastin, etc.) needed for cellular adhesion and viability. The composition may include sol–gel transformation with cells that will gel at higher temperatures.
WO 2011046519 A1	Polypeptide material composed of elastin-like segments and coiled-coil segments	Polypeptide material consisting of elastin-like segments, which are cross-linked via noncovalent interactions of coiled-coil segments, regulated by assembly and disassembly of the material, and additionally modified by functional domains to enhance specific cellular functions, such as growth, proliferation, and inhibition of microbial growth.
US 20130085099 A1	Therapeutic agents comprising ELP	The therapeutic agent consists of a therapeutic active component and an ELP, the latter contains certain peptide units of elastin protein and thus provide benefit (e.g., higher solubility, half-life, and stability) to the therapeutic active component

(*Continued*)

TABLE 9.3 (*Continued*) Patented Methods and Technologies Filed and Issued since 2008, in the Field of Elastin Regeneration and Repair

Patent Identifier	Patent Title	Elastin-Related Signaling Cues or Available Technologies
US 7803522 B2	Elastin-producing fibroblast formulations and methods of using the same	The formulation consists of fibroblasts that are stimulated to increase elastin or other matrix components by digests of mammalian elastin, certain plant extracts composed of ELP, or their synthetic counterparts.
EP 2419442 A1	3D matrices of human elastin-like polypeptides and method of preparation thereof	Biomimetic matrices composed of human ELP can be derived via enzymatic cross-linking of the polypeptides, which can be applied for biomedical or pharmaceutical applications for supporting cellular growth and the release of pharmacological active moieties.
US 20080107708 A1	Tropoelastin-based protoelastin biomaterials	The invention describes methods to fabricate biocompatible materials for vascular applications, where human recombinant tropoelastin and synthetic/natural biomaterials are utilized to form protoelastin. Being biocompatible, elastic, and strong, these materials are able to meet the wide requirements for vascular prosthesis.
WO 2014089610 A1	Scalable three-dimensional elastic construct manufacturing	The invention describes a method for production of elastic materials from tropoelastin, including application of heat in tropoelastin solution to fabricate elastic constructs.
US 20100106233 A1	Bionanocomposite for tissue regeneration and soft tissue repair	The method describes the scope of bionanocomposite as scaffolds for soft tissue regeneration where decellularized tissue (including collagen, elastin, and other matrix proteins) is cross-linked to nanomaterials, which retard the degradation of the tissue, improve the tissue strength, and promotes cellular functions, and so on.

(*Continued*)

TABLE 9.3 (*Continued*) Patented Methods and Technologies Filed and Issued since 2008, in the Field of Elastin Regeneration and Repair

Patent Identifier	Patent Title	Elastin-Related Signaling Cues or Available Technologies
US 7862564 B2	Method of remodeling stretch marks	The cosmetic method for skin regeneration in stretch marks includes application of thermal energy and forming successive regions of thermally treated tissue regions over the stretch marks and resulting in the reduction of stretch mark. Application of pulse energy between 1.5 and 3.5 J provided full epidermal regeneration and enhanced the fibroblastic activity for collagen and elastin regeneration.
US 20080312156 A1	*In situ* cross-linkable elastin-like polypeptides for defect filling in cartilaginous tissue repair	Cartilaginous defects filled by utilizing cross-linking agent such as amine-free hydroxyalkyl (preferably hydroxymethyl) phosphine and bioelastin polymer (composed of elastomeric units).
WO 2015021508 A1	Regeneration of damaged tissue	Prolonged contact of wound edge with tropoelastin or elastin-derived peptide will provide re-epithelialization of the wound. The study evaluated the impact of Integra dermal template with/without recombinant human tropoelastin on dermal regeneration of full thickness wound in pig models. After 2 weeks following the surgery, the regenerated dermis, containing the tropoelastin, led to improved wound repair with higher levels of elastin fibers.
US 7666829 B2	Compositions for elastogenesis and connective tissue treatment	Compositions of the invention include minerals (including the trivalent ions, manganese, and their salts) to enhance synthesis of connective tissue matrix (mainly collagen and elastin) and proliferation of HDF.
US 8142817 B2	Composition for restoration of age-related tissue loss in the face or selected areas of the body	A composition of growth factors (e.g., insulin, insulin-like growth factor, thyroid hormone, fibroblast growth factor, and estrogen) and HA (carrier) when injected in the dermal, hypodermal, or various regions of body can stimulate collagen, elastin, and fat cells. In addition, the composition enables to provide time-dependent release of growth factors in the tissue.

(Continued)

TABLE 9.3 (Continued)   Patented Methods and Technologies Filed and Issued since 2008, in the Field of Elastin Regeneration and Repair

Patent Identifier	Patent Title	Elastin-Related Signaling Cues or Available Technologies
US 20080306001 A1	Transcriptional modulation of ECM of dermal fibroblasts	Peptides (and compositions) and peptide mimetic (and methods) for preventing age-related skin conditions and interfere with inhibitory transcriptional regulators of aged fibroblasts to stimulate synthesis of ECM components, including collagen and elastin.
WO 2013044314 A1	*In vivo* synthesis of elastic fiber	The methods to restore tissue elasticity using composition of tropoelastin. It also details the delivery methods to enable the sustain release of tropoelastin in the tissues.
US 8859021 B2	Skin appearance through gene manipulation	Gene manipulation method via meroterpene for preventing and improving conditions of skin (preventing or reducing fine lines and wrinkles).
US 7674458 B2	Lysyl oxidase-like 1 (LOXL1) and elastogenesis	Methods to treat and prevent loss of elastic fibers by administering compounds that enhance LOXL1 activity (e.g., LOXL1 enhancers).
US 8367619 B2	Methods for promoting elastogenesis and elastin fiber formation by increasing tropoelastin expression	Methods to increase elastin fiber formation in a cell include contacting elastogenic cell with (a) a mutated biglycan polypeptide, (b) a versican V3 isoform polypeptide, and/or (c) metastatin (a hyaluronan-binding complex).
US 8221746 B2	Antioxidant for use in cosmetic, medicated, and pharmaceutical preparations	A cosmetic preparation and its application method, where 2,2-dimethyl chroman is utilized as a superoxide dismutase (SOD) mimetic, for preventing free radical-induced damage to skin cells and enhancing collagen and elastin synthesis.
US 8022195 B2	Vectors encoding cell growth and adhesion factors for simultaneous growth and adhesion of cells	Genetic manipulation of endothelial cells and SMCs to express or overexpress cell proliferation factors and cell adhesion factors (elastin, tropoelastin, fibronectin, etc.). Such genetically altered cells have wider implications to improve cellular seeding and functions on prosthetic grafts.

in vitro cultures and animal models. However, clinical translation of these technologies has occurred at a relatively slower pace, and the lag indicates the need for a bridge between laboratory successes and clinical applications. One solution that could help minimize this gap would be the establishment of appropriate universally acceptable *in vivo* and *in vitro* models to validate the devised technologies for prospective human applications (Couri et al. 2012). Such models should take into account the variations in the genetic and phenotypic make up of cells, tissues, and ECM in mammalian species, and the differences in the native elastin synthesis, cross-linking, deposition, orientation, and mechanical and biological properties.

Similarly, analysis of the expression patterns of tropoelastin, matrix elastin, and elastin-associated proteins in native versus experimental groups, developmental versus adult stages, *in vitro* versus *in vivo*, and across various species needs merit. This is particularly relevant for elastin regeneration because such proteins exhibit differential expression in the native tissues during prenatal, adolescent, and adult life (Votteler et al. 2013). Such information would be particularly helpful in understanding the differentiation of stem cells toward elastogenic cell lineages (SMCs, fibroblasts), as the evolution pattern of elastin and elastin-associated proteins can provide an index of the level of elastogenic differentiation. Besides, analysis of such a spatiotemporal expression of the proteins would help in screening and correlating the role of specialized molecules during specific elastogenic events. On a more encouraging note, start-up firms in the United States, Europe, and Asia are developing and refining protocols to fabricate elastin matrix scaffolds and tropoelastin building blocks for applications either as standalone or within consumer products (e.g., Elastagen Pty Ltd, KappaElastin, ConnecTiss, LLC., DermaPlus Inc., Induchem).

ACKNOWLEDGMENTS

C.K. acknowledges funding from the Cleveland State University and the US National Science Foundation (1337859). J.J. acknowledges funding support from the Cleveland State University and the Cellular and Molecular Medicine Specialization Program Fellowship to perform her doctoral dissertation.

REFERENCES

Allen, R. A., W. Wu, M. Yao, D. Dutta, X. Duan, T. N. Bachman, H. C. Champion, D. B. Stolz, A. M. Robertson, and K. Kim. 2014. Nerve regeneration and elastin formation within poly (glycerol sebacate)-based synthetic arterial grafts one-year post-implantation in a rat model. *Biomaterials* 35(1): 165–173.

Almine, J. F., D. V. Bax, S. M. Mithieux, L. Nivison-Smith, J. Rnjak, A. Waterhouse, S. G. Wise, and A. S. Weiss. 2010. Elastin-based materials. *Chem Soc Rev* 39(9): 3371–3379.

Alonso, D. and M. W. Radomski. 2003. The nitric oxide-endothelin-1 connection. *Heart Fail Rev* 8(1): 107–115.

Annabi, N., S. M. Mithieux, G. Camci-Unal, M. R. Dokmeci, A. S. Weiss, and A. Khademhosseini. 2013. Elastomeric recombinant protein-based biomaterials. *Biochem Eng J* 77: 110–118.

Attia-Vigneau, J., C. Terryn, S. Lorimier, J. Sandre, F. Antonicelli, and W. Hornebeck. 2014. Regeneration of human dermis by a multi-headed peptide. *J Invest Dermatol* 134(1): 58–67.

Babczyk, P., C. Conzendorf, J. Klose, M. Schulze, K. Harre, and E. Tobiasch. 2014. Stem cells on biomaterials for synthetic grafts to promote vascular healing. *J Clin Med* 3(1): 39–87.

Bartoli, M. A., F. E. Parodi, J. Chu, M. B. Pagano, D. Mao, B. T. Baxter, C. Buckley, T. L. Ennis, and R. W. Thompson. 2006. Localized administration of doxycycline suppresses aortic dilatation in an experimental mouse model of abdominal aortic aneurysm. *Ann Vasc Surg* 20(2): 228–236.

Bashur, C. A., R. R. Rao, and A. Ramamurthi. 2013. Perspectives on stem cell-based elastic matrix regenerative therapies for abdominal aortic aneurysms. *Stem Cells Transl Med* 2(6): 401–408.

Bashur, C. A., L. Venkataraman, and A. Ramamurthi. 2012. Tissue engineering and regenerative strategies to replicate biocomplexity of vascular elastic matrix assembly. *Tissue Eng Part B* 18(3): 203–217.

Baxter, B. T., W. H. Pearce, E. A. Waltke, F. N. Littooy, J. W. Hallett, K. C. Kent, G. R. Upchurch, E. L. Chaikof, J. L. Mills, and B. Fleckten. 2002. Prolonged administration of doxycycline in patients with small asymptomatic abdominal aortic aneurysms: Report of a prospective (Phase II) multicenter study. *J Vasc Surg* 36(1): 1–12.

Bonvallet, P. P., M. J. Schultz, E. H. Mitchell, J. L. Bain, B. K. Culpepper, S. J. Thomas, and S. L. Bellis. 2015. Microporous dermal-mimetic electrospun scaffolds pre-seeded with fibroblasts promote tissue regeneration in full-thickness skin wounds. *PLoS One* 10(3): e0122359.

Chen, J. Y., P. J. Tsai, H. C. Tai, R. L. Tsai, Y. T. Chang, M. C. Wang, Y. W. Chiou et al. 2013. Increased aortic stiffness and attenuated lysyl oxidase activity in obesity. *Arterioscler Thromb Vasc Biol* 33(4): 839–846.

Choi, J.-Y., S.-H. Kim, G.-J. Oh, S.-G. Roh, N.-H. Lee, and K.-M. Yang. 2014. Management of defects on lower extremities with the use of matriderm and skin graft. *Arch Plast Surg* 41(4): 337–343.

Couri, B. M., A. T. Lenis, A. Borazjani, M. F. R. Paraiso, and M. S. Damaser. 2012. Animal models of female pelvic organ prolapse: Lessons learned. *Expert Rev Obstet Gynecol* 7(3): 249–260.

Culav, E. M., C. H. Clark, and M. J. Merrilees. 1999. Connective tissues: Matrix composition and its relevance to physical therapy. *Phys Ther* 79(3): 308–319.

Dai, J., F. Losy, A. M. Guinault, C. Pages, I. Anegon, P. Desgranges, J. P. Becquemin, and E. Allaire. 2005. Overexpression of transforming growth factor-beta1 stabilizes already-formed aortic aneurysms: A first approach to induction of functional healing by endovascular gene therapy. *Circulation* 112(7): 1008–1015.

Dissaranan, C., M. A. Cruz, M. J. Kiedrowski, B. M. Balog, B. C. Gill, M. S. Penn, H. B. Goldman, and M. S. Damaser. 2014. Rat mesenchymal stem cell secretome promotes elastogenesis and facilitates recovery from simulated childbirth injury. *Cell Transplant* 23(11): 1395–1406.

Dong, X. R. and M. W. Majesky. 2012. Restoring elastin with microRNA-29. *Arterioscler Thromb Vasc Biol* 32(3): 548–551.

Franco, C., B. Ho, D. Mulholland, G. Hou, M. Islam, K. Donaldson, and M. P. Bendeck. 2006. Doxycycline alters vascular smooth muscle cell adhesion, migration, and reorganization of fibrillar collagen matrices. *Am J Pathol* 168(5): 1697–1709.

Hanemaaijer, R., H. Visser, P. Koolwijk, T. Sorsa, T. Salo, L. M. Golub, and V. W. van Hinsbergh. 1998. Inhibition of MMP synthesis by doxycycline and chemically modified tetracyclines (CMTs) in human endothelial cells. *Adv Dent Res* 12(2): 114–118.

Heise, R. L., A. Parekh, E. M. Joyce, M. B. Chancellor, and M. S. Sacks. 2012. Strain history and TGF-β1 induce urinary bladder wall smooth muscle remodeling and elastogenesis. *Biomech Model Mechanobiol* 11(1–2): 131–145.

Hughes, L. A., J. Gaston, K. McAlindon, K. A. Woodhouse, and S. L. Thibeault. 2015. Electrospun fiber constructs for vocal fold tissue engineering: Effects of alignment and elastomeric polypeptide coating. *Acta Biomater* 13: 111–120.

Ignarro, L. J., G. M. Buga, K. S. Wood, R. E. Byrns, and G. Chaudhuri. 1987. Endothelium-derived relaxing factor produced and released from artery and vein is nitric oxide. *Proc Natl Acad Sci USA* 84(24): 9265–9269.

Isenburg, J. C., D. T. Simionescu, B. C. Starcher, and N. R. Vyavahare. 2007. Elastin stabilization for treatment of abdominal aortic aneurysms. *Circulation* 115(13): 1729–1737.

Jiang, H. H., B. C. Gill, C. Dissaranan, M. Zutshi, B. M. Balog, D. Lin, and M. S. Damaser. 2013. Effects of acute selective pudendal nerve electrical stimulation after simulated childbirth injury. *Am J Physiol Renal Physiol* 304(3): F239–F247.

Kielty, C. M., M. J. Sherratt, and C. A. Shuttleworth. 2002. Elastic fibres. *J Cell Sci* 115(Pt 14): 2817–2828.

Kim, S. Y., K. C. Go, Y. S. Song, Y. S. Jeong, E. J. Kim, and B. J. Kim. 2014. Extract of the mycelium of T. matsutake inhibits elastase activity and TPA-induced MMP-1 expression in human fibroblasts. *Int J Mol Med* 34(6): 1613–1621.

Kothapalli, C. R. and A. Ramamurthi. 2009a. Copper nanoparticle cues for biomimetic cellular assembly of crosslinked elastin fibers. *Acta Biomater* 5(2): 541–553.

Kothapalli, C. R. and A. Ramamurthi. 2009b. Lysyl oxidase enhances elastin synthesis and matrix formation by vascular smooth muscle cells. *J Tissue Eng Regen Med* 3(8): 655–661.

Kothapalli, C. R. and A. Ramamurthi. 2010. Induced elastin regeneration by chronically activated smooth muscle cells for targeted aneurysm repair. *Acta Biomater* 6(1): 170–178.

Kozel, B. A., R. H. Knutsen, L. Ye, C. H. Ciliberto, T. J. Broekelmann, and R. P. Mecham. 2011. Genetic modifiers of cardiovascular phenotype caused by elastin haploinsufficiency act by extrinsic noncomplementation. *J Biol Chem* 286(52): 44926–44936.

Lannoy, M., S. Slove, L. Louedec, C. Choqueux, C. Journé, J. B. Michel, and M. P. Jacob. 2014. Inhibition of ERK1/2 phosphorylation: A new strategy to stimulate elastogenesis in the aorta. *Hypertension* 64(2): 423–430.

Lee, K. W., D. B. Stolz, and Y. Wang. 2011. Substantial expression of mature elastin in arterial constructs. *Proc Natl Acad Sci USA* 108(7): 2705–2710.

Li, S.-H., Z. Sun, L. Guo, M. Han, M. F. Wood, N. Ghosh, I. A. Vitkin, R. D. Weisel, and R. K. Li. 2012. Elastin overexpression by cell-based gene therapy preserves matrix and prevents cardiac dilation. *J Cell Mol Med* 16(10): 2429–2439.

Lim, J. Y, B. H. Choi, S. Lee, Y. H. Jang, J. S. Choi, and Y.M. Kim. 2013. Regulation of wound healing by granulocyte-macrophage colony-stimulating factor after vocal fold injury. *PLoS One* 8(1): e54256.

Lisa, N.-S. and W. Anthony. 2011. Elastin based constructs. In: Daniel Eberli (ed.), *Regenerative Medicine and Tissue Engineering – Cells and Biomaterials.* InTech.

Liu, J., W. Xiong, L. Baca-Regen, H. Nagase, and B. T. Baxter. 2003. Mechanism of inhibition of matrix metalloproteinase-2 expression by doxycycline in human aortic smooth muscle cells. *J Vasc Surg* 38(6): 1376–1383.

Lüscher, T. F. and G. Noll. 1994. Endothelium dysfunction in the coronary circulation. *J Cardiovasc Pharmacol* 24(3): S16–S26.

Merk, D. R., J. T. Chin, B. A. Dake, L. Maegdefessel, M. O. Miller, N. Kimura, P. S. Tsao et al. 2012. miR-29b participates in early aneurysm development in Marfan syndrome. *Circ Res* 110(2): 312–324.

Min, J. H., I. S. Yun, D. H. Lew, T. S. Roh, and W. J. Lee. 2014. The use of matriderm and autologous skin graft in the treatment of full thickness skin defects. *Arch Plast Surg* 41(4): 330–336.

Moore, J. and S. Thibeault. 2012. Insights into the role of elastin in vocal fold health and disease. *J Voice* 26(3): 269–275.

Palmer, R. M., A. G. Ferrige, and S. Moncada. 1987. Nitric oxide release accounts for the biological activity of endothelium-derived relaxing factor. *Nature* 327(6122): 524–526.

Patel, A., B. Fine, M. Sandig, and Mequanint. K. 2006. Elastin biosynthesis: The missing link in tissue-engineered blood vessels. *Cardiovas Res* 71(1): 40–49.

Pathi, S. D., J. F. Acevedo, P. W. Keller, A. H. Kishore, R. T. Miller, C. Y. Wai, and R. A. Word. 2012. Recovery of the injured external anal sphincter after injection of local or intravenous mesenchymal stem cells. *Obstet Gynecol* 119(1): 134–144.

Prall, A. K., G. M. Longo, W. G. Mayhan, E. A. Waltke, B. Fleckten, R. W. Thompson, and B. T. Baxter. 2002. Doxycycline in patients with abdominal aortic aneurysms and in mice: Comparison of serum levels and effect on aneurysm growth in mice. *J Vasc Surg* 35(5): 923–929.

Pyo, R., J. K. Lee, J. M. Shipley, J. A. Curci, D. Mao, S. J. Ziporin, T. L. Ennis, S. D. Shapiro, R. M. Senior, and R. W. Thompson. 2000. Targeted gene disruption of matrix metalloproteinase-9 (gelatinase B) suppresses development of experimental abdominal aortic aneurysms. *J Clin Invest* 105(11): 1641–1649.

Ramamurthi, A., Venkataraman. L., A. T. Lenis, B. M. Couri, and M. S. Damaser. 2012. Induced regenerative elastic matrix repair in LOXL1 knockout mouse cell cultures: Towards potential therapy for pelvic organ prolapse. *J Tissue Sci Eng* 3: 120.

Rnjak, J., S. G. Wise, S. M. Mithieux, and A. S. Weiss. 2011. Severe burn injuries and the role of elastin in the design of dermal substitutes. *Tissue Eng Part B* 17(2): 81–91.

Rock, M. J., S. A. Cain, L. J. Freeman, A. Morgan, K. Mellody, A. Marson, C. A. Shuttleworth, A. S. Weiss, and C. M. Kielty. 2004. Molecular basis of elastic fiber formation. Critical interactions and a tropoelastin-fibrillin-1 cross-link. *J Biol Chem* 279(22): 23748–23758.

Rossetti, D., M. G. Kielmanowicz, S. Vigodman, Y. P. Hu, N. Chen, A. Nkengne, T. Oddos, D. Fischer, M. Seiberg, and C. B. Lin. 2011. A novel anti-ageing mechanism for retinol: Induction of dermal elastin synthesis and elastin fibre formation. *Int J Cosmet Sci* 33(1): 62–69.

Salcedo, L., L. Lian, H.-H. Jiang, N. Sopko, M. Penn, M. Damaser, and M. Zutshi. 2012. Low current electrical stimulation upregulates cytokine expression in the anal sphincter. *Int J Colorectal Dis* 27(2): 221–225.

Sheng, L., M. Yang, Y. Liang, and Q. Li. 2013. Adipose tissue-derived stem cells (ADSCs) transplantation promotes regeneration of expanded skin using a tissue expansion model. *Wound Repair Regen* 21(5): 746–754.

Simmers, P., A. Gishto, N. Vyavahare, and C. R. Kothapalli. 2015. Nitric oxide stimulates matrix synthesis and deposition by adult human aortic smooth muscle cells within 3D cocultures. *Tissue Eng* 21(7–8): 1455–1470.

Sinha, A., A. Shaporev, N. Nosoudi, Y. Lei, A. Vertegel, S. Lessner, and N. Vyavahare. 2014. Nanoparticle targeting to diseased vasculature for imaging and therapy. *Nanomed Nanotech Biol Med* 10(5): 1003–1012.

Sivaraman, B., C. A. Bashur, and A. Ramamurthi. 2012. Advances in biomimetic regeneration of elastic matrix structures. *Drug Deliv Transl Res* 2(5): 323–350.

Sivaraman, B., G. Howard, and A. Ramamurthi. 2014. Localized therapeutic delivery from multifunctional magnetic nanoparticles for elastic matrix stabilization and repair. In *Society for Biomaterials*, Abstract#613.

Sivaraman, B. and A. Ramamurthi. 2013. Multifunctional nanoparticles for doxycycline delivery towards localized elastic matrix stabilization and regenerative repair. *Acta Biomater* 9(5): 6511–6525.

Sylvester, A., B. Sivaraman, P. Deb, and A. Ramamurthi. 2013. Nanoparticles for localized delivery of hyaluronan oligomers towards regenerative repair of elastic matrix. *Acta Biomater* 9(12): 9292–9302.

Tassabehji, M., K. Metcalfe, D. Donnai, J. Hurst, W. Reardon, M. Burch, and A. P. Read. 1997. Elastin: Genomic structure and point mutations in patients with supravalvular aortic stenosis. *Hum Mol Genet* 6(7): 1029–1036.

Uchinaka, A., N. Kawaguchi, Y. Hamada, S. Miyagawa, A. Saito, S. Mori, Y. Sawa, and N. Matsuura. 2012. Transplantation of elastin-secreting myoblast sheets improves cardiac function in infarcted rat heart. *Mol Cell Biochem* 368(1–2): 203–214.

Uitto, J., Q. Li, and Z. Urban. 2013. The complexity of elastic fibre biogenesis in the skin—A perspective to the clinical heterogeneity of cutis laxa. *Exp Dermatol* 22(2): 88–92.

Urban, Z. 2012. The complexity of elastic fiber biogenesis: The paradigm of cutis laxa. *J Invest Derm* 132(E1): E12–E14.

Votteler, M., D. A. Berrio, A. Horke, L. Sabatier, D. P. Reinhardt, A. Nsair, E. Aikawa, and K. Schenke-Layland. 2013. Elastogenesis at the onset of human cardiac valve development. *Development (Cambridge, England)* 140(11): 2345–2353.

Vučević, D., T. Radosavljević, D. Đorđević, D. Mladenović, and M. Vesković. 2014. The relationship between atherosclerosis and pulmonary emphysema. *Med Pregl* 67(7–8): 231–238.

Wills, A., M. M. Thompson, M. Crowther, R. D. Sayers, and P. R. F. Bell. 1996. Pathogenesis of abdominal aortic aneurysms—Cellular and biochemical mechanisms. *Eur J Vasc Endovasc Surg* 12(4): 391–400.

Wise, S. G., M. J. Byrom, A. Waterhouse, P. G. Bannon, M. K. C. Ng, and A. S. Weiss. 2011. A multilayered synthetic human elastin/polycaprolactone hybrid vascular graft with tailored mechanical properties. *Acta Biomater* 7(1): 295–303.

Zhang, P., A. Huang, M. Morales-Ruiz, B. C. Starcher, Y. Huang, W. C. Sessa, L. E. Niklason, and F. J. Giordano. 2012. Engineered zinc-finger proteins can compensate genetic haploinsufficiency by transcriptional activation of the wild-type allele: Application to Willams-Beuren syndrome and supra-valvular aortic stenosis. *Hum Gene Ther* 23(11): 1186–1199.

Zhong, J., N. Hu, X. Xiong, Q. Lei, and L. Li. 2011. A novel promising therapy for skin aging: Dermal multipotent stem cells against photoaged skin by acti-vation of TGF-β/Smad and p38 MAPK signaling pathway. *Med Hypotheses* 76(3): 343–346.

Zou, X. H., Y. L. Zhi, X. Chen, H. M. Jin, L. L. Wang, Y. Z. Jiang, Z. Yin, and H. W. Ouyang. 2010. Mesenchymal stem cell seeded knitted silk sling for the treatment of stress urinary incontinence. *Biomaterials* 31(18): 4872–4879.

Index

Note: Page numbers followed by f and t refer to figures and tables, respectively.